Asthma

METHODS IN MOLECULAR MEDICINE™

John M. Walker, SERIES EDITOR

55. **Hematologic Malignancies: *Methods and Techniques,*** edited by *Guy B. Faguet,* 2000
54. **Mycobacterium Tuberculosis Protocols,** edited by *Tanya Parish and Neil G. Stoker,* 2001
53. **Renal Cancer: *Methods and Protocols*,** edited by *Jack H. Mydlo,* 2001
52. **Atherosclerosis Methods and Protocols,** edited by *Angela F. Drew,* 2000
51. **Angiotensin Protocols,** edited by *Donna H. Wang,* 2000
50. **Colorectal Cancer: *Methods and Protocols,*** edited by *Steven M. Powell,* 2000
49. **Molecular Pathology Protocols,** edited by *Anthony A. Kileen,* 2000
48. **Antibiotic Resistance Methods and Protocols,** edited by *Stephen H. Gillespie,* 2000
47. **Ocular Molecular Biology Protocols,** edited by *Piroska Elizabeth Rakoczy,* 2000
46. **Angiogenesis: *Methods and Protocols,*** edited by *J. Clifford Murray,* 2000
45. **Hepatocellular Carcinoma: *Methods and Protocols,*** edited by *Nagy A. Habib,* 2000
44. **Asthma: *Mechanisms and Protocols,*** edited by *K. Fan Chung and Ian Adcock,* 2000
43. **Muscular Dystrophy: *Methods and Protocols,*** edited by *Katherine M. D. Bushby and Louise V. B. Anderson,* 2000
42. **Vaccine Adjuvants: P*reparation Methods and Research Protocols,*** edited by *Derek T. O'Hagan,* 2000
41. **Celiac Disease: *Methods and Protocols,*** edited by *Michael N. Marsh,* 2000
40. **Diagnostic and Therapeutic Antibodies,** edited by *Andrew J. T. George and Catherine E. Urch,* 2000
39. **Ovarian Cancer: *Methods and Protocols,*** edited by *John M. S. Bartlett,* 2000
38. **Aging Methods and Protocols,** edited by *Yvonne A. Barnett and Christopher R. Barnett,* 2000
37. **Electrochemotherapy, Electrogenetherapy, and Transdermal Drug Delivery: *Electrically Mediated Delivery of Molecules and Cells,*** edited by *Mark J. Jaroszeski, Richard Heller, and Richard Gilbert,* 2000
36. **Septic Shock Methods and Protocols,** edited by *Thomas J. Evans,* 2000
35. **Gene Therapy of Cancer: *Methods and Protocols*,** edited by *Wolfgang Walther and Ulrike Stein*, 2000
34. **Rotovirus Methods and Protocols,** edited by *James Gray and Ulrich Desselberger*, 2000
33. **Cytomegalovirus Protocols,** edited by *John Sinclair*, 2000
32. **Alzheimer's Disease: *Methods and Protocols,*** edited by *Nigel M. Hooper*, 1999
31. **Hemostasis and Thrombosis Protocols: *Methods in Molecular Medicine,*** edited by *David J. Perry and K. John Pasi*, 1999
30. **Vascular Disease: *Molecular Biology and Gene Therapy Protocols,*** edited by *Andrew H. Baker*, 1999
29. **DNA Vaccines: *Methods and Protocols,*** edited by *Douglas B. Lowrie and Robert Whalen,* 1999
28. **Cytotoxic Drug Resistance Mechanisms,** edited by *Robert Brown and Uta Böger-Brown,* 1999
27. **Clinical Applications of Capillary Electrophoresis,** edited by *Stephen M. Palfrey*, 1999
26. **Quantitative PCR Protocols,** edited by *Bernd Kochanowski and Udo Reischl,* 1999
25. **Drug Targeting,** edited by *G. E. Francis and Cristina Delgado,* 1999
24. **Antiviral Methods and Protocols,** edited by *Derek Kinchington and Raymond F. Schinazi,* 1999
23. **Peptidomimetics Protocols,** edited by *Wieslaw M. Kazmierski,* 1999
22. **Neurodegeneration Methods and Protocols,** edited by *Jean Harry and Hugh A. Tilson,* 1999
21. **Adenovirus Methods and Protocols,** edited by *William S. M. Wold,* 1998
20. **Sexually Transmitted Diseases: *Methods and Protocols,*** edited by *Rosanna Peeling and P. Frederick Sparling,* 1999
19. **Hepatitis C Protocols,** edited by *Johnson Yiu-Nam Lau,* 1998
18. **Tissue Engineering,** edited by *Jeffrey R. Morgan and Martin L. Yarmush,* 1999

METHODS IN MOLECULAR MEDICINE™

Asthma

Mechanisms and Protocols

Edited by

K. Fan Chung and Ian Adcock

Imperial College School of Medicine, London, UK

Humana Press Totowa, New Jersey

999 Riverview Drive, Suite 208
Totowa, New Jersey 07512

This publication is printed on acid-free paper. ∞
ANSI Z39.48-1984 (American Standards Institute) Permanence of Paper for Printed Library Materials.

Cover design by Patricia F. Cleary.

For additional copies, pricing for bulk purchases, and/or information about other Humana titles, contact Humana at the above address or at any of the following numbers: Tel.: 973-256-1699; Fax: 973-256-8341; E-mail: humana@mindspring.com; Website: http://humanapress.com

Printed in the United States of America. 10 9 8 7 6 5 4 3 2 1

Library of Congress Cataloging in Publication Data

Main entry under title:

Methods in molecular medicine™.

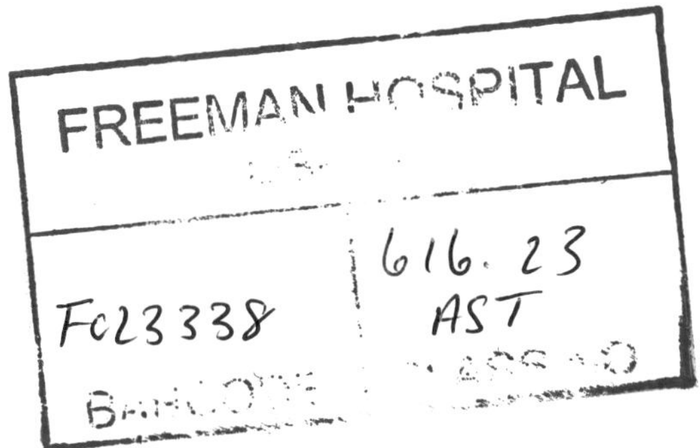

Preface

Asthma has rapidly become one of the most common chronic illnesses of the Western world, and its prevalence continues to rise, with the proportion of patients with more severe diseases also increasing. Faced with this problem, more researchers are focusing on the causes, mechanisms, and pathophysiology of asthma. The major hopes are that more effective drugs will become available and that preventive measures can be instituted. Increasingly, molecular and cell biology approaches are being used to characterize and understand the mechanisms of the inflammatory process that is typical of the asthmatic airway. This volume on *Asthma: Mechanisms and Protocols* in the *Methods in Molecular Medicine* series provides an overview of the molecular mechanisms involved in asthma by providing extensive protocols that are being used in asthma research. Briefly, it covers details of methods for obtaining cells from the airways, analysis of gene and protein expression in the limited clinical samples from asthmatic airways, use of molecular and cellular tools for studying cytokine expression and release, studies of asthma-related genes and genetic polymorphisms, and understanding the effects of asthma treatments. With such coverage, the volume ties in several disciplines, including allergy and immunology, cell biology, pharmacology, and histology. We have continued in the spirit of the series to provide a bench book for day-to-day use. We hope that those who have little or no experience in the field of asthma research will find the book a useful starting point, and eventually come to use the volume on a daily basis. This volume would not have been possible without the contribution of all those excellent investigators who took time away from their bench to write about their methods. We thank them.

K. Fan Chung
Ian Adcock

Contents

Contributors

IAN M. ADCOCK • *National Heart and Lung Institute, Imperial College School of Medicine, London, UK*

FRANÇOIS AUGER • *Centre de Pneumologie de L'Hopital Laval, Ste Foy, Quebec, Canada*

PETROS BAKAKOS • *Southampton General Hospital, Southampton, UK*

PETER J. BARNES • *National Heart and Lung Institute, Imperial College School of Medicine, London, UK*

NEVILLE BERKMAN • *Institute of Pulmonology, Hadassah University Hospital, Jerusalem, Israel*

BRUCE S. BOCHNER • *Department of Medicine, Johns Hopkins Allergy and Asthma Center, Johns Hopkins University Medical School, Baltimore, MD*

LOUIS-PHILIPPE BOULET • *Centre de Pneumologie de L'Hopital Laval, Ste Foy, Quebec, Canada*

KATHLEEN BRENNAN • *Division of Pulmonary Critical Care Medicine, Department of Medicine, Temple University School of Medicine, Philadelphia, PA*

JAMILA CHAKIR • *Centre de Pneumologie de L'Hopital Laval, Ste Foy, Quebec, Canada*

POTA CHRISTODOULOPOULOS • *Meakins-Christie Laboratories, Montreal, Quebec, Canada*

K. FAN CHUNG • *National Heart and Lung Institute, Imperial College School of Medicine, London, UK*

DAVID CICCOLELLA • *Division of Pulmonary Critical Care Medicine, Department of Medicine, Temple University School of Medicine, Philadelphia, PA*

PATRICIA M. DE SOUZA • *National Heart and Lung Institute, Imperial College School of Medicine, London, UK*

JANE C. DEWAR • *National Asthma Campaign, Department of Medicine, University Hospital, Queens Medical Centre, Nottingham, UK*

JEAN DUBÉ • *Centre de Pneumologie de L'Hopital Laval, Ste Foy, Quebec, Canada*

ANTHONY J. FREW • *Southampton General Hospital, Southampton, UK*

JACK GAULDIE • *Department of Pathology, McMaster University, Hamilton, Ontario, Canada*

Lucie Germain • *Centre de Pneumologie de L'Hopital Laval, Ste Foy, Quebec, Canada*
Mark A. Giembycz • *National Heart and Lung Institute, Imperial College School of Medicine, London, UK*
Francine Goulet • *Centre de Pneumologie de L'Hopital Laval, Ste Foy, Quebec, Canada*
Stuart A. Green • *Pulmonary/Critical Care Medicine, University of Cincinnati, OH*
Ian P. Hall • *National Asthma Campaign, Department of Medicine, University Hospital, Queens Medicial Centre, Nottingham, UK*
Qutayba Hamid • *Meakins-Christie Laboratories, Montreal, Quebec, Canada*
Stephen T. Holgate • *Immunopharmacology Group, Southampton General Hospital, Southampton, UK*
Kazuhiro Ito • *National Heart and Lung Institute, Imperial College School of Medicine, London, UK*
Matthias John • *Klinik für Innere Medizin, University Hospital Charite, Berlin, Germany*
Hannu Kankaanranta • *National Heart and Lung Institute, Imperial College School of Medicine, London, UK*
Steven G. Kelsen • *Division of Pulmonary Critical Care Medicine, Department of Medicine, Temple University School of Medicine, Philadelphia, PA*
Stephen J. Lane • *UMDS Division of Medicine, Department of Allergy and Respiratory Medicine, Guy's Hospital, London, UK*
Mark Larché • *National Heart and Lung Institute, Imperial College School of Medicine, London, UK*
Michel Laviolette • *Centre de Pneumologie de L'Hopital Laval, Ste Foy, Quebec, Canada*
Aili L. Lazaar • *Pulmonary and Critical Care Division, Department of Medicine, University of Pennsylvania School of Medicine, Philadelphia, PA*
Tak H. Lee • *UMDS Division of Medicine, Department of Allergy and Respiratory Medicine, Guy's Hospital, London, UK*
Sam Lim • *Klinik für Innere Medizin, University Hospital Charite, Berlin, Germany*
Mark A. Lindsay • *National Heart and Lung Institute, Imperial College School of Medicine, London, UK*
Jacqueline Madden • *Southampton General Hospital, Southampton, UK*
Judith C. W. Mak • *National Heart and Lung Institute, Imperial College School of Medicine, London, UK*
Adel H. Mansur • *Department of Respiratory Medicine, City General Hospital, Stoke on Trent, UK*

JOHN F. J. MORRISON • *Department of Respiratory Medicine, City General Hospital, Stoke on Trent, UK*

YUTAKA NAKAMURA • *Meakins-Christie Laboratories, Montreal, Quebec, Canada*

ROBERT NEWTON • *National Heart and Lung Institute, Imperial College School of Medicine, London, UK*

REYNOLD A. PANETTIERI, JR. • *Pulmonary and Critical Care Division, Department of Medicine, University of Pennsylvania School of Medicine, Philadelphia, PA*

LISA M. SCHWIEBERT • *University of Alabama, Birmingham, AL*

MARTIN R. STÄMPFLI • *Department of Pathology, McMaster University, Hamilton, Ontario, Canada*

MARCIA L. TAYLOR • *Department of Medicine, Johns Hopkins Allergy and Asthma Center, Johns Hopkins University Medical School, Baltimore, MD*

AMANDA P. WHEATLEY • *National Asthma Campaign, Department of Medicine, University Hospital, Queens Medical Centre, Nottingham, UK*

SUSAN J. WILSON • *Immunopharmacology Group, Southampton General Hospital, Southampton, UK*

REEN WU • *University of California, Davis, CA*

ZHOU XING • *Department of Pathology, McMaster University, Hamilton, Ontario, Canada*

Asthma

1

Asthma

Application of Cell and Molecular Biology Techniques to Unravel Causes and Pathophysiological Mechanisms

Fan Chung and Ian Adcock

1. Introduction

The condition termed "asthma" has been difficult to define satisfactorily. Much of this problem arises from poor understanding of its causes, natural history, and pathophysiology, and also from a lack of a specific marker(s) of the disease. To the clinician, the diagnosis of asthma is not difficult in most cases, particularly if patients present early with symptoms of intermittent wheeze and chest tightness, and if their symptoms respond to particular treatments, such as β-adrenergic agonists. Early definitions of asthma included the presence of airway obstruction that could spontaneously reverse with treatment, and also the increased narrowing of the airways to non-specific bronchoconstrictor stimuli, i.e., bronchial hyperresponsiveness (BHR). The essential elements of this definition were useful in separating asthma from other conditions, such as chronic bronchitis, chronic obstructive pulmonary disease, and emphysema, which could sometimes be diagnostically confused with asthma. More recently, the definition of asthma has been enhanced by the recognition that the airway submucosa of patients with asthma are chronically inflamed with a typical inflammatory infiltrate, and that inflammatory processes are important causes of the chief characteristics of asthma: airway obstruction and BHR. In addition, the loss of reversibility of airway obstruction as a long-term effect of the chronic inflammatory process is recognized:

From: *Methods in Molecular Medicine, vol. 44: Asthma: Mechanisms and Protocols*
Edited by: K. F. Chung and I. Adcock

> Asthma is a common and chronic inflammatory condition of the airways whose cause is not completely understood. As a result of inflammation the airways are hyperresponsive and they narrow easily in response to a wide range of stimuli. This may result in coughing, wheezing, chest tightness, and shortness of breath and these symptoms are often worse at night. Narrowing of the airways is usually reversible, but in some patients with chronic asthma the inflammation may lead to irreversible airflow obstruction. Characteristic pathological features include the presence in the airway of inflammatory cells, plasma exudation, oedema, smooth muscle hypertrophy, mucus plugging, and shedding of the epithelium *(1)*.

This working definition of asthma has helped to concentrate research work on the characteristics of this inflammatory response, the potential causes, and the mechanisms underlying this response. To address these issues, a number of molecular and cell biological techniques have been applied. For the researcher new to the field of asthma, it is important to first describe some of the epidemiological and clinical aspects of the disease, prior to a description of the cellular and molecular aspects.

2. Epidemiology of Asthma

Asthma is one of the most common chronic diseases worldwide. Prevalence studies have centered on asking for a history of intermittent wheeze, and, on the basis of this, the prevalence of asthma in childhood has been reported to be up to 40% in some areas of the United Kingdom, Australia, New Zealand, and Ireland; in other less affluent countries, such as Indonesia, China, India, and Ethiopia, this may be as low as 3% *(2)*. In adults, prevalence rates are more difficult to assess, particularly with the potential confusion of asthma with chronic bronchitis, but up to 25% of adults questioned, aged 20–44 yr, reported wheeze in the preceding 6 mo; in the United Kingdom, only 5.7% reported an attack of asthma in the previous 12 mo *(3)*. In several Western countries, the prevalence of asthma among children has increased *(4)*. Factors underlying this increase are unclear.

The likelihood of diagnosed asthma is increased by the presence of atopy, as measured by positive skin-prick tests or elevated serum immunoglobulin E (IgE) levels, by home exposure to passive cigarette smoke, by lower respiratory tract infections, and by the presence of reduced lung function. The increased prevalence of asthma may be caused by changes in indoor or outdoor environment, and may involve aeroallergens, particularly house dust mites. It is possible that the increased prevalence of allergy and asthma may be caused by the synergistic action of air pollution or tobacco smoking with allergic sensitization *(5)*. Passive smoking in infancy may predispose to allergic sensitization to common aeroallergens *(6)*. Urbanization has also been correlated with increases in prevalence of asthma in some countries *(7)*. Data from Ethiopia indicate that westernization is associated with the appearance and increase in asthma and that this may occur within a relatively short period of time (10 yr)

(8). One possibility is that changes in the pattern of childhood infections through westernization may influence the development of atopy through changes in specific T-cell responses favoring the production of cytokines from T-helper type-2 lymphocytes (Th2), such as interleukin 2 (IL-4) and IL-5, with a reduction in Th1 cytokines, such as IFN interferon-γ. For example, children with measles infection are less likely to be atopic than those receiving measles immunization ***(9)***, and there is an inverse relationship between tuberculin responses and atopy ***(10)***. Dietary factors have also been implicated ***(11)***.

In addition to prevalence, the severity of asthma appears to have increased, as shown by the increase in hospital admissions for asthma and in the use of anti-asthma drugs, such as β-agonists and inhaled steroids ***(12–14)***. Mortality, however, is generally low, accounting for approx 5/100,000 population in 1990 in England and Wales. Although the mortality rates have been generally stable, there have been substantial but transient increases in some countries, such as New Zealand, in the late 1970s ***(15)***. Several reasons underlie continuing asthma mortality rates, including the overall increase in severity, thus augmenting the pool of patients at risk of death; failure to use appropriate medication, because of health care professionals not evaluating the severity of disease properly; poor access to medical care; and iatrogenic causes ***(16–19)***.

3. Natural History

There are relatively few cohort studies that have examined the natural history of asthma. Between 30 and 70% of children with asthma become markedly improved or become symptom-free by early adulthood, but significant disease will persist in about 30% ***(20,21)***. Some may experience asymptomatic periods, before developing wheeze again as adults ***(22)***. Among predictors of persistent wheezing from childhood to adulthood are low lung function in childhood and persistent BHR ***(23)***. The more severe the asthma in childhood, the more severe is the asthma in adulthood ***(20,24)***. Asthma can also start later in life, usually associated with a nonatopic background. Often, these asthmatics are smokers, and therefore their condition may be confused with chronic bronchitis or emphysema.

Asthmatics experience a more rapid decline in the lung function measurement of forced expiratory volume in the first second (FEV_1) than nonasthmatics, and smoking asthmatics have the greatest decline in FEV_1 ***(25,26)***, which may reflect an irreversible process that occurs in asthma, and, although asthma is predominantly a disease of reversible airway obstruction, it may become irreversible ***(27)***.

4. Presentation of Asthma

Presentation of asthma can vary from patient to patient. Asthma may be intermittent, with mild to severe episodes that may necessitate treatment. These

Table 1
Different Types of Asthma

Different Types of Asthma
Atopic or nonatopic
Early onset (childhood) or late onset (adult)
Nocturnal
Exercise-induced
Aspirin-induced
Occupational
Seasonal
Cough variant
Acute severe
Chronic severe
Asthma deaths
Fixed irreversible
Brittle
Corticosteroid-resistant
Corticosteroid-dependent

episodes may be provoked by an upper respiratory viral infection or by an exposure to an allergen to which the asthmatic is sensitive. Some cases of asthma may be entirely seasonal, such as pollen-induced asthma in the summer months. In children, exercise frequently provokes bronchoconstriction. Occupational asthma, induced by specific chemicals or proteins encountered at the workplace following sensitization, may also present in relation to exposures at work. Severe episodes of asthma may occur very rapidly sometimes over a period of a few minutes (brittle asthma), and may be life-threatening. Asthma may also present with persistent chronic symptoms, often characterized by worse symptoms at night or on waking in the morning. Some asthmatics develop exacerbations of their asthma when taking aspirin and other nonsteroidal anti-inflammatory drugs. These patients often develop asthma later in life, and have concomitant rhinosinusitis and nasal polyps.

4.1. Different Types of Asthma

Given the varied presentation and course of the disease, it is not surprising that asthma has been clinically classified in various ways, such as on the basis of provoking factors, severity, pattern of asthma attacks, and even on response to available treatments (**Table 1**). However, there is no real classification on the basis of molecular mechanisms, because there is currently poor understanding of these mechanisms. One central question is whether there are different types of asthma, or whether there is only one central mechanism with varying severity and interaction with other exogenous factors to create a varied presentation and course. For example, in terms of the cellular inflammation in the airway submucosa found in atopic and nonatopic asthma, there does not appear to be any striking difference *(28)*. However, the aspirin-sensitive asthmatic appears to have an increased activity of the leukotriene (LT) C4 synthase, compared to the nonaspirin-sensitive asthmatic *(29)*. Classification according to severity is probably most useful, since this can be used to determine not only the amount of treatment a particular patient may need, but may also be used to relate to the degree of inflammatory abnormalities in the airways. For example, using a clinical score of severity, there is a significant positive correlation between the number of eosinophils in bronchial biopsies or bronchoalveolar lavage (BAL) fluid and the clinical severity of asthma *(30)*. However, the measurement of severity is not clearly established. A useful characterization of severity is to use a combination of measurements of symptoms and lung function, and the number of acute attacks of asthma experienced.

5. Chronic Inflammation of Asthma

It has been recognized for a long time that patients who die of asthma attacks have grossly inflamed airways, with occlusion of the airway lumen by a tenacious plug made of plasma proteins exuded from airway vessels and mucus glycoproteins *(31)*. The airway wall is oedematous and infiltrated with inflammatory cells predominantly composed of eosinophils, lymphocytes and neutrophils. Over the past 15 yr, it has been possible to examine the airways of asthmatic patients, using rigid bronchoscopy under general anesthesia, but more usually using a fiberoptic bronchoscope, which can be undertaken with sedation. Studies of the bronchial mucosa of patients with mild and even asymptomatic asthma have established asthma as a chronic inflammatory disease of the airways, characterized by an airway submucosal infiltration of lymphocytes and eosinophils, epithelial shedding, subepithelial reticular fibrosis, and edema *(30,32–35)*. Immunostaining using the monoclonal antibody EG2, which specifically stains the cleaved, secreted form of eosinophil cationic protein, has identified increased numbers of activated eosinophils, both within the submucosal and the epithelial mucosal layers. A consistent increase in $CD25^+$ (IL-2 receptor-bearing) cells, representing activated T-lymphocytes in the bronchial submucosa of extrinsic asthmatics, has been shown *(35)*. An increase in activated monocytes, probably recruited from the circulating blood compartment, has also been reported in bronchial mucosal biopsies *(36)*. An increase in the number of mast cells has also been demonstrated *(32)*. BAL of the lower airways, with 0.9% saline solution, usually yields an excess of eosinophils, mast cells, and T-lymphocytes, with evidence of activation of macrophages *(30,37)*. Alveolar macrophages from asthmatics express an excess of various markers on their surface as determined by flow cytometric analysis, including

CD16, CD18, CD32, CD44, histocompatibility leukocyte antigen (HLA) Class 1, HLA-DR, and HLA-DQ *(38)*.

Recent studies in patients with more severe disease indicate that there is an eosinophilic inflammation that involves not only the mucosa of the proximal airways, but also the more distal airways, together with the alveolar inflammation *(39)*. In addition, there appears to be a predominance of neutrophils in more severe asthmatic patients needing high doses of oral corticosteroids *(40)*. This has also been confirmed in the examination of expectorates obtained from such patients, following induction with inhaled hypertonic saline *(41)*.

5.1. Airway Wall Remodeling

Together with the cellular abnormalities, there are changes indicative of an ongoing repair process *(42)*. There is an increase in the number of myofibroblasts in the subepithelial areas *(43)*, together with an increase in the thickness of the lamina reticularis, which is composed of collagen, types III and V, and fibronectin *(44)*. There has been some dispute as to the presence of shedding of the airway epithelium. It is likely that the epithelium is more fragile and likely to shed with the slightest trauma in asthma *(45)*. The proportion of the bronchial wall area occupied by mucous glands is increased in the lungs of fatal cases of asthma *(46–48)*; an increase in the number of goblet cells in the airway epithelium of mild asthmatics has been reported *(34)*.

In the lungs of patients with fatal asthma, the area of airway smooth muscle (ASM) is substantially increased in both large and small airways *(47–51)*. Detailed morphometric analysis indicates the presence of two distinct patterns of smooth muscle thickening: in those cases in which the process is confined to the central airways, and those in which the changes involve the whole bronchial tree *(51)*. In the first pattern, the increase in ASM occurs from hyperplasia; in the latter pattern, there is predominant hyperplasia *(52)*. An excess of blood vessels in the airways of patients with asthma is also reported *(53)*.

Alterations in the resident cells of the airways therefore constitute airway wall remodeling, and this altered structure may result in altered lung function, in a number of ways. With an increased thickening of the airways resulting from an increase in the amount of ASM, the degree of smooth muscle shortening required to occlude the airways would be expected to be lower *(54)*. An increase in the adventitial area could also lead to uncoupling of the distending forces of parenchymal recoil from the forces that narrow the airways *(55)*. Thus, these factors may contribute to the airway hyperresponsiveness of asthma. How the other remodeling features of the airways relate to airflow obstruction is not clear. Finally, structural cells must now be considered as potential important sources of cytokines. For example, ASM cells are capable of releasing several chemokines, including regulated on actuation normal T-cell expressed and secreted (RANTES), IL-8, eotaxin, and macrophage chemoattractant protein-1 (MCP-1) and -3, and granulocyte-macrophage colony-stimulating factor (GM-CSF) together with prostoglandin E_2 (PGE2) ***(56–58)*** which indicates that the ASM may participate in the inflammatory response.

5.2. Overexpression of Cytokines

Increased gene expression of IL-3, IL-4, IL-5, and GM-CSF, presumably in T-lymphocytes, has been observed in mucosal biopsies ***(59)***. Elevated numbers of mRNA cells for IL-3, IL-4, IL-5, and GM-CSF in BAL fluid of symptomatic asthmatic patients were found, compared to asymptomatic subjects ***(60)***. However, there were no differences in the expression of IL-2 and IFN-γ, indicating that there was a predominance of cytokines derived from Th2, such as IL-3, IL-4, and IL-5, rather than from Th1-lymphocytes, such as IFN-γ and IL-2. An increase in the number of cells in bronchial biopsies of asthmatics expressing the IL-5 receptor has been reported, mostly on eosinophils ***(61)***.

IL-5 is an important cytokine, involved as an eosinophil-differentiating factor, particularly on late-committed eosinophil precursors ***(62,63)***, and can prolong the survival of eosinophils ***(64)***. IL-4 is important in the class switch of B-cells to the synthesis of IgE and promotes the development of Th2-like $CD4^+$ T-cells ***(65,66)***. Factors identified as consisting of IL-5 and GM-CSF activities in BAL fluid from patients with asthma can prolong eosinophil survival; GM-CSF appears to be the most important contributor ***(67)***, and is predominantly expressed in airway epithelium and macrophages ***(68,69)***. IL-5 and GM-CSF can prime eosinophils, e.g., to increase the release of granule-associated proteins, such as eosinophil-derived neurotoxin and eosinophil cationic protein (ECP) from stimulated eosinophils ***(70,71)***. GM-CSF can also enhance the production of leukotrienes from eosinophils ***(72)***.

Increased mRNA expression of the chemoattractant cytokine, RANTES, and eotaxin has been reported, particularly in the airway epithelium ***(73,74)***. These chemokines are important in causing the chemotaxis of inflammatory cells, such as T-cells, monocytes, and eosinophils, into the airway submucosa, with eotaxin being very selective for eosinophils. Cooperation between IL-5 and chemokines, such as eotaxin, has been described in terms of eosinophil mobilization from the bone marrow and to the airways ***(75,76)***. Such cooperation may occur in terms of the development of BHR ***(77)***. The airway epithelium of patients with asthma also expresses another chemokine, MCP-1, compared to airway epithelium from nonasthmatic subjects. Thus, release of chemokines, such as RANTES and eotaxin, and other cytokines, such as IL-5 and GM-CSF, may lead to the recruitment of eosinophils to the airways, with prolonged survival, which are activated to release LTs and eosinophilic proteins. Eosinophilic proteins may in turn damage airway epithelium and contribute to BHR.

Alveolar macrophages obtained by BAL from patients with mild asthma release more proinflammatory cytokines, such as GM-CSF, IL-8, MIP-1α, tumor necrosis factor-α (TNF-α), IL-1, and IFN-γ *(78–80)*. Lymphocytes and alveolar macrophages from BAL of asthmatic patients demonstrate an augmented expression of TNF-α, IL-6, and GM-CSF following allergen challenge *(81,82)*. Increased amounts of IL-1, IL-6, and GM-CSF have been measured in bronchoalveolar fluid of patients with symptomatic asthma, and the source of these cytokines appears to be epithelial cells (ECs) and macrophages *(83)*. Normally, airway macrophages are poor at antigen presentation, and suppress T-cell proliferative responses, possibly via the release of cytokines, such as receptor antagonist (IL-1[ra]), but in asthma there is evidence for reduced suppression after exposure to allergen *(84,85)*. The expression of IL-1ra in the airway epithelium is reduced in asthma *(86)*. Both GM-CSF and IFN-γ increase the ability of macrophages to present allergen and express HLA-DR *(87)*. IL-1 is important in activating T-lymphocytes, and is an important co-stimulator of the expansion of Th2 cells after antigen presentation *(88)*. Airway macrophages may be an important source of first-wave cytokines, such as IL-1, TNF-α, and IL-6, which may be released on exposure to inhaled allergens via the low-affinity IgE receptors (FcεRII). These cytokines may then act on ECs to release a second wave of cytokines, including GM-CSF, IL-8, and RANTES, which then amplifies the inflammatory response and leads to an influx of secondary cells, such as eosinophils, which themselves may release multiple cytokines. Mast cells can also express IL-4, IL-5, IL-6, and TNF-α in asthma *(89)*.

Cytokines may exert an important regulatory effect on the expression of adhesion molecules, both on endothelial cells of the bronchial circulation and on airway ECs. IL-4 increases the expression of vascular cell adhesion molecule-1 (VCAM-1) on endothelial cells and ECs, which may be important for the regulation of eosinophil and lymphocyte trafficking *(90)*. On the other hand, IL-1 and TNF-α increase the expression of intercellular adhesion molecule-1 (ICAM-1) in both vascular endothelium and airway epithelium *(91)*. Following allergen challenge, there is increased expression of ICAM-1 and E-selectin, with no increase in VCAM-1 in asthmatic biopsies *(92)*. In asthmatics, E-selectin, ICAM-1, and VCAM-1 can be detected in atopic, but not in nonatopic asthmatics *(93–95)*. ICAM-1 expression is generally increased in the airway epithelium of patients with asthma *(96,97)*. The importance of the integrin, very late antigen-4 (VLA4), has been demonstrated in several animal models of airway eosinophilia *(77,98)*.

5.3. Transcription Factors in Asthma

Increased gene expression in asthma raises the possibility that there is increased activation of transcription factors that bind to regulatory sequences, usually on the 5'-upstream promoter region of target genes, to increase or decrease transcription. Transcription factors are involved in the regulation of expression of cytokine genes, and play an important role in the long-term regulation of cell function, growth, and differentiation. c-*fos*, a nuclear proto-oncogene and constituent of the transcriptional activator protein, AP-1, has been shown to be overexpressed in the airway epithelium of patients with asthma ***(99)***. Overexpression of c-*fos* in circulating blood mononuclear cells of patients with steroid-resistant asthma has been described ***(100)***.

Nuclear factor κB (NF-κB) is another family of transcription factors important in the induction of a wide array of genes, including chemokines, cytokines, enzymes, receptors, and stress proteins. It consists of dimeric complexes composed of various members, but the p50/p65 heterodimer is usually the most abundant of the transactivating complexes. NF-κB DNA-binding activity in cells, such as macrophages from induced sputum, and in biopsies of mild asthmatic patients, is increased, and the expression of this transcription factor was increased in the airway epithelium of patients with mild asthma ***(101)***. The epithelium in asthma has been the site of enhanced expression of several proteins, including cytokines such as GM-CSF, RANTES, and MCP-1, enzymes such as inducolde macrophages-type nitric oxide synthase (iNOS) and cytochrome oxidase-2, and adhesion molecules such as ICAM-1 ***(68,73,93,102–104)***, and the transcriptional control of these genes is partly dependent on NF-κB activation. A crucial role for NF-κB has been demonstrated in the p50(–/–) knockout mice which were defective in their capacity to mount an allergic eosinophil response because of lack of production of the Th2 cytokine, IL-5, and the chemokine, eotaxin ***(105)***. Other transcription factors of interest include GATA3, which is also expressed in the Th2, but not Th1, cells, and is crucial for activation of IL-5 promoter gene by different stimuli. Ectopic expression of GATA-3 is sufficient to drive IL-5, but not IL-4, gene expression ***(106)***.

5.4. Inflammatory Mediators in Asthma

Many different mediators have been implicated in asthma and possess a variety of effects on the airways that could account for the pathophysiological features of asthma (**Figs. 1** and **2**). Mediators, such as histamine, PGs, and LTs, contract ASM, increase microvascular leakage, cause airway mucus secretion, and attract inflammatory cells ***(107)***. The role of individual mediators in asthma is not clear. Recently, much attention has been given to the cysteinyl-LTs LTC4, LTD4, and LTE4, which are potent constrictors of human airways and can induce BHR ***(108,109)***. In addition, other effects of cysteinyl-LTs have been described, including chemotactic effects on eosinophils, and a permissive effect on ASM proliferation ***(110,111)***. Potent LTD4 antagonists protect against exercise- and allergen-induced bronchoconstriction, indicating the contribu-

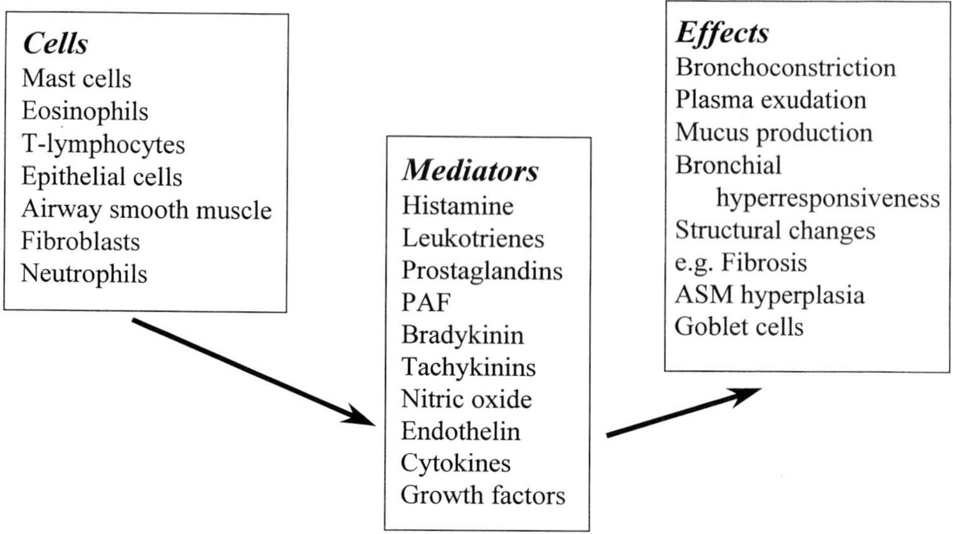

Fig. 1. Cellular sources, inflammatory mediators, and effects of mediators involved in asthma.

tion of LTs to bronchoconstrictor responses ***(112)***. Treatment of asthmatic patients with LT-receptor antagonists or LT-biosynthesis inhibitors improves lung function and symptoms ***(113,114)***. The clinical significance of the other properties of LTs is currently unclear.

Histamine was one of the first mediators implicated in asthma, but its contribution in asthma is unclear, because potent histamine H1-receptor antagonists have not shown any benefit in asthma. It is likely that they do contribute to the pathophysiology of asthma, since combination of a LT antagonist with that of a potent H1-antagonist causes more protection of allergen-induced early- and late-phase responses than the LT antagonist given alone ***(115)***. Platelet-activating factor (PAF), which is produced by eosinophils, and which has proinflammatory effects on inflammatory cells, such as neutrophils and eosinophils, is also released during asthmatic episodes, such as after exposure to allergen ***(116)***. Potent PAF-receptor antagonists do not appear to have provided benefit in patients with asthma ***(117,118)***.

Other mediators have also been implicated in asthma. Products of the cyclooxygenase enzyme pathway include PGs and thromboxane. PGD_2 and PGF2α, and thromboxane may facilitate the release of acetylcholine from cholinergic nerves, to augment bronchoconstriction ***(119–121)***. PGE_2, on the other hand, may have antibronchoconstrictor properties, and protects against exercise- and allergen-induced bronchoconstriction ***(122,123)***. Neuropeptides, such as sub-

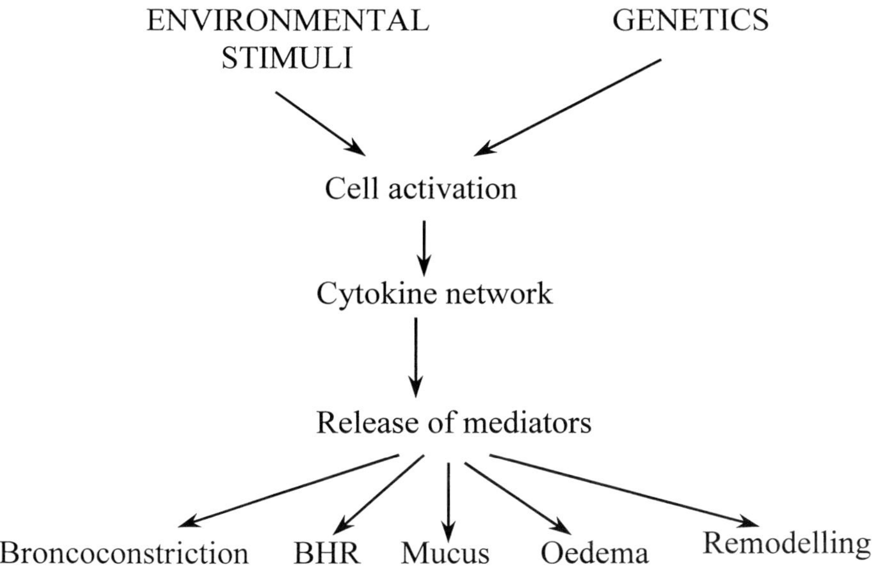

Fig. 2. Release of mediators in asthma is likely to be the final pathway of interaction between cell activation and cytokine network.

stance P, neurokinin A, and calcitonin-gene-related peptide, may be released from sensitized inflammatory nerves in the airways, which increase and extend the ongoing inflammatory response ***(124)***. Neuropeptides may influence immune cells involved in asthma ***(125)***. Kinins, such as bradykinin, are generated from α_2-globulin precursor proteins, kininogens. Bradykinin is generated in the airways following allergen challenge, and also during common viral infections ***(126–128)***. Bradykinin can cause bronchoconstriction, mucus secretion, and plasma exudation in the airways ***(129–131)***, and activates sensory C-fibers ***(132)***, with concomitant release of neuropeptides, and may therefore enhance neural reflexes in the airways ***(133)***.

Endothelins are potent peptide mediators that are potent vasoconstrictors and bronchoconstrictors, and they also induce ASM cell and fibroblast proliferation ***(134)***. An increase in endothelin immunoreactivity has been reported in asthmatic airways, and endothelin is released during segmental allergen challenge ***(135,136)***. Therefore, endothelins could be involved in the chronic inflammatory response of asthma. Other potential mediators of airway wall remodeling include transforming growth factor-β, which has been observed to be increased in BAL fluid in asthma ***(137)***, and which is overexpressed in eosinophils in the bronchial submucosa ***(138)***.

Nitric oxide (NO) is produced by the action of the enzymes, NOSs, and the increased expression of inducible NOS in the airway epithelium of patients with asthma ***(102)*** is likely to underlie the increased levels of NO in exhaled breath ***(139)***. The role of NO as a mediator of asthma remains unclear. Its direct effect as an ASM relaxant is small. NO is a potent vasodilator that may lead to an increase in plasma exudation ***(140)***. It may influence the development of a Th2 response with eosinophilia ***(141)***.

6. Pathophysiology: Initiating Events and Sustaining Events

There is little knowledge of the molecular events that predispose to asthma and the processes that sustain the chronic inflammatory process (**Fig. 2**); in addition, the crucial aspects of the inflammatory process that leads to a given clinical phenotype of asthma have not been unraveled. Twin studies ***(142,143)*** indicate that between 35 and 75% of the susceptibility to asthma is explained by genetic influences. The clinical manifestation of asthma in a particular individual will depend on the combination of genetic predisposition and environmental exposure. Asthma is a polygenic disease, and genes linked to asthma may be identified either by a process known as positional cloning or by examining candidate genes. Because of the close association of asthma with atopy, genes predisposing to atopy have been looked for. Various genetic loci have been linked to atopy, including FcεRIβ, the high-affinity receptor for IgE on chromosome 11q; the 5q23–31 region on chromosome 5, which contains several molecules, such as IL-3, 4, 5, 9, 12b, and 13, and the β2-adrenergic receptor (β-AR); and the IL-4 receptor on chromosome 16 ***(144–148)***. Genetic linkage between IgE responses and microsatellites from the T-cell receptor α/δ region has been demonstrated, indicating that a locus in that region is modulating IgE responses ***(149)***. Linkage of BHR and total serum IgE has been shown to several markers on chromosome 5 ***(146)***. The glutamic acid-27 polymorphism on the β_2-AR has been associated with reduced bronchial responsiveness ***(150)***. Systematic whole-genome screens for genes predisposing to asthma have been carried out, with the following traits used: atopy, skin-prick tests, total serum IgE, blood eosinophil count, and bronchial responsiveness. Potential linkages have been identified on chromosomes 4, 6, 7, 11, 13, and 16 ***(151)***, which indicates that the genetic predisposition to asthma may be very complex.

Although these genes may be involved in initiating asthma, there are other genes that may be involved in determining the clinical phenotype or the severity of the disease. For example, certain genes may be involved in airway remodeling or in the expression of inflammation in the airways, such as IL-10 or TNF-α ***(152)***. In addition, certain genes may be important in the response to environmental factors.

The development of sensitization to various allergens is generally regarded as occurring prior to the development of asthma, and therefore this has been taken to mean that exposure to these allergens causes asthma. Thus, the degree

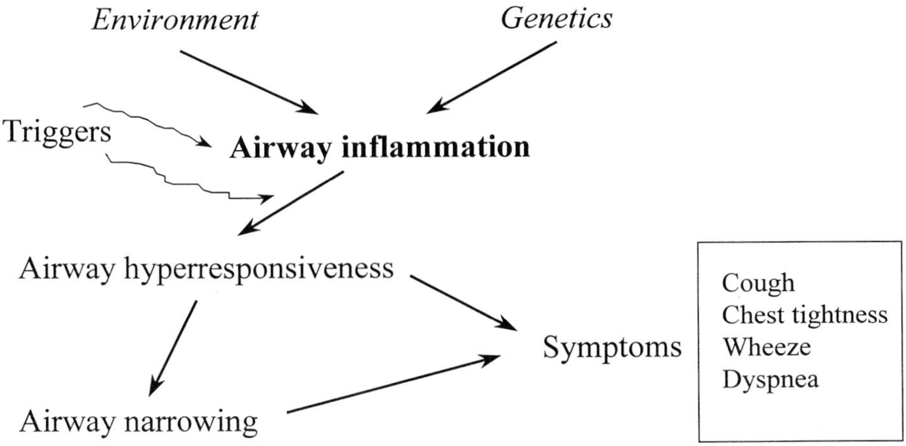

Fig. 3. Interactions between environmental and genetic factors in the induction of chronic inflammation in asthma, leading to airway hyperresponsiveness and narrowing, which underlie the clinical presentation.

of exposure to house dust mites during the first 2 yr of life was associated with the likelihood of developing asthma up to the age of 11 yr ***(153)***. However, it is still possible that patients who are susceptible to asthma are also more susceptible to the allergic response. Other theories about the causation of asthma have been put forward, particularly regarding an imbalance of the Th1/Th2 toward a Th2 response. There is the concept of a sensitization window during infancy, when exposure to allergen predisposes toward the development of long-term Th2-skewed allergen-specific immunological memory ***(154)***. Tolerance to repeated low-level inhaled aeroallergens may involve the activation of additional subsets of T-cells or other cells that act as suppressor cells. These cells may cause Th2–Th1 switch, or suppress both Th1 and Th2 responses. The failure of this process to occur naturally in atopic individuals is likely to result from a combination of allergic genetic predisposition and persistent stimulation by aeroallergens at a critical phase of immune maturation ***(155)***. Repeated aeroallergen stimulation may perpetuate a Th2/IgE response, and stimulate a Th2 response indefinitely ***(156)***.

Although these predisposing and sustaining factors are implicated, it remains to be understood how these translate into the initiation and continuation of chronic airway inflammation (**Figs. 2** and **3**). In addition, how chronic inflammatory changes relate to the typical changes of asthma (symptoms, BHR, and so on) need to be understood.

One area of interest is the study of how allergen-activated T-lymphocytes differentiate into Th2 lymphocytes, because this appears to be of central importance in the early stages of asthma. Allergen is not sufficient to initiate this cascade of events, and T-cells need a co-stimulatory signal which is provided to the T-cell through interaction with cells specialized in antigen capture and presentation, particularly dendritic cells. Two co-stimulatory signals, CD80 and CD86, bind to a receptor on T-cells, termed CD28 ***(157)***. Dendritic cells and macrophages express CD80 and CD86. Th2 immune responses may be preferentially activated by CD86; Th1 immune responses are regulated by CD80. Specific blockade of CD80 at the time of intranasal allergen challenge blocks allergic inflammation in the mouse ***(158)***.

7. Acute Exacerbation of Asthma

Asthma exacerbations are the major cause of morbidity and mortality in asthma. The initial pathology of asthma was described from patients who have died of severe status asthmaticus. More recent description of patients who have died suddenly of a severe episode describes the presence of a neutrophilic inflammation in the airways, with little evidence of intraluminal obstruction ***(159)***. Respiratory virus infections precipitate acute exacerbations of asthma in all age groups. In school children, a respiratory virus was associated with at least 80% of all exacerbations, and 50% of all viruses detected were rhinoviruses (RVs) ***(160)***. Asthmatic subjects infected with RV-16 ***(161)*** have increased levels of IL-8 in nasal lavage, together with increased levels of ECP. There is increased intraepithelial eosinophil numbers in bronchial biopsies during experimental RV infection of asthmatic subjects ***(162)***; in addition, there were $CD4^+$ and $CD8^+$ T-lymphocyte accumulations in the submucosa. Allergen-induced eosinophil numbers were increased in bronchial lavage from atopic individuals during a RV infection ***(163)***. The eosinophil recruitment may involve the release of chemokines, such as RANTES, and there is evidence for a role for the transcription factor, NF-κB, in the induction of IL-6 by RV ***(164)***.

8. Difficult Therapy-Resistant Asthma

Although the therapy of asthma with bronchodilator drugs, such as β-agonist, and anti-inflammatory drugs, such as corticosteroids, is usually successful in controlling the disease in most patients with asthma, a small proportion do not respond, even when using maximal doses of these therapies ***(165)***. Such patients make up a heterogeneous group, often labeled corticosteroid-dependent or corticosteroid-resistant, because of partial or lack of response to corticosteroids. There may be several reasons for this poor response. The cellular inflammatory response may be different from that found in milder patients. In severe patients needing corticosteroid therapy, a cellular infiltrate of eosinophils and neutrophils was observed in both proximal and peripheral airways ***(40)***. This has been confirmed by examination of induced sputum samples from similar patients ***(41)***. Another possibility is that there are excessive structural changes in the airways, such as an excessive amount of ASM or collagen deposition, leading to excessive airway narrowing and decreased response to the anti-inflammatory effects of corticosteroids. There is no current evidence for or against this possibility. Alternatively, these patients have an intrinsic defect in their response to corticosteroids (*see* Chapter 21). This particular group of patients is in desperate need of newer, more effective, therapies.

9. Research into Cell and Molecular Biology of Asthma

It is clear that there will be increasing need for research into the cell and molecular biology of asthma (**Table 2**). Issues that are of importance include the capacity for structural cells to produce inflammatory proteins, dendritic and other cells in antigen processing and presentation, the role of T-cells and their subtypes, the ability of cells such as eosinophils and neutrophils to be activated by cytokines, their apoptotic profiles during inflammation, the role of the epithelium in orchestrating inflammation in the airways submucosa, and the relationship of the inflammation with clinical phenotype. In addition to cellular inflammation the process of remodeling of the airways needs to be understood. There is little information regarding the cellular mechanisms because it is not possible to obtain enough material from patients' airways for adequate studies of the structural cells and matrix proteins. How some of these cells, particularly the structural cells, such as the airway epithelium, respond to external stimuli, such as viruses and allergens and components of air pollution, are unknown. Because the cells from asthmatic patients appear to behave differently from those of nonasthmatic patients, it is of importance to ultimately obtain information on cells derived from asthmatic patients. In this context, examination of the genes expressed by these cells, compared to nonasthmatic cells, may yield important differences. The predisposition to asthma/allergy, and to developing particular patterns of asthma, will continue to be studied. On the molecular level, one important aspect is to investigate whether there is a defect in transcriptional control of several inflammatory or anti-inflammatory genes in asthma. This may only be present in certain cells.

These areas of research continue to be pursued at present. Regarding the examination of cells involved in the chronic airway inflammation of asthma, it would be best to examine airway cells, rather than circulating white cells. However, it may not be possible to obtain sufficient cells from the airways and lungs by such techniques as BAL. For example, many studies have reported results on purified populations of T-cells, monocytes and eosinophils from circulating blood (e.g., ***166,167***); however, it is not known at present whether these data also reflect similar behavior in the airways. Certain structural cells such as ASM cells, fibroblasts, and ECs may be obtained from lung tissues

Table 2
Cells for Study of Cell Molecular Biology of Asthma

Circulating blood cells for FACS analysis/purification of cells
Eosinophils
Neutrophils
Monocytes
T-lymphocytes
Bronchial biopsies (asthmatic or normal)
Immunohistology
In situ hybridization
RT-PCR
Explant cultures for epithelium and fibroblasts (myofibroblasts)
BAL cells (asthmatic or normal)
Alveolar macrophages
T-cells
(Mast cells)
Bronchial brushings for ECs (asthmatic or normal)
Lung tissues from cancer surgery or lung-transplant programs
Primary cultures of ECs, ASM, fibroblasts, mucus cells, dendritic cells
Cell lines
Epithelium: A549, BEAS-2B, 16HBE
Monocytes/macrophages
Eosinophils
T-cells
Endothelial cells
Experimental conditions of asthma
Stable mild to moderately severe asthma
Asthma following exposure to single or multiple doses of allergen
Upper respiratory tract infections
Asthma following treatment with inhaled or oral corticosteroid therapy

FACS, fluorescence-activated cell sorter.

obtained from patients undergoing surgical resections, or from donors in lung transplant programs, and placed in culture. Use of bronchial biopsies obtained via the fiberoptic bronchoscope has been useful in localizing various inflammatory genes or their products, particularly under conditions of allergen exposure or of upper respiratory virus infections. Application of reverse transcription polymerase chain reaction (RT-PCR), *in situ* hybridization, and immunohistochemical techniques are now generally used. Bronchial biopsies can also be cultured to obtain, under specific conditions, primary EC or fibroblast cell cultures, with cells preserving any intrinsic abnormalities. T-cells have been cloned from BAL cells. Recently, the less-invasive method of obtaining airway cells by inducing sputum production following inhalation of hypertonic saline has become widespread in the assessment of airway inflammation. However, it is not possible to culture the cells in induced sputum (e.g., macrophages) with any degree of certainty. For studies of more fundamental relevance to the mechanisms of asthmatic inflammation, cell lines continue to be used in such studies as the transcriptional control of certain inflammatory genes in the airway epithelium. Finally, animal models will continue to be examined in order to understand mechanisms. The most interesting examples are those of transgenic or knockout mice, which have provided useful insights into the role of various cytokines or transcription factors in the pathogenesis of allergic inflammation. Similarly, the transfer of particular genes to specific cells of the airways, e.g., the airway epithelium, has thrown light on some molecular mechanisms.

References

1. British Thoracic Society (1993) Guidelines for the management of asthma: a summary. *Br. Med. J.* **306,** 776–782.
2. International Study of Asthma and Allergies in Childhood (ISAAC) Steering Committee (1998) Worldwide variation in prevalence of symptoms of asthma, allergic rhinoconjunctivitis, and atopic eczema: ISAAC. *Lancet* **351,** 1225–1232.
3. Anonymous (1996) Variations in the prevalence of respiratory symptoms, self-reported asthma attacks, and use of asthma medication in the European Community Respiratory Health Survey (ECRHS). *Eur. Respir. J.* **9,** 687–695.
4. Kaur, B., Anderson, H. R., Austin, J., Burr, M., Harkins, L. S., Strachan, D. P., and Warner, J. O. (1998) Prevalence of asthma symptoms, diagnosis, and treatment in 12–14 year old children across Great Britain (international study of asthma and allergies in childhood, ISAAC UK). *Br. Med. J.* **316,** 118–124.
5. Martinez, F. D., Morgan, W. J., Wright, A. L., Holberg, C. J., and Taussig, L. M. (1988) Diminished lung function as a predisposing factor for wheezing respiratory illness in infants. *N. Engl. J. Med.* **319,** 1112–1117.
6. Murray, A. B. and Morrison, B. J. (1992) Effect of passive smoking on asthmatic children who have and who have not had atopic dermatitis. *Chest* **101,** 16–18.
7. Andrae, S., Axelson, O., Bjorksten, B., Fredriksson, M., and Kjellman, N. I. (1988) Symptoms of bronchial hyperreactivity and asthma in relation to environmental factors. *Arch. Dis. Child* **63,** 473–478.
8. Yemaneberhan, H., Bekele, Z., Venn, A., Lewis, S., Parry, E., and Britton, J. (1997) Prevalence of wheeze and asthma and relation to atopy in urban and rural Ethiopia. *Lancet* **350,** 85–90.
9. Shaheen, S. O., Aaby, P., Hall, A. J., Barker, D. J., Heyes, C. B., Shiell, A. W., and Goudiaby, A. (1996) Measles and atopy in Guinea-Bissau. *Lancet* **347,** 1792–1796.

10. Shirakawa, T., Enomoto, T., Shimazu, S., and Hopkin, J. M. (1997) Inverse association between tuberculin responses and atopic disorder. *Science* **275,** 77–79.
11. Demissie, K., Ernst, P., Gray Donald, K., and Joseph, L. (1996) Usual dietary salt intake and asthma in children: a case-control study. *Thorax* **51,** 59–63.
12. Keating, G., Mitchell, E. A., Jackson, R., Beaglehole, R., and Rea, H. (1984) Trends in sales of drugs for asthma in New Zealand, Australia, and the United Kingdom, 1975–81. *Br. Med. J. Clin. Res. Ed.* **289,** 348–351.
13. Mullally, D. I., Howard, W. A., Hubbard, T. J., Grauman, J. S., and Cohen, S. G. (1984) Increased hospitalizations for asthma among children in the Washington, D. C. area during 1961–1981. *Ann. Allergy* **53,** 15–19.
14. Anderson, H. R., Bailey, P., and West, S. (1980) Trends in the hospital care of acute childhood asthma 1970–8: a regional study. *Br. Med. J.* **281,** 1191–1194.
15. Sears, M. R. and Rea, H. H. (1987) Patients at risk of dying of asthma: New Zealand experience. *J. Allergy Clin. Immunol.* **80,** 477–481.
16. Johnson, A. J., Nunn, A. J., Somner, A. R., Stableforth, D. E., and Stewart, C. J. (1984) Circumstances of death from asthma. *Br. Med. J. Clin. Res. Ed.* **288,** 1870–1872.
17. Rea, H. H., Scragg, R., Jackson, R., Beaglehole, R., Fenwick, J., and Sutherland, D. C. (1986) Case-control study of deaths from asthma. *Thorax* **41,** 833–839.
18. Sears, M. R., Rea, H. H., Fenwick, J., Beaglehole, R., Gillies, A. J., Holst, P. E., et al. (1986) Deaths from asthma in New Zealand. *Arch. Dis. Child* **61,** 6–10.
19. Crane, J., Pearce, N., and Flatt, A. E. A. (1989) Prescribed fenoterol and death from asthma in New Zealand, 1981–83: case-control study. *Lancet* **i,** 917–922.
20. Mcnicol, K. N., Macnicol, K. N., and Williams, H. B. (1973) Spectrum of asthma in children. I. Clinical and physiological components. *Br. Med. J.* **4,** 7–11.
21. Williams, H. and Mcnicol, K. N. (1969) Prevalence, natural history, and relationship of wheezy bronchitis and asthma in children. An epidemiological study. *Br. Med. J.* **4,** 321–325.
22. Strachan, D. P., Butland, B. K., and Anderson, H. R. (1996) Incidence and prognosis of asthma and wheezing illness from early childhood to age 33 in a national British cohort. *Br. Med. J.* **312,** 1195–1199.
23. Roorda, R. J., Gerritsen, J., van Aalderen, W. M., Schouten, J. P., Veltman, J. C., Weiss, S. T., and Knol, K. (1993) Risk factors for the persistence of respiratory symptoms in childhood asthma. *Am. Rev. Respir. Dis.* **148,** 1490–1495.
24. Martin, A. J., Landau, L. I., and Phelan, P. D. (1982) Asthma from childhood at age 21: the patient and his disease. *Br. Med. J. Clin. Res. Ed.* **284,** 380–382.
25. Peat, J. K., Woolcock, A. J., and Cullen, K. (1987) Rate of decline of lung function in subjects with asthma. *Eur. J. Respir. Dis.* **70,** 171–179.
26. Lange, P., Parner, J., Vestbo, J., Schnohr, P., and Jensen, G. (1998) 15-year follow-up study of ventilatory function in adults with asthma. *N. Eng. J. Med.* **339,** 1194–2000.
27. Finucane, K. E., Greville, H. W., and Brown, P. J. (1985) Irreversible airflow obstruction. Evolution in asthma. *Med. J. Aust.* **142,** 602–604.
28. Humbert, M., Durham, S. R., Ying, S., Kimmitt, P., Barkans, J., Assoufi, B., et al. (1996) IL-4 and IL-5 mRNA and protein in bronchial biopsies from

patients with atopic and nonatopic asthma: evidence against "intrinsic" asthma being a distinct immunopathologic entity. *Am. J. Respir. Crit. Care Med.* **154,** 1497–1504.

29. Cowburn, A. S., Sladek, K., Soja, J., Adamek, L., Nizankowska, E., Szczeklik, A., et al. (1998) Overexpression of leukotriene C4 synthase in bronchial biopsies from patients with aspirin-intolerant asthma. *J. Clin. Invest.* **101,** 834–846.
30. Bousquet, J., Chanez, P., Lacoste, J. Y., Barneon, G., Ghavanian, N., Enander, I., et al. (1990) Eosinophilic inflammation in asthma. *N. Engl. J. Med.* **323,** 1033–1039.
31. Dunnill, M. S. (1960) Pathology of asthma with special reference to changes in the bronchial mucosa. *J. Clin. Pathol.* **13,** 27–33.
32. Djukanovic, R., Wilson, J. W., Britten, K. M., Wilson, S. J., Walls, A. F., Roche, W. R., Howarth, P. H., and Holgate, S. T. (1990) Quantitation of mast cells and eosinophils in the bronchial mucosa of symptomatic atopic asthmatics and healthy control subjects using immunohistochemistry. *Am. Rev. Respir. Dis.* **142,** 863–871.
33. Laitinen, L. A., Heino, M., Laitinen, A., Kava, T., and Haahtela, T. (1985) Damage of the airway epithelium and bronchial reactivity in patients with asthma. *Am. Rev. Respir. Dis.* **131,** 599–606.
34. Laitinen, L. A., Laitinen, A., and Haahtela, T. (1993) Airway mucosal inflammation even in patients with newly diagnosed asthma. *Am. Rev. Respir. Dis.* **147,** 697–704.
35. Azzawi, M., Bradley, B., Jeffery, P. K., Frew, A. J., et al. (1990) Identification of activated T lymphocytes and eosinophils in bronchial biopsies in stable atopic asthma. *Am. Rev. Respir. Dis.* **142,** 1407–1413.
36. Poston, R., Chanez, P., Lacoste, J. Y., Litchfield, P., Lee, T. H., and Bousquet, J. (1992) Immunohistochemical characterization of the cellular infiltration of asthmatic bronchi. *Am. Rev. Respir. Dis.* **145,** 918–921.
37. Flint, K. C., Leung, K. B. P., Huspith, B. N., Brostoff, J., Pearce, F. L., and Johnson, N. M. (1985) Bronchoalveolar mast cells in extrinsic asthma: mechanism for the initiation of antigen specific bronchoconstriction. *Br. Med. J.* **291,** 923–927.
38. Viksman, M. Y., Liu, M. C., Bickel, C. A., Schleimer, R. P., and Bochner, B. S. (1997) Phenotypic analysis of alveolar macrophages and monocytes in allergic airway inflammation. I. Evidence for activation of alveolar macrophages, but not peripheral blood monocytes, in subjects with allergic rhinitis and asthma. *Am. J. Respir. Crit. Care Med.* **155,** 858–863.
39. Kraft, M., Djukanovic, R., Wilson, S., Holgate, S. T., and Martin, R. J. (1996) Alveolar tissue inflammation in asthma. *Am. J. Respir. Crit. Care Med.* **154,** 1505–1510.
40. Wenzel, S. E., Szefler, S. J., Leung, D. Y. M., Sloan, S. I., Rex, M. D., and Martin, R. J. (1997) Bronchoscopic evaluation of severe asthma: persistent inflammation associated with high dose glucocorticoids. *Am. J. Respir. Crit. Care Med.* **156,** 737–743.

41. Jatakanon, A., Mohamed, J. B., Lim, S., Maziak, W., Chung, K. F., and Barnes, P. J. (1998) Neutrophils may contribute to the pathogenesis of airway inflammation in steroid dependent intractable asthma. *Am. J. Respir. Crit. Care Med.* **157,** A875.
42. Redington, A. E., and Howarth, P. H. (1997) Airway wall remodelling in asthma. *Thorax* **52,** 310–312.
43. Brewster, C. E. P., Howarth, P. H., Djukanovic, R., Wilson, J., Holgate, S. T., and Roche, W. R. (1990) Myofibroblasts and subepithelial fibrosis in bronchial 'asthma'. *Am. J. Resp. Cell Mol. Biol.* **3,** 507–511.
44. Roche, W. R., Beasley, R., Williams, J. H. and Holgate, S. T. (1989) Subepithelial fibrosis in the bronchi of asthmatics. *Lancet* **1,** 520–524.
45. Jeffery, P. K., Wardlaw, A. J., Nelson, F. C., Collins, J. V., and Kay, A. B. (1989) Bronchial biopsies in asthma:an ultrastructural, quantiative study and correlation with hyperreactivity. *Am. Rev. Respir. Dis.* **140,** 1745–1753.
46. Glynn, A. A. and Michaels, L. (1960) Bronchial biopsy in chronic bronchitis and asthma. *Thorax* **15,** 142–153.
47. Dunnill, M. S., Massarella, G. R., and Anderson, J. A. (1969) Comparison of the quantitative anatomy of the bronchi in normal subjects, in status asthmaticus, in chronic bronchitis, and in emphysema. *Thorax* **24,** 176–179.
48. Takizawa, T. and Thurlbeck, W. M. (1971) Muscle and mucous gland size in the major bronchi of patients with chronic bronchitis, asthma, and asthmatic bronchitis. *Am. Rev. Respir. Dis.* **104,** 331–336.
49. Heard, B. E. and Hossain, S. (1972) Hyperplasia of bronchial muscle in asthma. *J. Pathol.* **110,** 319–331.
50. Hossain, S. (1973) Quantitative measurement of bronchial muscle in men with asthma. *Am. Rev. Respir. Dis.* **107,** 99–109.
51. Ebina, M., Yaegashi, H., Chiba, R., Takahashi, T., Motomiya, M., and Tanemura, M. (1990) Hyperreactive site in the airway tree of asthmatic patients revealed by thickening of bronchial muscles. A morphometric study. *Am. Rev. Respir. Dis.* **141,** 1327–1332.
52. Ebina, M., Takahashi, T., Chiba, T., and Motomiya, M. (1993) Cellular hypertrophy and hyperplasia of airway smooth muscle underlying bronchial asthma. *Am. Rev. Respir. Dis.* **148,** 720–726.
53. Li, X. and Wilson, J. W. (1997) Increased vascularity of the bronchial mucosa in mild asthma. *Am. J. Respir. Crit. Care Med.* **156,** 229–233.
54. James, A. L., Pare, P. D., and Hogg, J. C. (1989) Mechanics of airway narrowing in asthma. *Am. Rev. Respir. Dis.* **139,** 242–246.
55. Moreno, R. H., Hogg, J. C., and Pare, P. D. (1986) Mechanics of airway narrowing. *Am. Rev. Respir. Dis.* **133,** 1171–1180.
56. John, M., Au, B. T., Jose, P. J., Lim, S., Saunders, M., Barnes, P. J., et al. (1998) Expression and release of interleukin-8 by human airway smooth muscle cells: inhibition by Th-2 cytokines and corticosteroids. *Am. J. Respir. Cell Mol. Biol.* **18,** 84–90.
57. John, M., Hirst, S. J., Jose, P. J., Robichaud, A., Berkman, N., Witt, C., et al. (1997) Human airway smooth muscle cells express and release RANTES in

response to Th-1 cytokines: regulation by Th-2 cytokines and corticosteroids. *J. Immunol.* **158,** 1841–1847.

58. Saunders, M. A., Mitchell, J. A., Seldon, P. M., Yacoub, M. H., Barnes, P. J., Giembycz, M. A., and Belvisi, M. G. (1997) Release of granulocyte-macrophage colony stimulating factor by human cultured airway smooth muscle cells: suppression by dexamethasone. *Br. J. Pharmacol.* **120,** 545–546.
59. Hamid, Q., Azzawi, M., Ying, S., Moqbel, R., Wardlaw, A. J., Corrigan, C. J., et al. (1991) Expression of mRNA for interleukins in mucosal bronchial biopsies from asthma. *J. Clin. Invest.* **87,** 1541–1546.
60. Robinson, D. S., Hamid, Q., Ying, S., Tsicopoulos, A., Barkans, J., Bentley, A. M., et al. (1992) Predominant TH2-like bronchoalveolar T-lymphocyte population in atopic asthma. *N. Engl. J. Med.* **326,** 298–304.
61. Yasruel, Z., Humbert, M., Kotsimbos, T. C., Ploysongsang, Y., Minshall, E., Durham, S. R., et al. (1997) Membrane-bound and soluble alpha IL-5 receptor mRNA in the bronchial mucosa of atopic and nonatopic asthmatics. *Am. J. Respir. Crit. Care Med.* **155,** 1413–1418.
62. Clutterbuck, E. J., Hirst, E. M., and Sanderson, C. J. (1989) Human interleukin-5 (IL-5) regulates the production of eosinophils in human bone marrow cultures: comparison and interaction with IL-1, IL-3, IL-6 and GM-CSF. *Blood* **73,** 1504–1512.
63. Lopez, A. F., Sanderson, C. J., Gamble, J. R., Campbell, H. D., Young, I. G., and Vadas, M. A. (1988) Recombinant human interleukin 5 is a selective activator of human eosinophil function. *J. Exp. Med.* **167,** 219–224.
64. Yamaguchi, Y., Hayashi, Y., Sugama, Y., miura, Y., Kasuhara, T., Kitamura, S., et al. (1988) Highly purified murine interleukin 5 (IL-5) stimulates eosinophil function and prolongs in vitro survival. IL-5 as an eosinophil factor. *J. Exp. Med.* **167,** 1737–1740.
65. Le Gros, G., Ben-Sasson, S. Z., Seder, R. A., Finkelman, F. D., and Paul, W. E. (1990) Generation of interleukin 4 (IL-4)-producing cells in vivo and in vitro: IL-2 and IL-4 are required for in vitro generation of IL-4-producing cells. *J. Exp. Med.* **172,** 921–929.
66. Swain, S. L., Weinberg, A. D., English, M., and Huston, G. (1990) IL-4 directs the development of Th2–like helper effectors. *J. Immunol.* **145,** 3796–3806.
67. Park, C. S., Choi, Y. S., Ki, S. Y., Moon, S. H., Jeong, S. W., Uh, S. T., and Kim, Y. H. (1998) Granulocyte macrophage colony-stimulating factor is the main cytokine enhancing survival of eosinophils in asthmatic airways. *Eur. Respir. J.* **12,** 872–878.
68. Sousa, A. R., Poston, R. N., Lane, S. J., Narhosteen, J. A., and Lee, T. H. (1993) Detection of GM-CSF in asthmatic bronchial epithelium and decrease by inhaled corticosteroids. *Am. Rev. Respir. Dis.* **147,** 1557–1561.
69. Broide, D. H. and Firestein, G. S. (1991) Endobronchial allergen challenge: demonstration of cellular source of granulocyte macrophage colony-stimulating factor by in situ hybridization. *J. Clin. Invest.* **88,** 1048–1053.
70. Fujisawa, T., Abu-Ghazaleh, R., Kita, H., Sanderson, C. J., and Gleich, G. J. (1990) Regulatory effect of cytokines on eosinophil degranulation. *J. Immunol.* **144,** 642–646.

71. Tai, P. C. and Spry, C. J. (1990) Effects of recombinant granulocyte-macrophage colony-stimulating factor (GM-CSF) and interleukin-3 on the secretory capacity of human blood eosniophils. *Clin. Exp. Immunol.* **80,** 426–434.
72. Gilberstein, D. S., Owen, W. F., Gasson, J. C., Di Persio, J. F., Golde, D. W., Bina, J. C., et al. (1986) Enhancement of human eosinophil cytotoxicity and leukotriene synthesis by biosynthetic (recombinant) pneulocyte-macrophage colony-stimulating factor. *J. Immunol.* **137,** 3290–3294.
73. Berkman, N., Krishnan, V. L., Gilbey, T., Newton, R., O'Connor, B. J., Barnes, P. J., and Chung, K. F. (1996) Expression of RANTES mRNA and protein in airways of patients with mild asthma. *Am. J. Respir. Crit. Care Med.* **154,** 1804–1811.
74. Ying, S., Robinson, D. S., Meng, Q., Rottman, J., Kennedy, R., Ringler, D. J., et al. (1997) Enhanced expression of eotaxin and CCR3 mRNA and protein in atopic asthma. Association with airway hyperresponsiveness and predominant co-localization of eotaxin mRNA to bronchial epithelial and endothelial cells. *Eur. J. Immunol.* **27,** 3507–3516.
75. Collins, P. D., Griffiths-Johnson, D. A., Jose, P. J., Williams, T. J., and Marleau, S. (1995) Cooperation between interleukin-5 and the chemokine,eotaxin, to induce eosinophil accumulation in vivo. *J. Exp. Med.* **182,** 1169–1174.
76. Palframan, R. T., Collins, P. D., Severs, N. J., Rothery, S., Williams, T. J., and Rankin, S. M. (1998) Mechanisms of acute eosinophil mobilization from the bone marrow stimulated by interleukin 5: the role of specific adhesion molecules and phosphatidylinositol 3-kinase. *J. Exp. Med.* **188,** 1621–1632.
77. Hisada, T., Hellewell, P., Teixeira, M. M., Malm, M. G. K., Salmon, M., Huang, T., and Chung, K. F. (1999) α_4-integrin dependent eotaxin-induction of bronchial hyperresponsiveness and eosinophil migration in IL-5 transgenic mice. *Am. J. Respir. Cell. Mol. Biol.* **20,** 992–1000.
78. John, M., Lim, S., Seybold, J., Jose, P., Robichaud, A., O'Connor, B., Barnes, P. J., and Chung, K. F. (1998) Inhaled corticosteroids increase interleukin-10 but reduce macrophage inflammatory protein-1α, granulocyte-macrophage colony-stimulating factor and interferon-γ release from alveolar macrophages in asthma. *Am. J. Respir. Crit. Care Med.* **157,** 256–262.
79. Hallsworth, M. P., Soh, C. P. C., Lane, S. J., Arm, J. P., and Lee, T. H. (1994) Selective enhancement of GM-CSF, TNF-α, IL-1β and IL-8 production by monocytes and macrophages of asthmatic subjects. *Eur. Respir. J.* **7,** 1096–1102.
80. Cembrzynska-Norvak, M., Szklarz, E., Inglot, A. D., and Teodorczyk-Injeyan, J. A. (1993) Elevated release of TNF-α and interferon-gamma by bronchoalveolar leukocytes from patients with bronchial asthma. *Am. Rev. Respir. Dis.* **147,** 291–295.
81. Broide, D. H. and Firestein, G. S. (1991) Endobronchial allergen challenge in asthma. Demonstration of cellular source of granulocyte-macrophage colony stimulating factor by in situ hybridization. *J. Clin. Invest.* **88,** 1048–1053.
82. Gosset, P., Tsicopoulos, A., Wallaert, B., Vannimenus, C., Joseph, M., Tonnel, A. B., and Capron, A. (1991) Increased secretion by tumor necrosis factor a and interleukin 6 by alveolar macrophages consecutive to the development of the late asthmatic reaction. *J. Allergy Clin. Immunol.* **88,** 561–571.

83. Broide, D. H., Lotz, M., Cuomo, A. J., Coburn, D. A., Federman, E. C., and Wasserman, S. I. (1992) Cytokines in symptomatic asthmatic airways. *J. Allergy Clin. Immunol.* **89,** 958–967.
84. Spiteri, M., Knight, R. A., Jeremy, J. Y., Barnes, P. J., and Chung, K. F. (1994) Alveolar macrophage-induced suppression of T-cell hyperresponsiveness in bronchial asthma is reversed by allergen exposure. *Eur. Resp. J.* **7,** 1431–1438.
85. Aubus, P., Cosso, B., Godard, P., Miche, F. B., and Clot, J. (1984) Decreased suppressor cell activity of alveolar macrophages in bronchial asthma. *Am. Rev. Respir. Dis.* **130,** 875–878.
86. Sousa, A. R., Lane, S. J., Nakhosteen, J. A., Lee, T. H., and Poston, R. N. (1996) Expression of interleukin-1 beta (IL-1beta) and interleukin-1 receptor antagonist (IL-1ra) on asthmatic bronchial epithelium. *Am. J. Respir. Crit. Care Med.* **154,** 1061–1066.
87. Fischer, H. G., Frosch, S., Reske, K., and Reske-Kunz, A. B. (1988) Granulocyte-macrophage colony-stimulating factor activates macrophages derived from bone marrow cultures to synthesis of MHC class II molecules and to augmented antigen presentation function. *J. Immunol.* **141,** 3882–3888.
88. Chang, T. L., Shea, C. H., Urioste, S., Thompson, R. C., Boom, W. H., and Abbas, A. K. (1990) Heterogeneity of helper/inducer T lymphocytes: lymphokine production and lymphokine responsiveness. *J. Immunol.* **145,** 2803–2808.
89. Bradding, P., Roberts, J. A., Britten, K. M., Montefort, S., Djukanovic, R., Mueller, R., Heusser, C. H., et al. (1994) Interleukin-4, -5 and -6 and tumor necrosis factor-α in normal and asthmatic airways: evidence for the human mast cell as a source of these cytokines. *Am. J. Respir. Cell Mol. Biol.* **10,** 471–480.
90. Schleimer, R. P., Sterbinsky, C. A., Kaiser, C. A., Bickel, D. A., Klunk, K., Tomioka, K., et al. (1992) Interleukin-4 induces adherence of human eosinophils and basophils but not neutrophils to endothelium: association with expression of VCAM-1. *J. Immunol.* **148,** 1086–1092.
91. Tosi, M. F., Stark, J. M., Smith, C. W., Hamedani, A., Gruenert, D. C., and Infeld, M. D. (1992) Induction of ICAM-1 expression on human airway epithelial cells by inflammatory cytokines: effects on neutrophil-epithelial cell adhesion. *Am. J. Respir. Cell Mol. Biol.* **7,** 214–221.
92. Montefort, S., Gratziou, C., Goulding, D., Polosa, R., Haskard, D. O., Howarth, P. H., Holgate, S. T., and Carroll, M. P. (1994) Bronchial biopsy evidence for leukocyte infiltration and upregulation of leukocyte-endothelial cell adhesion molecules 6 hours after local allergen challenge of sensitized asthmatic airways. *J. Clin. Invest.* **93,** 1411–1421.
93. Gosset, P., Tillie Leblond, I., Janin, A., Marquette, C. H., Copin, M. C., Wallaert, B., and Tonnel, A. B. (1995) Expression of E-selectin, ICAM-1 and VCAM-1 on bronchial biopsies from allergic and non-allergic asthmatic patients. *Int. Arch. Allergy Immunol.* **106,** 69–77.
94. Ohkawara, Y., Yamauchi, K., Maruyama, N., Hoshi, H., Ohno, I., Honma, M., et al. (1995) In situ expression of the cell adhesion molecules in bronchial tissues from asthmatics with air flow limitation: in vivo evidence of VCAM- 1/VLA-4 interaction in selective eosinophil infiltration. *Am. J. Respir. Cell Mol. Biol.* **12,** 4–12.

95. Fukuda, T., Fukushima, Y., Numao, T., Ando, N., Arima, M., Nakajima, H., et al. (1996) Role of interleukin-4 and vascular cell adhesion molecule-1 in selective eosinophil migration into the airways in allergic asthma. *Am. J. Respir. Cell Mol. Biol.* **14,** 84–94.
96. Bentley, A. M., Durham, S. R., Robinson, D. S., Menz, G., Storz, C., Cromwell, O., Kay, A. B., and Wardlaw, A. J. (1993) Expression of endothelial and leukocyte adhesion molecules interacellular adhesion molecule-1, E-selectin, and vascular cell adhesion molecule-1 in the bronchial mucosa in steady-state and allergen-induced asthma. *J. Allergy Clin. Immunol.* **92,** 857–868.
97. Vignola, A. M., Campbell, A. M., Chanez, P., Bousquet, J., Paul Lacoste, P., Michel, F. B., and Godard, P. (1993) HLA-DR and ICAM-1 expression on bronchial epithelial cells in asthma and chronic bronchitis. *Am. Rev. Respir. Dis.* **148,** 689–694.
98. Abraham, W. M., Sielczak, M. W., Ahmed, A., Cortes, A., Lauredo, I. T., Kim, J., et al. (1994) Alpha 4-integrins mediate antigen-induced late bronchial responses and prolonged airway hyperresponsiveness in sheep. *J. Clin. Invest.* **93,** 776–787.
99. Demoly, P., Basset-Seguin, N., Chanez, P., Campbell, A. M., Gauthier-Rouvriere, C., Godard, P., Michel, R., and Bousquet, J. (1992) C-fos proto-oncogene expression in bronchial biopsies of asthmatics. *Am. J. Resp. Cell. Mol. Biol.* **7,** 128–133.
100. Adcock, I. M., Lane, S. J., Brown, C. R., Lee, T. H., and Barnes, P. J. (1995) Abnormal glucocorticoid receptor-activator protein 1 interaction in steroid-resistant asthma. *J. Exp. Med.* **182,** 1951–1958.
101. Hart, L. A., Krishnan, V. L., Adcock, I. M., Barnes, P. J., and Chung, K. F. (1998) Activation and localisation of transcription factor, nuclear factor-kB, in asthma. *Am. J. Respir. Crit. Care Med.* **158,** 1585–1592.
102. Hamid, Q., Springall, D. R., Riveros-Moreno, V., Chanez, P., Howarth, P., Redington, A., et al. (1993) Induction of nitric oxide synthase in asthma. *Lancet* **342,** 1510–1514.
103. Shannon, V. R., Chanez, P., Bousquet, J., and Holtzman, M. J. (1993) Histochemical evidence for induction of arachidonate 15-lipoxygenase in airway disease. *Am. Rev. Respir. Dis.* **147,** 1024–1028.
104. Sousa, A. R., Lane, S. J., Nakhosteen, J. A., Yoshimura, T., Lee, T. H., and Poston, R. N. (1994) Increased expression of the monocyte chemoattractant protein-1 in bronchial tissues from asthmatic subjects. *Am. J. Resp. Cell Mol. Biol.* **10,** 142–147.
105. Yang, L., Cohn, L., Zhang, D. H., Homer, R., Ray, A., and Ray, P. (1998) Essential role of nuclear factor kappaB in the induction of eosinophilia in allergic airway inflammation. *J. Exp. Med.* **188,** 1739–1750.
106. Zhang, D. H., Yang, L., and Ray, A. (1998) Differential responsiveness of the IL-5 and IL-4 genes to transcription factor GATA-3. *J. Immunol.* **161,** 3817–3821.
107. Barnes, P. J., Chung, K. F., and Page, C. P. (1998) Inflammatory mediators of asthma: an update. *Pharmacol. Rev.* **50,** 515–596.

108. Davidson, A. B., Lee, T. H., Scanlon, P. D., Solway, J., McFadden, E. R., Ingram, R. H., et al. (1987) Bronchoconstrictor effects of leukotriene E4 in normal and asthmatic subjects. *Am. Rev. Respir. Dis.* **135,** 500–504.
109. Arm, J. P., Spur, B. W., and Lee, T. H. (1988) Effects of inhaled leukotriene E4 on the airway responsiveness to histamine in subjects with asthma and normal subjects. *J. Allergy Clin. Immunol.* **82,** 654–660.
110. Bischoff, S. C., Krieger, M., Brunner, T., and Dahinden, C. A. (1992) Monocyte chemotactic protein 1 is a potent activator of human basophils. *J. Exp. Med.* **175,** 1271–1275.
111. Panettieri, R. A., Tan, E. M., Ciocca, V., Luttmann, M. A., Leonard, T. B., and Hay, D. W. (1998) Effects of LTD4 on human airway smooth muscle cell proliferation, matrix expression, and contraction In vitro: differential sensitivity to cysteinyl leukotriene receptor antagonists. *Am. J. Respir. Cell Mol. Biol.* **19,** 453–461.
112. Chung, K. F. (1995) Leukotriene receptor antagonists and biosynthesis inhibitors: potential breakthrough in asthma therapy. *Eur. Respir. J.* **8,** 1203–1213.
113. Spector, S. L., Smith, L. J., and Glass, M. (1994) Effects of six weeks of therapy with oral doses of ICI **204,219,** a leukotriene D4 receptor antagonist, in subjects with bronchial asthma. *Am. J. Respir. Crit. Care Med.* **150,** 618–623.
114. Noonan, M. J., Chervinsky, P., Brandon, M., Zhang, J., Kundu, S., McBurney, J., and Reiss, T. F. (1998) Montelukast, a potent leukotriene receptor antagonist, causes dose-related improvements in chronic asthma. Montelukast Asthma Study Group. *Eur. Respir. J.* **11,** 1232–1239.
115. Roquet, A., Dahlen, B., Kumlin, M., Ihre, E., Anstren, G., Binks, S., and Dahlen, S. E. (1997) Combined antagonism of leukotrienes and histamine produces predominant inhibition of allergen-induced early and late phase airway obstruction in asthmatics. *Am. J. Respir. Crit. Care Med.* **155,** 1856–1863.
116. Chung, K. F. (1992) Platelet-activating factor in inflammation and pulmonary disorders. *Clin. Sci.* **83,** 127–138.
117. Kuitert, L. M., Angus, R. M., Barnes, N., Barnes, P. J., Bone, M. C., Chung, K. F., et al. (1995) Effect of a novel potent platelet-activating factor antagonist, Modipafant, in clinical asthma. *Am. J. Respir. Crit. Care Med.* **151,** 1331–1335.
118. Spence, D. P., Johnston, S. L., Calverley, P. M., Dhillon, P., Higgins, C., Ramhamadany, E., et al. (1994) Effect of the orally active platelet-activating factor antagonist WEB 2086 in the treatment of asthma. *Am. J. Respir. Crit. Care Med.* **149,** 1142–1148.
119. Chung, K. F., Evans, T. W., Graf, P. D., and Nadel, J. A. (1985) Modulation of cholinergic neurotransmission in canine airways by thromboxane-mimetic U 46619. *Eur. J. Pharmacol.* **117,** 373–375.
120. Fuller, R. W., Dixon, C. M. S., Dollery, C. T., and Barnes, P. J. (1986) Prostaglandin D2 potentiates airway responses to histamine and methacholine. *Am. Rev. Respir. Dis.* **133,** 252–254.
121. Walters, E. H., Parrish, R. W., Bevan, C., and Smoth, A. P. (1981) Induction of bronchial hypersensitivity: evidence for a role of prostaglandins. *Thorax* **36,** 571–574.

122. Melillo, E., Woolley, K. L., Manning, P. J., Watson, R. M., and O'Byrne, P. M. (1994) Effect of inhaled PGE2 on exercise-induced bronchoconstriction in asthmatic subjects. *Am. J. Respir. Crit. Care Med.* **149,** 1138–1141.
123. Pavord, I. D., Wong, C. S., Williams, J., and Tattersfield, A. E. (1993) Effect of inhaled prostaglandin E2 on allergen-induced asthma. *Am. Rev. Respir. Dis.* **148,** 87–90.
124. Barnes, P. J., Baraniuk, J. N., and Belvisi, M. G. (1991) Neuropeptides in the respiratory tract. Part 1. *Am. Rev. Respir. Dis.* **144,** 1187–1198.
125. Daniele, R. P., Barnes, P. J., Goetzl, E. J., Nadel, J., O'Dorisio, S., Kiley, J., and Jacobs, T. (1992) NHLBI workshop summaries. Neuroimmune interactions in the lung. *Am. Rev. Respir. Dis.* **145,** 1230–1235.
126. Christiansen, S. C., Proud, D., and Sarnoff, R. B. (1992) Elevation of tissue kallikrein and kinin in the airways of asthmatic subjects after endobronchial allergen challenge. *Amer. Rev. Resp. Dis.* **145,** 900–905.
127. Liu, M. C., Hubbard, W. C., Proud, D., Stealey, B. A., Galli, S. J., Kagey Sobotka, A., Bleecker, E. R., and Lichtenstein, L. M. (1991) Immediate and late inflammatory responses to ragweed antigen challenge of the peripheral airways in allergic asthmatics. Cellular, mediator, and permeability changes. *Am. Rev. Respir. Dis.* **144,** 51–58.
128. Proud, D., Naclerio, R. M., Gwaltney, J. M., and Hendley, J. O. (1990) Kinins are generated in nasal secretions during natural rhinovirus colds. *J. Infect. Dis.* **161,** 120–123.
129. Molimard, M., Martin, C. A., Naline, E., Hirsch, A., and Advenier, C. (1994) Contractile effects of bradykinin on the isolated human small bronchus. *Am. J. Respir. Crit. Care Med.* **149,** 123–127.
130. Berman, A. R., Liu, M. C., Wagner, E. M., and Proud, D. (1996) Dissociation of bradykinin-induced plasma exudation and reactivity in peripheral airways. *Am. J. Respir. Crit. Care Med.* **154,** 418–423.
131. Baker, A. P., Hillegrass, L. M., Holden, D. A., and Smith, W. J. (1977) Effect of kallidin, substance P, and other basic polypeptides on the production of respiratory macromolecules. *Am. Rev. Respir. Dis.* **115,** 811–817.
132. Kaufman, M. P., Coleridge, H. M., Coleridge, J. C. G., and Baker, D. G. (1980) Bradykinin stimulates afferent vagal C-fibers in intrapulmonary airways of dogs. *J. Appl. Physiol.* **48,** 511–517.
133. Barnes, P. J. (1986) Asthma as an axon reflex. *Lancet* **i,** 242–245.
134. Hay, D. W., Henry, P. J., and Goldie, R. G. (1996) Is endothelin-1 a mediator in asthma? *Am. J. Respir. Crit. Care Med.* **154,** 1594–1597.
135. Redington, A. E., Springall, D. R., Meng, Q. H., Tuck, A. B., Holgate, S. T., Polak, J. M., and Howarth, P. H. (1997) Immunoreactive endothelin in bronchial biopsy specimens: increased expression in asthma and modulation by corticosteroid therapy. *J. Allergy Clin. Immunol.* **100,** 544–552.
136. Redington, A. E., Springall, D. R., Ghatei, M. A., Madden, J., Bloom, S. R., Frew, A. J., et al. (1997) Airway endothelin levels in asthma: influence of endobronchial allergen challenge and maintenance corticosteroid therapy. *Eur. Respir. J.* **10,** 1026–1032.

137. Redington, A. E., Madden, J., Frew, A. J., Djukanovic, R., Roche, W. R., Holgate, S. T., and Howarth, P. H. (1997) Transforming growth factor-β 1 in asthma. Measurement in bronchoalveolar lavage fluid. *Am. J. Respir. Crit. Care Med.* **156,** 642–647.
138. Minshall, E. M., Leung, D. Y. M., Martin, R. J., Song, Y. L., Cameron, L., Ernst, P., and Hamid, Q. (1997) Eosinophil-associated TGFβ1 mRNA expression and airways fibrosis in asthma. *Am. J. Respir. Cell. Mol. Biol.* **17,** 326–333.
139. Kharitonov, S. A., Yates, D., Robbins, R. A., Logan-Sinclair, R., Shinebourne, E. A., and Barnes, P. J. (1994) Increased nitric oxide in exhaled air of asthmatic patients. *Lancet* **343,** 133–135.
140. Kuo, H. P., Liu, S., and Barnes, P. J. (1992) Effect of endogenous nitric oxide on neurogenic plasma exudation in guinea-pig airways. *Eur. J. Pharmacol.* **221,** 385–388.
141. Taylor Robinson, A. W., Phillips, R. S., Severn, A., Moncada, S., and Liew, F. Y. (1993) Role of TH1 and TH2 cells in a rodent malaria infection. *Science* **260,** 1931–1934.
142. Harris, J. R., Magnus, P., Samuelson, S. O., and Tambs, K. (1997) No evidence for effects of family environment on asthma. A retrospective study of Norwegian twins. *Am. J. Respir. Crit. Care Med.* **156,** 43–49.
143. Nieminen, M. M., Kaprio, J., and Koskenvuo, M. (1991) A population-based study of bronchial asthma in adult twin pairs. *Chest* **100,** 70–75.
144. Sandford, A. J., Shirakawa, T., Moffatt, M. F., Daniels, S. E., Ra, C., Faux, J. A., et al. (1993) Localisation of atopy and beta subunit of high-affinity IgE receptor (Fc epsilon RI) on chromosome 11q. *Lancet* **341,** 332–334.
145. Doull, I. J., Lawrence, S., Watson, M., Begishvili, T., Beasley, R. W., Lampe, F., Holgate, T., and Morton, N. E. (1996) Allelic association of gene markers on chromosomes 5q and 11q with atopy and bronchial hyperresponsiveness. *Am. J. Respir. Crit. Care Med.* **153,** 1280–1284.
146. Postma, D. S., Bleecker, E. R., Amelung, P. J., Holroyd, K. J., Xu, J., Panhuysen, C. I., Meyers, D. A., and Levitt, R. C. (1995) Genetic susceptibility to asthma—bronchial hyperresponsiveness coinherited with a major gene for atopy. *N. Engl. J. Med.* **333,** 894–900.
147. Marsh, D. G., Neely, J. D., Breazeale, D. R., Ghosh, B., Freidhoff, L. R., Ehrlich Kautzky, E., et al. (1994) Linkage analysis of IL4 and other chromosome 5q31.1 markers and total serum immunoglobulin E concentrations. *Science* **264,** 1152–1156.
148. Walley, A. J. and Cookson, W. O. (1996) Investigation of an interleukin-4 promoter polymorphism for associations with asthma and atopy. *J. Med. Genet.* **33,** 689–692.
149. Moffatt, M. F., Hill, M. R., Cornelis, F., Schou, C., Faux, J. A., Young, R. P., et al. (1994) Genetic linkage of T-cell receptor alpha/delta complex to specific IgE responses. *Lancet* **343,** 1597–1600.
150. Hall, I. P., Wheatley, A., Wilding, P., and Liggett, S. B. (1995) Association of Glu 27 beta 2-adrenoceptor polymorphism with lower airway reactivity in asth-

matic subjects. Association of Glu 27 β_2-adrenoceptor polymorphism with lower airway reactivity in asthmatic subjects. *Lancet* **345,** 1213–1214.

151. Daniels, S. E., Bhattacharrya, S., James, A., Leaves, N. I., Young, A., Hill, M. R., et al. (1996) Genome-wide search for quantitative trait loci underlying asthma. *Nature* **383,** 247–250.
152. Moffatt, M. F. and Cookson, W. O. (1997) Tumour necrosis factor haplotypes and asthma. *Hum. Mol. Genet.* **6,** 551–554.
153. Sporik, R., Holgate, S. T., Platts-Mills, T. A. E., and Cogswell, J. J. (1990) Exposure to house-dust mite allergen (Der p I) and the development of asthma in childhood. *N. Engl. J. Med.* **323,** 502–507.
154. Holt, P. G., McMenamin, C., and Nelson, D. (1990) Primary sensitisation to inhalant allergens in infancy. *Ped. Allergy Immunol.* **1,** 3–13.
155. Bjorksten, B. (1994) Risk factors in early childhood for the development of atopic diseases. *Allergy* **49,** 400–407.
156. Holt, P. G. and Sly, P. D. (1997) Allergic respiratory disease: strategic targets for primary prevention during childhood. *Thorax* **52,** 1–4.
157. Lenschow, D. J., Walunas, T. L., and Bluestone, J. A. (1996) CD28/B7 system of T cell costimulation. *Annu. Rev. Immunol.* **14,** 233–258.
158. Harris, N., Peach, R., Naemura, J., Linsley, P. S., Le Gros, G., and Ronchese, F. (1997) CD80 costimulation is essential for the induction of airway eosinophilia. *J. Exp. Med.* **185,** 177–182.
159. Sur, S., Crotty, T. B., Kephart, G. M., Hyma, B. A., Colby, T. V., Reed, C. E., Hunt, L. W., and Gleich, G. J. (1993) Sudden-onset fatal asthma: A distinct entity with few eosinophils and relatively more neutrophils in the airway submucosa? *Am. Rev. Resp. Dis* **148,** 713–719.
160. Johnston, S. L., Pattemore, P. K., Sanderson, G., Smith, S., Lampe, F., Josephs, L., et al. (1995) Community study of role of viral infections in exacerbations of asthma in 9–11 year old children. *Br. Med. J.* **310,** 1225–1229.
161. Grunberg, K., Timmers, M. C., Smits, H. H., de Klerk, E. P., Dick, E. C., Spaan, W. J., Hiemstra, P. S., and Sterk, P. J. (1997) Effect of experimental rhinovirus 16 colds on airway hyperresponsiveness to histamine and interleukin-8 in nasal lavage in asthmatic subjects in vivo. *Clin. Exp. Allergy* **27,** 36–45.
162. Fraenkel, D. J., Bardin, P. G., Sanderson, G., Lampe, F., Johnston, S. L., and Holgate, S. T. (1995) Lower airways inflammation during rhinovirus colds in normal and in asthmatic subjects. *Am. J. Respir. Crit. Care Med.* **151,** 879–886.
163. Calhoun, W. J., Dick, E. C., Schwartz, L. B., and Busse, W. W. (1994) Common cold virus, rhinovirus **16,** potentiates airway inflammation after segmental antigen bronchoprovocation in allergic subjects. *J. Clin. Invest.* **94,** 2200–2208.
164. Zhu, Z., Tang, W., Ray, A., Wu, Y., Einarsson, O., Landry, M. L., Gwaltney, J. and Elias, J. A. (1996) Rhinovirus stimulation of interleukin-6 in vivo and in vitro: evidence for nuclear factor-kB-dependent transcriptional activation. *J. Clin. Invest.* **97,** 421–430.
165. Chung, K. F. and Godard, P. (1999) Difficult therapy-resistant asthma: report of a task force. *Eur. Respir. J.* **13,** 1198–1208.

166. Chanez, P., Dent, G., Yukawa, T., Barnes, P. J., and Chung, K. F. (1990) Generation of oxygen free radicals from blood eosinophils from asthma patients after stimulation with PAF or phorbol ester. *Eur. Respir. J.* **3,** 1002–1007.
167. Lim, S., John, M., Seybold, J., Taylor D., Witt, D., Barnes, P. J., and Chung, K. F. (2000) Increased interleukin 10 and macrophage inflammatory protein-1α release from blood monocytes ex-vivo during late phase response to allergen in asthma. *Allergy*, in press.

2

Culture of Normal Human Airway Epithelial Cells and Measurement of Mucin Synthesis and Secretion

Reen Wu

1. Introduction

The plasticity of conducting airway epithelia is well recognized *(1–3)*. Under normal conditions, the epithelia express mucociliary function, which is the first pulmonary defense mechanism against inhaled air pollutants. Aberrance in this function is either the cause or one of the major contributors to the pathogenesis of various pulmonary diseases, such as asthma and bronchitis. To exert this vital defense function, mucus-secreting cell types of surface epithelium and submucosal gland synthesize and secrete a high-mol-wt mucous glycoprotein, mucin, which is responsible for the viscoelastic property of the surface mucus layer. Secreted mucus, which is able to trap air pollutants and microorganisms, is steadily removed from the airway surface by ciliary escalation. Overall, the coordinated mucociliary function helps to maintain homeostasis in airway lumen.

However, changes in airway epithelial cell (EC) differentiation are frequently observed *(1–3)*, including the development of squamous and mucous cell metaplasia, as well as hypermucus secretion. The nature of these changes is not entirely clear. In addition, conducting airway epithelium also plays a pivotal role in the initiation and development of bronchogenic carcinoma *(2)*. Most bronchogenic cancers are epithelial in origin. An uncontrolled cell proliferation of a certain EC type may lead to the development of a certain type of lung cancer. Because of the plasticity of epithelium, tracing the original cell type that initiates carcinogenic development is most difficult. These difficulties suggest a great need to understand the nature of airway EC differentiation and how it is regulated.

To achieve these goals, progress has been made in culturing differentiated airway ECs from human tissues in a well-defined culture environment *(4,5)*,

From: *Methods in Molecular Medicine, vol. 44: Asthma: Mechanisms and Protocols*
Edited by: K. F. Chung and I. Adcock

and for mucin quantitation *(6)*. The primary culture system of hamster tracheal ECs is the first in vitro demonstration of new mucous cell differentiation *(7,8)* and ciliogenesis *(9)*. This success mostly results from the development of serum-free, hormone-supplemented medium and the use of collagen gel substratum for cultivation. However, this similar culture condition was unable to allow primary human airway ECs to achieve new ciliogenesis in culture, except for mucous cell differentiation. It was not until the development of an air–liquid interface culture system that new ciliogenesis could be demonstrated in human cells *(10,11)*. The first part of this chapter describes the procedures involved in the isolation of human airway ECs *(12)*, the culture condition for serial cultivation of human airway ECs, and the air–liquid interface system to achieve mucociliary differentiation; the second half describes how mucin secretion and synthesis are quantified by a double-sandwich enzyme-linked, immunosorbent assay (ELISA) method.

Hypersecretion of mucin and the hypertrophy of mucous cell type are two clinical hallmarks associated with various airway diseases and infections *(13,14)*. There are biochemical *(15,16)* and immunological methods *(6,17)* to measure these abnormalities: The biochemical method requires the fractionation of samples by gel filtration *(15)* and centrifugation, prior to the quantitation; for the immunological method, no preparation is needed. The biochemical separation method is based on the biochemical properties of mucin, which include the following characteristics: high mol wt, highly glycosylated and *O*-glycosidic linkage, and high buoyant density. The immunological approach is based on the specificity of the antibody (Ab), which must be able to recognize purified mucin and mucus-secreting granules at the morphological level *(6,17,18)*. However, with few exceptions, Abs generated are specific for the carbohydrate portion of high-mol-wt mucous glycoprotein. The heterogeneous structure of mucous carbohydrate chains is well recognized, including differences in length, branching unit, and terminal sugar. Therefore, it is necessary to characterize the specificity of the epitope of Ab used in the study. The author and colleagues have extensively characterized both human mucin-specific 17B1 and 17Q2 monoclonal antibodies (MAbs), before the application of these Abs for mucin ELISA *(6,18)*, and have observed that the epitopes for both Abs are not determined by blood group antigen or terminal sugar, nor are they affected by enzymes specific to various proteoglycans. However, the activity of the epitope was reduced by half by endo-β-galactosidase *(6)*. The nature of this effect is not clear. Nevertheless, the result suggests that the epitope of these mucin-specific Abs may involve the structure at or near the nonsulfated galactosidic bond, such as Gal(β1–4)Glc in lacto-*N*-tetraose, the structure of which is the major backbone structure in mucin. Thus, these studies confirm the specificity of these two Abs on the carbohydrate chains of human mucin.

Using these Abs, a double-sandwich ELISA method ***(6)*** was developed to quantify the amount of human mucin in various samples. The basic approach in this ELISA method is, first, to trap mucin antigen in the liquid sample by the purified immunoglobin of these MAbs, then to quantify the amount of mucin trapped on the microplate with an alkaline phosphatase-conjugated, mucin-specific Ab. Because there are many epitope sites in mucin, a single mucin-specific Ab is used for both the trapping and detecting steps. The author and others have used this ELISA system to determine the amount of mucin secreted in culture and in various biological specimens. Some of these studies have led to the conclusion that the serum mucin level can be used as a diagnostic indicator that is correlated with the severity of the airway diseases, cystic fibrosis ***(19)***, and acute respiratory distress syndrome ***(20)***.

2. Materials

2.1. Human Airway EC Culture

2.1.1. Serial Cultivation

1. Minimum essential medium (MEM) from Gibco-BRL (Grand Island, NY) containing 50 U/L penicillin and 50 µg/L streptomycin (Sigma, St. Louis, MO), 50 mg/L gentamicin (Irvine Scientific, Santa Ana, CA), 1.98 g/L $NaHCO_3$, and 15 m*M* HEPES, pH 7.2.
2. 0.1% Protease solution: 0.1 g Sigma's type 14 protease in 100 mL MEM medium. This solution should be sterilized by filtering through 0.2-µm sterile filter membrane, then stored at –20°C until use.
3. Fetal bovine serum (FBS) (Sigma, or any other qualified commercial company).
4. Equal volumes of Dulbecco Modified Eagle's Medium (DMEM) and Ham's F12 nutrient medium are mixed, containing similar concentrations of penicillin, streptomycin, gentamicin, and 15 m*M* HEPES buffer as MEM, except $NaHCO_3$ at 2.45 g/L.
5. Airway serum-free, hormone-supplemented medium: DMEM–F12 medium is supplemented with 5 µg/mL insulin (Sigma), 5 µg/mL transferrin (Sigma), 10 ng/mL epidermal growth factor (Upstate Biotechnology, Lake Placid, NY), 0.5 µ*M* dexamethasone (Sigma), 20 ng/mL cholera toxin (List Biochemical, Campbell, CA), 15 µg/mL bovine hypothalamus extract, (30 n*M* all-*trans*-retinoic acid, 5 mg/mL bovine serum albumin (BSA) (Sigma), 0.3 m*M* $MgCl_2$, 0.4 m*M* $MgSO_4$, and 1.05 m*M* $CaCl_2$ (*see* **Note 1**).
6. 0.1% Trypsin (Sigma)–ethylene diamine tetraacetic acid (EDTA) (1 m*M*), stored at 4°C.
7. 1 mg/mL soybean trypsin-inhibitor (Sigma), stored at 4°C.

2.1.2. Differentiation of Human Airway ECs in Culture

1. Collagen gel substratum preparation: Collagen gel solution is prepared by mixing 3 mg/mL Vitrogen solution (Collagen, Palo Alto, CA) with an alkaline–F12

solution at 4:1 vol ratio under cold (4°C) conditions. The alkaline–F12 solution is prepared by mixing 1 *N* NaOH with 5X F12 medium at a ratio of 1:2.
2. Transwell chamber (ICN).
3. Humidified CO_2-37°C incubator.

2.2. Mucin Quantitation

2.2.1. Preparation of Standard Human Mucin Antigen

1. Protease inhibitor solution: 200 m*M* *p*-phenylmethylsulfonyl fluoride (PMSF) dissolved in methanol, toxic, and stored at 4°C.
2. CsCl density gradient centrifugation: 250,000*g*, for 48 h.
3. Sepharose CL-2B column (Pharmacia, Piscataway, NJ)
4. Elution buffer: Phosphate-buffered saline (PBS) solution is added with 0.1% sodium dodecyl sulfate and 3% β-mercaptoethanol.
5. Dialysis solution: PBS and water.

2.2.2. Quantitation of Mucin by Double-Sandwich ELISA Method

1. 17Q2 (or 17B1) immunoglobulin G (IgG) solution (Babco, Berkeley, CA): IgG of 17Q2 (17B1) is purified by affinity chromatography in a protein G-agarose column. Briefly, 2–5 mL 17Q2 (17B1) ascite fluids are passed through a protein G-agarose column at pH 8.0. The column is then washed several times with 0.01 *M* Tris-Cl, pH 8.0. After extensive washing, IgG of 17Q2 (17B1) is eluted from the column by a pH 3.0 buffer. After extensive dialysis against 2–3 changes of cold PBS, IgG concentration is adjusted to 1 mg/mL, and stored at –20°C.
2. Alkaline phosphatase-conjugated IgG solution: Conjugation is carried out by mixing 2 mg (2 mL) 17Q2 (17B1) IgG and 5 mg alkaline phosphatase (Sigma) in the presence of 0.06% glutaraldehyde. After an overnight conjugation at cold temperatures, the mixture is extensively dialyzed against PBS. After dialysis, the mixture is adjusted to a final solution containing 200 μg/mL IgG and 2 mg/mL BSA, and stored at 4°C.
3. Coating solution: 0.05 *M* sodium carbonate, pH 9.0, stored at 4°C.
4. Washing solution: PBS–Tween-20 (0.05%), filtered, and stored at room temperature.
5. Phosphate substrate solution: *p*-nitrophenyl phosphate, disodium (Sigma) at 1 mg/mL in 10% diethanolamine solution (pH 9.8). Freshly prepared at room temperature.
6. Immulon II 96-well plate (Dynatech, Alexandria, VA).
7. 3 *N* NaOH.
8. MR600 Microplate reader (Dynatech) or equivalent model from other manufacturer.

3. Methods

3.1. Growth and Differentiation of Human Airway ECs in Culture

Primary culture of human airway ECs is widely used as an in vitro model for various studies related to airway diseases, bronchogenic cancer, environmental air pollutant effects, and cell differentiation. ECs are dissociated from air-

Table 1
Effects of Culture Conditions on Cell Differentiation of Cultured Airway ECs

Culture conditions	Mucous cell differentiation	Ciliogenesis
Tissue culture dish	+	–
Collagen gel substratum	++	–
Transwell chamber/air–liquid interface	+++	++
Transwell chamber/CG/air–liquid interface	++++	++++

way tissue by protease (*see* **Note 2**). These ECs rapidly adhere to the culture surface of various tissue culture wares. With the development of defined hormone-supplemented culture medium, human airway ECs can be serially cultivated. This procedure yields ECs obtained from the distal region of airway tree, which is isolated by microdissection. Despite serial cultivation, ECs are largely squamous ones, expressing keratinization and cornification. To achieve mucociliary differentiation, at least three additional culture conditions are needed. First, vitamin A or one of its retinoid derivatives is essential for all of the differentiation to occur in vitro. The second requirement is to maintain the culture under an air–liquid interface condition. Finally, the use of collagen gel substratum can further maximize the differential potential. **Table 1** summarizes the extent of EC differentiation under various culture conditions.

3.1.1. Serial Cultivation of Human Airway ECs

Human airway tissues can be obtained from local and national programs related to consent autopsy, organ transplant, and routine biopsy services. These tissues are immersed in serum-free MEM with various antibiotics, such as penicillin, streptomycin, and gentamicin, and shipped to the lab cold. Treating these tissues immediately upon arrival with further washing and cleaning is advisable, because it can further minimize the contamination in culture (*see* **Note 3**).

1. These tissues are immersed in 0.1% protease solution in MEM overnight at 4°C or for 1 h at 37°C (*see* **Note 4**).
2. After protease treatment, epithelial sheets are flushed away from tissue with ice-cold 10% FBS–MEM medium, and the cold cell suspension is then centrifuged at 200*g* for 5 min (*see* **Note 5**).
3. The cell pellets are then suspended in the airway serum-free, hormone-supplemented culture medium at $0.1–1 \times 10^6$ cells/mL. Normally, the initial seeding density is at least 1×10^4 cells/cm^2 of culture surface area. Dishes are incubated in a CO_2 incubator at 37°C and 5% CO_2 (*see* **Note 6**).
4. Medium change is carried out every other day.

5. A confluent culture with a cell density of approx 1–5 × 10^5 cells/cm^2 is achieved within 7–10 d of incubation (*see* **Note 7**).
6. For subculturing, confluent dishes are treated with trypsin–EDTA solution at room temperature, or at 37°C, until cell detachment occurs. An equal or slightly higher volume of trypsin-inhibitor solution is added to stop further trypsinization (*see* **Note 8**).
7. The cell suspension is centrifuged, and cell pellets are suspended in the culture medium with a density of 1 × 10^5 cells/mL.
8. Cells are plated at a density of 1 × 10^4 cells/cm^2. Human airway ECs can be routinely passaged 3–5×, with a total of approx 25 population doublings, until senescence is reached.

3.1.2. Expression of Mucociliary Differentiation in Culture (see **Note 9**)

1. ICN's Transwell chamber well is coated with freshly prepared collagen gel solution at 0.2 mL/cm^2 surface area. Incubate at 37°C for 30–60 min until gel forms.
2. ECs, obtained from protease-treated tissues, are suspended in the airway serum-free, hormone-supplemented medium, and pipeted on the chamber well.
3. After 1-d incubation, the medium at the upper chamber well of Transwell is removed and replaced with new serum-free, hormone-supplemented medium.
4. The outer and lower part of the Transwell chamber is also filled with airway culture medium.
5. Maintain the immersed culture condition with a periodic medium change for 5–7 d, then change the immersed culture condition to an air–liquid interface, by removing the apical culture medium and incubating the culture in a well-humidified CO_2 incubator.
6. After 7–10 d of air–liquid interface culturing, a mucociliary epithelium is formed in culture.

3.2. Mucin ELISA

3.2.1. Preparation of Referenced Mucin

1. Sputum mucus or secreted culture media collected from human airway cultures are treated with DNase and hyaluronidase in the presence of 1–2 m*M* PMSF protease-inhibitor solution.
2. After overnight treatment, the mixture is heat-denatured in the presence of 1% SDS and 3% β-mercaptoethanol.
3. Powdered CsCl is added to the mixture until a density of 1.5 g/mL is achieved.
4. The mixture is centrifuged at 30,000 rpm for 48 h. Fractions having a density greater than 1.5 g/mL are collected and pooled. The collected mixture is dialyzed against PBS.
5. The mixture is further fractionated in a preparative Sepharose CL-2B column, which has been equilibrated with the eluting solution of PBS–0.1%SDS–3% β-mercaptoethanol.

6. Void volume peak fractions are collected and further fractionated in a new Sepharose CL-2B column. Void volume fractions are collected and dialyzed against PBS and water, with 2–3 changes.
7. A small but sufficient amount of solution is subjected to amino-acid-analysis. The amino acid analyzed results provide both necessary information regarding the mucin nature of the preparation and information regarding the content.
8. Based on this information, references of mucin are prepared at 0.5, 1, 2, 4, 8, and 16 ng/mL levels.

3.2.2. Double-Sandwich Mucin ELISA Method

1. Immulon microplate wells are coated with purified 17Q2 (17B1) IgG, at 0.2 µg/well in coating buffer, and incubated at 37°C for 1 h under an airtight cover (*see* **Note 10**).
2. After washing with PBS–Tween-20 (0.05%) solution, 200 µL of various standard mucin (0.5–16 ng/mL), and unknown samples at different dilutions, are added to each well. The reaction is carried out at 37°C under an airtight cover for 1–2 h (*see* **Notes 11** and **12**).
3. Microplate wells are washed with PBS–Tween-20 (0.05%), then each well is treated with 200 µL diluted alkaline phosphatase-conjugated 17Q2 (17B1) IgG solution at 1 µg/mL IgG and 10 µg/mL BSA in PBS–Tween-20 (0.05%).
4. After further incubation at 37°C for 1 h under an airtight cover, wells are washed with PBS–Tween-20, and 200 µL phosphate substrate solution is added to each well for color development.
5. The reaction can be stopped by the addition of 50 µL 3 *N* NaOH to each well.
6. Developed color in the plate is read at 405 nm wavelength in an MR600 microplate reader.

4. Notes

1. Bovine hypothalamus extract is prepared according to the procedure described by Maciag et al. ***(21)***. Commercial sources, such as endothelial cell growth supplement from Collaborative Research (Waltham, MA), are also suitable. The concentration used in the culture should be predetermined, because preparation of the extract can be variable, and the biological activity is variable from lot to lot.
2. General safety and ethical rules for acquiring human tissue for research should be followed.
3. Microorganism contamination in human airway tissues, especially those from autopsy, is a major problem in preventing the development of a successful and uncontaminated primary culture. Generally, the fresher the tissue from an organ donor patient, the less contamination. The initial step of cleaning and treatments with various antibiotics on tissues can vastly improve the contamination problem.
4. Tissues are viable for several days, when immersed in the culture medium under cold condition (4°C).
5. Protease-dissociated EC preparation has a viability greater than 95%, and tissues can be repeatedly treated with protease to ensure a complete recovery of all ECs from tissue.

6. Seeding density less than the recommended 1×10^4 cells/cm^2 has a difficult time in achieving confluency and in subsequently performing serial cultivation.
7. Low calcium medium, such as LHC-9 ***(5)*** and the commercial media from Clonetics (San Diego, CA), such as the bronchial EC growth medium and small airway EC growth medium, are suitable for serial cultivation of airway ECs. Within the low-calcium medium (<0.1 m*M* Ca^{2+}), ECs multiply and maintain basal appearance. However, these low-calcium media are not suitable for airway ECs to grow on collagen gel substratum nor to express mucociliary differentiation.
8. Cells grown on tissue culture wares are easily used for serial cultivation by trypsin–EDTA solution; cells plated on collagen gel substratum are difficult to use.
9. Mucous cell differentiation in culture can be assessed at the level of mucin secretion, and the mucous cell population can be identified by mucin-specific Ab.
10. Primary IgG coating may be variable, depending on the quality of the microplate well. Excessive coating reduces the sensitivity of the assay; less coating traps less mucin and shortens the linearity of reference mucin.
11. The presence of detergents and reducing agents in the sample should be kept to a minimum, or <0.1% and 1 m*M* levels, respectively.
12. Protease inhibitor should be included during mucin ELISA for samples known to be contaminated with protease, such as sputum ***(19,20)***.

References

1. Basbaum, C. and Jany, B. (1990) Plasticity in the airway epithelium. *Am. J. Physiol. (Lung Cell Mol. Physiol.)* **259,** L38–L46.
2. Jetten, A. M. (1993) Proliferation and differentiation in normal and neoplastic tracheobronchial epithelial cells, in *Lung Cancer and Differentiation: Implications for Diagnosis and Treatment* (Bernal, S. D. and Hesketh, P. J., eds.), Marcel Dekker, New York, pp. 3–43.
3. Wu, R. (1997) Growth and differentiation of tracheobronchial epithelial cells, in *Lung Growth and Development* (McDonald, J. A., ed.), Marcel Dekker, New York, pp. 211–241.
4. Wu, R. (1986) In vitro differentiation of airway epithelial cells, in *In Vitro Models of Respiratory Epithelium* (Schiff, L. J., ed.), CRC, Boca Raton, FL, pp. 1–26.
5. Lechner, J. F., Stoner, G. D., Yoakum, G. H., Willey, J. C., Grafstrom, R. C., Mastui, T., LaVeck, M. A., and Harris, C. C. (1986) In vitro carcinogenesis studies with human tracheobronchial tissues and cells, in *In Vitro Models of Respiratory Epithelium* (Schiff, L. J., ed.), CRC, Boca Raton, FL, pp. 143–159.
6. Lin, H., Carlson, D. M., St. George, J. A., Plopper, C. G., and Wu, R. (1989) An ELISA method for the quantitation of tracheal mucins from human and nonhuman primates. *Am. J. Respir. Cell Mol. Biol.* **1,** 41–48.
7. Wu, R., Nolan, E., and Turner, C. (1985) Expression of tracheal differentiated functions in a serum-free hormone-supplemented medium. *J. Cell. Physiol.* **125,** 167–181.
8. Kim, K. C., Rearick, J. I., Nettesheim, P., and Jetten, A. M. (1985) Biochemical characterization of mucin secreted by hamster tracheal epithelial cells in primary culture. *J. Biol. Chem.* **260,** 4021–4027.

9. Lee, T. C., Wu, R., Brody, A. R., Barrett, J. C., and Nettesheim, P. (1983) Growth and differentiation of hamster tracheal epithelial cells in culture. *Exp. Lung Res.* **6,** 27–45.
10. Whitcutt, M. J., Adler, K. B., and Wu, R. (1988) A biphasic chamber system for maintaining polarity of differentiation of cultured respiratory tract epithelial cells. *In Vitro Cell. Dev. Biol.* **24,** 420–428.
11. de Jong, P. M., van Strekenburg, M. A. J. A., Hesseling, S. C., Kempenaar, J. A., Mulder, A. A., Mommaas, A. M., Dijkman, J. H., and Ponec, M. (1994) Ciliogenesis in human bronchial epithelial cells cultured at the air-liquid interface. *Am. J. Respir. Cell Mol. Biol.* **10,** 271–277.
12. Wu, R., Martin, W. R., St. George, J. A., Plopper, C. G., Kurland, G., Last, J. A., et al. (1990) Expression of mucin synthesis and secretion in human tracheobronchial epithelial cells grown in culture. *Am. J. Respir. Cell Mol. Biol.* **3,** 467–478.
13. Aikawa,T., Shimura, S., Hidetada, S., Ebina, M., and Takishima, T. (1992) Marked globet cell hyperplasia with mucus accumulation in the airways of patients who died of severe acute asthma attack. *Chest* **101,** 916–921.
14. Larivee, P., Levine, S. J., Rieves, R. D., and Shelhamer, J. H. (1994) Airway inflammation and mucus hypersecretion, in *Airway Secretion: Physiological Bases for the Control of Mucus Hypersecretion* (Shimura, S. and Takishima, T., eds.), Marcel Dekker, New York, pp. 469–511.
15. Cheng, P. W., Sherman, J. M., Boat, T. F., and Margaret, B. (1981) Quantitation of radiolabeled mucous glycoproteins secreted by tracheal explants. *Anal. Biochem.* **117,** 301–306.
16. Nordman, H., Davies, J. R., Herrmann, A., Karlsson, N. G., Hansson, G. C., and Carlstedt, I. (1997) Mucus glycoproteins from pig gastric mucosa: identification of different mucin populations from the surface epithelium. *Biochem. J.* **326,** 903–910.
17. Basbaum, C. B., Chow, A., Macher, B. A., Finkneiner, W. E., Viessiere, D., and Foresberg, L. S. (1986) Tracheal carbohydrate antigens identified by monoclonal antibodies. *Arch. Biochem. Biophys.* **249,** 363–373.
18. St. George, J. A., Cranz, D. L., Zicker, S., Etchison, J. R., Dungworth, D. L., and Plopper, C. G. (1985) An immunohistochemical characterization of rhesus monkey respiratory secretions using monoclonal antibodies. *Am. Rev. Respir. Dis.* **132,** 556–563.
19. Robinson, C. B., Martin, W. R., Ratliff, J. L., Holland, P. V., Wu, R., and Cross, C. E. (1993) Elevated levels of serum mucin-associated antigen in adult patients with cystic fibrosis. *Am. Rev. Respir. Dis.* **148,** 385–389.
20. Shih, J. Y., Yang, S. C., Yu, C. J., Wu, H. D., Liaw, Y. S., Wu, R., and Yang, P. C. (1997) Elevated serum levels of mucin-associated antigen in patients with acute respiratory distress syndrome. *Am. J. Respir. Crit. Care Med.* **156,** 1467–1472.
21. Maciag, T. S., Cerumdolo, S., Ilsley, P., Kelley, P., and Forand, P. (1979) An endothelial cell growth factor from bovine hypothalamus: identification and partial characterization. *Proc. Natl. Acad. Sci. USA* **76,** 5674–5678.

3

Brush Biopsy and Culture of Airway Epithelial Cells

β-*Adrenoceptor System Function*

Steven G. Kelsen, David Ciccolella, and Kathleen Brennan

1. Introduction

Stimulation by catecholamine agonists of the β-adrenergic coupled adenylyl cyclase (βAR-AC) system, expressed on human tracheobronchial epithelial cells (ECs), elicits a variety of cellular responses that favorably affect airway function, the intensity of the inflammatory reaction, and even the integrity of the epithelial lining ***(1–6)***. For example, β-agonist-stimulated production of second messenger, cyclic adenosine monophosphate (cAMP), enhances salt and water exchange ***(2)***, ciliary beating ***(3)***, mucus secretion by goblet cells ***(1,4)***, proliferation of airway ECs ***(5)***, and protection against free radical induced injury ***(6)***.

Previous studies examining βAR expression and the functional coupling of the receptor to cAMP production in human airway epithelium have been performed in cultured cells, or in cells freshly harvested at autopsy or at thoracotomy from subjects with airway disease ***(7–9)***. Unfortunately, however, a variety of confounding effects may influence the biologic properties of cells obtained postmortem (e.g., premortem medication, stress, variable ischemia time). Likewise, use of tissues obtained from subjects undergoing thoracotomy (usually for bronchogenic carcinoma) is of concern, because occult airway disease may be present, even in areas remote from sites of obvious pathology. Use of a relatively noninvasive way of harvesting tracheobronchial ECs from living donors circumvents limitations inherent in autopsy and thoracotomy specimens, allows repeated studies in the same subject, and, perhaps most important, allows cells from subjects with a variety of airway diseases to be studied immediately after removal from the body.

From: *Methods in Molecular Medicine, vol. 44: Asthma: Mechanisms and Protocols*
Edited by: K. F. Chung and I. Adcock

The authors describe here a relatively noninvasive method of obtaining tracheobronchial ECs from living donors ***(10,11)***, involving brushing the luminal surface of the airway under direct vision using a fiberoptic bronchoscope. The method is well tolerated and yields a large number of cells of all three major cell subtypes (i.e., ciliated, secretory, basal), which comprise approximately two-thirds of the yield. The mix of cells appears to be similar in the same healthy subject over time, which is of importance for serial studies. Finally, the acutely dissociated cells are metabolically active, express a highly functioning βAR-AC system, and grow well in culture over multiple passages ***(10,11)***.

2. Materials

2.1. Cell Procurement and Isolation

1. Flexible fiberoptic bronchoscope.
2. 75 mg meperidine.
3. 0.6 mg atropine intramuscularly.
4. Lidocaine solution (2% and 4%) and gel.
5. Sleeved catheter brushes (Mill-Rose Labs, Mentor, OH, model no. 149R) with 3-mm-long nylon bristles extending 12 mm from the tip.
6. Minimal essential medium (MEM) or Ham's F12 nutrient medium supplemented with 10% fetal bovine serum.
7. 10-mL sterile polystyrene conical tubes.

2.2. Cell Preparation and Identification

1. 100-μm Nitex filter (Tetko, Elmsford, NY).
2. 50 μg/mL DNase.
3. 1X Trypsin–sodium ethylenediamine tetraacetic acid (EDTA) 0.5 g trypsin and 0.2 g/L EDTA Hank's balanced salt solution (HBSS) (Sigma cats. no. T-5775).
4. Serum-free Ham's F12 medium.
5. Hemocytometer.
6. Trypan blue (0.4%) exclusion dye.
7. Vortex.
8. Glass slides.
9. 10% Formalin.
10. Alcian blue/basic fuchsin stain.
11. Microscope with oil immersion (×100) capabilities.

2.3. Cell Culture Techniques

1. Medium 1: (Ham's F12 supplemented with [per mL]: 25 ng epidermal growth factor; 5 μg transferrin; 5 μg insulin; 40 ng cholera toxin; 5 mg bovine hypothalamic extract; 1 μg hydrocortisone; 100 U penicillin; 100 μg streptomycin) or Medium 2: (LHC-9 complete medium [Biofluids, Bethesda, MD]).

2. CO_2 incubator (37°C in a 5% CO_2–95% air mixture).
3. Culture dishes (35 or 100 mm), either collagen-coated or uncoated.
4. Phase-contrast microscope.
5. Cell culture hood with ultraviolet (UV) light.
6. Human placental collagen type IV (Sigma).
7. Glacial acetic acid.
8. 0.2-µ*M* sterile filters.
9. Vortex.

2.4. cAMP Assay Using a Radioimmunoassay

1. 12 × 75 mm glass test tubes.
2. 13 × 100 mm ore glass test tube.
3. Double-distilled water.
4. Absorbant paper for blotting.
5. cAMP[^{125}I] radioimmunoassay (RIA) kit (adenosine 3',5' cyclic monophosphate) (New England Nuclear [NEN],). The kit includes one vial cAMP antiserum complex, lyophilized; two vials cAMP [^{125}I]-tracer, 1 mL (concentrate); two vials cAMP carrier serum, lyophilized; one vial cAMP standard, lyophilized; one vial cAMP buffer, 25 mL (concentrate); one bottle cAMP precipitator, 100 mL.
6. 1X Phosphate-buffered saline (PBS).
7. 300 µ*M* isobutylmethylxanthine (IBMX).
8. 300 µ*M* ascorbic acid.
9. 10 µ*M* isoproterenol.
10. 10 µ*M* indomethacin.
11. Airway ECs: 100,000–200,000 cells/tube in 440 µL PBS.
12. Shaking water bath at 37°C.
13. 1.2 *M* perchloric acid.
14. 7.5% sodium bicarbonate.

2.5. β-Binding Assay/Scatchard Analysis

1. ^{125}I-iodopindolol (Dupont, NEN).
2. Alprenolol (10 m*M* Stock).
3. 10 m*M* Tris-HCl, 2 m*M* $MgCl_2$, pH 7.4.
4. 1X PBS.
5. Polypropylene tubes/test tube rack.
6. Airway ECs: 100–200,000 cells/tube in 100 µL PBS.
7. Temperature-controlled shaker bath.
8. Brandel cell harvester (Brandel, Gaithersburg, MD).
9. Whatman GF/B fired filter paper (Brandel).
10. γ-counter.
11. Graffit software for analysis of binding data ***(10,11)***.

3. Methods

3.1. EC Harvest

Bronchoscopy has been used to collect both airway and alveolar cells in many lung diseases, especially asthma ***(10–12)***. Both the central airways (trachea, mainstem bronchi or right middle lobe bronchus, and lingular bronchus) and more peripheral airways can be brushed. However, the composition of EC types and cell number differs in the central vs peripheral airways. In general, both the percentage of columnar cells and total cell number are greater when brushing is performed in the central airways.

In general, standard preparation of the subject is used to perform bronchoscopy, with the caveat that use of lidocaine is minimized below the vocal cords (*see* **Note 1**). Regarding safety issues of bronchoscopy in subjects with asthma in whom life-threatening airway obstruction may be induced with this procedure, guidelines have been published ***(12)*** delineating patient characteristics, asthma severity, and preparations to be used so that the procedure can be performed safely.

1. Subjects are premedicated with intramuscular injection of 75 mg meperidine and 0.6 mg atropine 45–60 min prior to the procedure.
2. Local anesthesia of the nasal cavity is achieved with topical application of 2% viscous lidocaine.
3. The bronchoscope is inserted, so that the distal tip is positioned at the desired level of the airway to be sampled.
4. A sleeved catheter is introduced via the sampling channel of the bronchoscope, and the brush is exposed and rubbed against the surface of the airway wall, in a twirling motion under direct visual guidance. The brush is then retracted and the dissociated cells are recovered by gently vortexing the brush in a 10-mL polystyrene tube containing 8 mL medium on ice (*see* **Subheading 2.1.6.**) for several seconds. (Either MEM or the supplemented Ham's F12 media can be used for initial cell collection and transport. Use of Ham's F12 media has the advantage that the cells can be cultured in this media.) The maneuver is repeated ~10× at each location. A separate brush is used for each new site. Cell yield approximates $0.5–5 \times 10^6$ viable cells per site.
5. After a site is brushed 10 times, the brush is cut off into a 10-mL polystyrene conical tube containing ice-cold media. Residual cells adherent to the brush are removed with a sterile curet.

3.2. Cell Preparation and Identification

1. Working in the culture hood under sterile conditions, transfer cells to a 50-mL sterile conical plastic tube on ice. The cell suspension is filtered through a 100-μm sterile Nitex filter (or sterile gauze) to remove mucus. The cells are then treated with 50 μg/mL DNase for 10 min at 4°C, to prevent clumping.

2. The cells are centrifuged at 150*g* for 10 min, and the pellet is resuspended in ice-cold, serum-free Ham's F12 medium.
3. To eliminate dead cells and increase the percentage of viable cells, the cell pellet is exposed to 1 mL 1X trypsin–EDTA for 1–3 min at 37 °C in the CO_2 incubator. Trypsin activity is quenched by exposing cells to a 2X volume of serum.
4. Cells are washed twice with PBS, and then resuspended in 1–2 mL PBS (depending on the size of the cell pellet) for counting.
5. Cell number and viability are determined by mixing 25-μL cell suspension with 75 μL trypan blue (0.4%) exclusion dye.
6. To identify the subtypes of cells, aliquots of cells were smeared on glass slides and fixed with 10% formalin and stained with alcian blue/basic fuchsin.

3.3. Cell Culture

In the authors' hands, cells grow well on a collagen (human type IV collagen) or collagen–Vitrogen matrix in LHC-9 medium (***10***; **Fig. 1**). In general, cells reach confluence in 10–20 d, and can be passaged successfully 2–4× before becoming extremely undifferentiated or experiencing growth arrest. However, under identical conditions, cell growth varies markedly across individuals. Under ideal conditions, repeated passage can amplify cell yield as much as 10–20-fold.

The expression of cytokeratin can be used to confirm the epithelial nature of the cultured cells. However, this is generally not necessary, because contamination of the EC sample with other cell types (e.g., inflammatory cells or fibroblasts) is usually not a problem, given the superficial nature of the biopsy. Although some white blood cells may be present in samples obtained from subjects with inflammatory airway diseases, such as asthma, they do not attach or reproduce on a collagen matrix.

If keratin cytochemistry is desired, cells are grown on glass culture slides and reacted with polyclonal antibodies (Abs) against human keratins ***(10,13)***.

1. To coat dishes or wells with collagen (recipe for ~100 dishes), mix 13 mg type IV human placental collagen with 26 mL ddH_2O and 52 μL glacial acetic acid. Vortex, and place in water bath at 37°C, until completely dissolved (~ 1 h).
2. Add 78 mL ddH_2O to the collagen solution and sterile-filter with a 0.2-μm filter.
3. Add 1 mL/100-mm dish (or 0.5 mL for 35-mm well) in sterile cell culture hood.
4. Place in CO_2 incubator overnight at 37°C to fix collagen surface layer, then remove all possible collagen with a pipet and expose to UV light in hood overnight, to induce collagen crosslinking.
5. To seed culture plates, ECs are resuspended in either medium 1 or 2, and added in a seeding density of $0.05–0.1 \times 10^6$ cells/cm^2 to collagen-coated surfaces.
6. The cells are then incubated at 37°C in a 5% CO_2-95% air mixture, and medium is changed after 24 h, and then every 48 h until cells reach confluence (10–20 d). Viable cells should attach to the dish within 12 h after plating. Excessive red

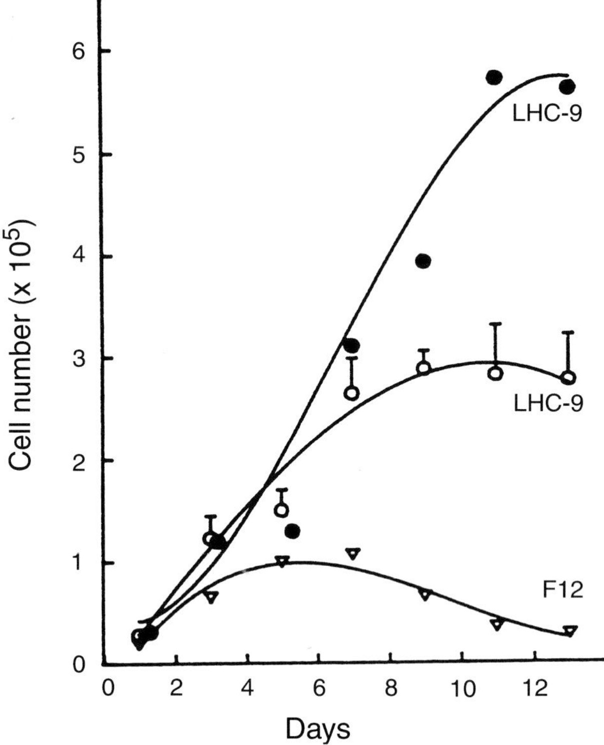

Fig. 1. Growth curves of HAECs harvested by brushing and grown in primary culture. Cells were plated at a density of 5000/cm^2 and grown in LHC-9 or Ham's F12 medium in 35-mm dishes precoated with collagen gel (open symbols) or collagen coat, as described in Methods.

blood cells, if present, can be removed 24 h after plating by washing the dish twice with 10 mL Delbecco's Minimal Essential Media (DMEM).

7. At confluence, cells can harvested for passage using 1X trypsin–EDTA, freezing in liquid nitrogen, or study.

3.4. cAMP Assay

In human airway epithelial cells (HAECs), intracellular cAMP levels control a variety of differentiated cell functions (e.g., ion transport, ciliary beat frequency, secretion of macromolecules, and so on). Intracellular cAMP levels, in turn, are increased by stimulation of the β-adrenergic receptor and subsequent activation of adenyl cyclase. Accordingly, HAECs are induced to produce cAMP by treatment with βAR (e.g., isoproterenol) or by agents that stimulate adenylyl cyclase directly (e.g., forskolin). cAMP levels can then be measured using a double Ab RIA technique, or, more recently, by sandwich enzyme immunoassay (EIA). The sensitivity and accuracy of the two methods appear to be similar. The EIA, which is based on a colorometric assay (tetramethylbenzidine) catalyzed by horseradish peroxidase, may be read using a microtiter plate reader (Amersham, Buckinghamshire, UK, Biotrak cellular communication assays). The EIA appears to be faster and simpler to perform than the RIA. However, since the authors have greater experience with the RIA, this method will be described in detail. Of note, the cAMP stimulation is standard, regardless of which cAMP assay method is employed.

3.4.1. cAMP Stimulation

1. HAECs are resuspended at a concentration of 1×10^5 cell in 400 µL PBS, and preincubated with 300 µ*M* ascorbic acid, 300 µ*M* IBMX and 10 µ*M* indomethacin for 15–30 min on ice. (IBMX inhibits phosphodiesterases, which break down cAMP; ascorbic acid prevents oxidation of isoproterenol; and indomethacin prevents release of prostaglandins (PG), which also stimulate cAMP production by the PGE_2 receptor) (*see* **Note 2**).
2. 12 × 75-mm glass tubes, kept on ice, are treated with 40 µL PBS (no stimulation), isoproterenol, or forskolin. Cells are then added in a volume of 400 µL, and the tubes incubated for 15 min in a shaking water bath at 37°C (*see* **Note 3**).
3. Cells are lysed and reactions quenched by rapid addition of 200 µL 1.2 *M* perchloric acid. After standing on ice for 3 min, tubes are neutralized with 400 µL 7.5% sodium bicarbonate (*see* **Note 4**).
4. The tubes are then vortexed and centrifuged at 250*g* for 20 min at 4°C, and supernatants are then ready for cAMP assay.

3.4.2. cAMP Radioimmunoassay

1. Samples assayed for cAMP content may be assayed by a double-Ab RIA using [^{125}I]cAMP tracer (Rainen, NEN-DuPont, Boston). Samples are diluted 1:2 with cAMP assay buffer in 12 × 75-mm glass tubes.
2. For each assay, a cAMP standard curve is required. Standard cAMP concentrations are prepared in 12 × 75-mm glass tubes ***(20)***, as shown in the **Table 1**. To make the initial 50 p*M*/mL concentration, add 50 µL cAMP stock to 4950 µL cAMP assay buffer. Serially dilute the remaining tubes to make the final concentrations.
3. Sample (and standard containing) tubes are treated according to the protocol in **Table 2**, and prepared in duplicate. Label 2 *N* 12 × 75-mm glass tubes for samples, to run assay in duplicate. Deliver 25 µL cAMP assay buffer to each tube, then add 25 µL sample. The total sample volume will be 50 µL (*see* **Note 5**).
4. After addition of all reagents, vortex tubes, and seal tightly (cover with parafilm or stoppers).
5. Incubate tubes for 16–18 h at 4°C, to allow the Ab to complex with the cAMP.
6. After incubation, deliver 250 µL precipitating solution to all tubes, except total count tubes, and vortex.

Table 1
cAMP Standard Concentrations

Tube	μL	cAMP assay Buffer (μL)	Final concentration (p*M*/mL)
A	50 cAMP standard stock	4950 μL	50
B	500 A	500 μL	25
C	500 B	750 μL	10
D	500 C	500 μL	5
E	500 D	500 μL	2.5
F	500 E	750 μL	1.0
G	500 F	500 μL	0.5

Table 2
cAMP Assay: Standards and Unknowns

Tubes	cAMP assay buffer (μL)	Standards (μL)	Sample (μL)	Working tracer[a] (μL)	Antiserum complex (μL)
Total count	–	–	–	50	–
Blank	100	–	–	50	–
0 Standard	50	–	–	50	50
G	–	50	–	50	50
F	–	50	–	50	50
E	–	50	–	50	50
D	–	50	–	50	50
C	–	50	–	50	50
B	–	50	–	50	50
A	–	50	–	50	50
Samples (1:2) dilution	25	–	25	50	50

[a]Working tracer is 50% [^{125}I]-tracer and 50% carrier serum.

7. Centrifuge tubes at 1200*g* for 15 min at 4°C. A white precipitate will be seen. Decant, and drain the supernatant by inverting glass tubes for 2 min over blotting paper. After draining supernatant, return the tubes to upright position, and count in a γ-counter.
8. The cAMP concentration of the sample (assessed from the radioactivity of the precipitate) is determined by interpolation from the standard curve.

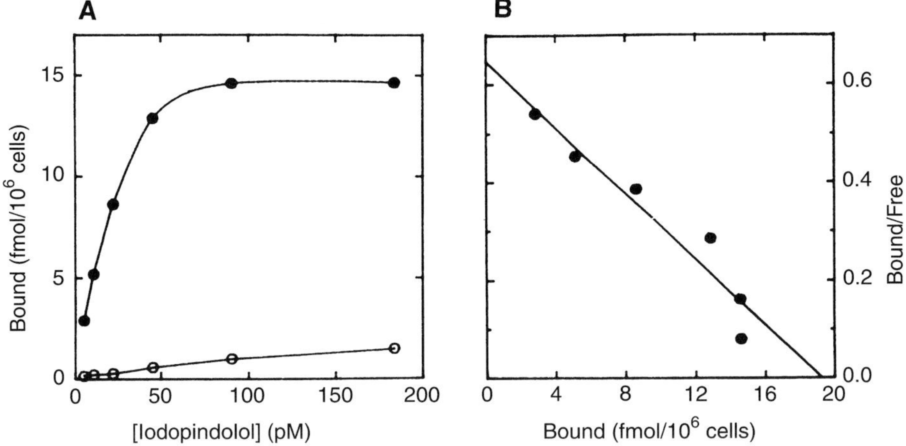

Fig. 2. **(A)** Saturation binding curve of [^{125}I]-iodopindolol to cultured human tracheocytes from a single representative experiment. Data were obtained using the methods outlined in the text. **(B)** Scatchard plot of data shown in **(A)** B_{max} = 19 fmol/ 10^6 cells; K_d = 29.7 p*M*.

3.5. β-Binding Assay/Scatchard Analysis

Receptor density (B_{max}) and equilibrium binding affinity (K_d) of βAR, expressed by HAECs, can be assessed by conventional radioligand binding, using a βAR subtype, nonselective antagonist.

In the method described below, cells undergo hypotonic lysis, making both surface and intracellular receptors available to the hydrophobic ligand used, i.e., [^{125}I]-iodopindolol. The authors have used the radioligand, [^{125}I]-iodopindolol, because it has high activity and specificity for the βAR. B_{max} and K_d are assessed by exposing cells to a wide range of radioligand concentrations in the presence and absence of a cold nonsubtype specific, βAR antagonist, to block all available specific sites. Specific binding is assessed by subtracting binding data in the presence (nonspecific binding) from binding in the absence (total binding) of a single, supersaturating concentration of cold ligand (e.g., alprenolol 40 μ*M*) to block all specific sites (**Fig. 2**). The highest concentration of radioligand used should be sufficient to saturate all available binding sites (i.e., ~10× the equilibrium binding concentration of ~25 p*M*).

B_{max} and K_d are calculated from the total and nonspecific binding data from a conventional Scatchard plot, generated using commercially available, windows-based, computer software (e.g., the Graffit program) ***(13)*** (**Fig. 2**).

1. **Table 3** is a generic design for each concentration of [^{125}I]-iodopindolol used. Generally, 7–9 concentrations, ranging from 5 to 350 p*M*, are used to adequately define

Table 3
βAR Binding Assay

	Pindolol (μL)	10 m*M* Tris (μL)	Stock alprenolol (μL)	Cells (μL)
Total binding	300	100	–	100
Nonspecific binding	300	–	100	100
Reference	300	–	–	–

the curves generated. Reference tubes are used to calculate the [^{125}I]-iodopindolol concentration (i.e., radioactive counts [cpm] divided by 1850 = pindolol concentration in p*M*).

2. Number polypropylene tubes and keep on ice.
3. Mix [^{125}I]-iodopindolol in 10 m*M* Tris-HCl, 2 m*M* $MgCl_2$, pH 7.4. Make serial dilutions of [^{125}I]-iodopindolol using 10 m*M* Tris-HCl–$MgCl_2$ solution, as needed. To achieve an initial supersaturating concentration of free [^{125}I]-iodopindolol (e.g., ~350 p*M*) in 500 μL final vol, add sufficient [^{125}I]-iodopindolol to 10 m*M* Tris-2 m*M* HCl–$MgCl_2$ to achieve ~650,000 cpm/300 μL vol.
4. Mix alprenolol (final concentration, 40 μ*M*) in 10 m*M* Tris-HCl, 2 m*M* $MgCl_2$. Use frozen stock (10 m*M* at –20°C). Add 100 μL dilute alprenolol to all nonspecific tubes.
5. Make up cell suspension (100,000–200,000 cells/100 μL in PBS) for each tube, in sufficient volume for all sample tubes.
6. Add 100 μL cells (100,000–200,000/100 μL) to each tube, except reference, then vortex vigorously.
7. Incubate tubes (except reference) in shaker (40 cpm) for 2 h at 28°C. Use special 48-tube (12 × 4) tube rack made for Brandel harvester.
8. Quench reaction by filtering samples through Whatman GF/C paper, using a Brandel harvester. Do not filter reference tubes. Wash filters 3× to separate bound from free iodopindolol.
9. Remove filter paper from Brandel harvester, and place in clean polypropylene tubes for counting in γ-counter (2 min).
10. Retain tubes/filters for 1–2 d before discarding, in case repeat counting is necessary.

4. Notes

1. Lidocaine decreases cell viability. In fact, concentrations of lidocaine >0.1% markedly diminished cell viability in vitro ***(10)***. Hence, minimizing lidocaine use below the vocal cords improves viability of the isolated cells. In the absence of lidocaine below the vocal cords, and following trypsin–EDTA treatment, cell viability is typically 85–95%.
2. For optimal results, both ascorbic acid and isoproterenol should be made fresh and kept on ice. Isoproterenol should also be kept wrapped in aluminum foil,

because it is light-sensitive. Indomethicin can be kept as a frozen 10 m*M* stock solution. Dilutions of isoproterenol or forskolin, and so on, can be made with distilled water or with PBS.

3. To simplify and standardize HAEC exposure to control or drugs, it is best to determine the total number of cells needed for the experiment, using 1×10^5 cells in 400 µL PBS/tube. Dilute the total cells to the final concentration in PBS. Add ascorbic acid, IBMX, and indomethacin to the cell suspension, and incubate on ice. While cells are incubating, add ligands (e.g., PBS [basal], isoproterenol, PGE_2, forskolin, and so on). Once incubation is completed, aliquot 400 µL cell suspension (1×10^5 cells) per tube, then place tubes in shaking water bath.
4. After cAMP production is quenched with perchloric acid/sodium bicarbonate, and samples are centrifuged, the cAMP RIA can be performed immediately, or samples tightly sealed and refrigerated at 4°C for 5–7 d prior to assay.
5. In the authors' modification of the Rianen RIA, all volumes have been reduced by 50%, i.e., sample volume is 50 µL, working tracer is 50 µL, and so on.

References

1. Nijkamp, F. P., Engels, F., Henricks, P. A. J., and Vanoosterhout, A. J. M. (1992) Mechanisms of β-adrenergic receptor regulation in lungs and its implications for physiological responses. *Physiol. Rev.* **72,** 323–366.
2. Smith, P. L., Welsh, M. J., Stoff, S. J., and Frizzell, R. A. (1982) Chloride secretion by canine tracheal epithelium: role of intracellular cAMP levels. *J. Memb. Biol.* **70,** 215–226.
3. Sanderson, M. J. and Dirksen, E. R. (1989) Mechanosensitive and β-adrenergic control of the ciliary beat frequency of mammalian respiratory tract cells in culture. *Am. Rev. Respir. Dis.* **139,** 432–440.
4. Barnes, P. J., Chung, K. F., and Page, C. P. (1988) Inflammatory mediators and asthma. *Pharmacol. Rev.* **40,** 49–84.
5. Wiley, J., Laveck, M. A., McClendon, I. A., and Lechner, J. F. (1985) Relationship of ornithine decarboxylase activity and cAMP metabolism to proliferation of normal human bronchial epithelial cells. *J. Cell Physiol.* **124,** 207–212.
6. Koyama, S., Rennard, S. I., Claasen, L., and Robins, R. A. (1991) Dibutryly cAMP, prostaglandin E_2, and antioxidants protect cultured bovine bronchial epithelial cells from endotoxin. *Am. J. Physiol.* **261,** L126–L132.
7. Davis, P. B., Silski, C. L., Kercsmar, C. M., and Infeld, M. D. (1990) Beta adrenergic receptors on human tracheal epithelial cells in primary culture. *Am. J. Physiol.* **258,** C71–C76.
8. Kercsmar, C. M., Infeld, M. D., Silski, C. L., and Davis, P. B. (1990) Adenosine 3:5' monophosphate synthesis by human tracheal epithelial cells. *Am. J. Respir. Cell Mol. Biol.* **2,** 33–39.
9. Penn, R., Kelsen, S. G., and Benovic, J. L. (1994) Regulation of β-agonist and prostaglandin E_2-mediated adenylyl cyclase activity in human airway epithelial cells. *Am. J. Respir. Cell Mol. Biol.* **11,** 496–505.

10. Kelsen, S. G., Mardini, I. A., Zhou, S., Benovic, J. L., and Higgins, N. C. (1992) Technique to harvest viable tracheobronchial epithelial cells form living human donors. *Am. J. Respir. Cell Mol. Biol.* **7,** 66–72.
11. Kelsen, S. G., Higgins, N. C., Zhou, S., Mardini, I. A., and Benovic, J. L. (1995) Expression and function of the beta-adrenergic receptor-coupled adenylyl cyclase system on human airway epithelial cells. *Am. J. Respir. Crit. Care Med.* **152,** 1774–1783.
12. Smith, D. L. and Deshazo, R. D. (1993) Bronchoalveolar lavage in asthma. An update and perspective. *Am. Rev. Respir. Dis.* **148,** 523–532.
13. O'Guin, W. M., Schermer, S., and Sun, T. (1990) Immunofloresecnce staining of keratin filaments in cultured epithelial cells. *J. Tissue Culture Methods* **9,** 123–128.
13. Scatchard, G. (1949) Attraction of proteins for small molecules and ions. *Ann. NY Acad. Sci.* **51,** 660–672.

4

Isolation and Characterization of Human Airway Fibroblasts in Culture

Jamila Chakir, Jean Dubé, Michel Laviolette, Francine Goulet, Lucie Germain, François Auger, and Louis-Philippe Boulet

1. Introduction

Asthma is considered an airway inflammatory disorder characterized by variable airflow obstruction and airway hyperresponsiveness *(1)*. The inflammatory component of asthma has been studied extensively over the past few years, but, more recently, the potential contribution of airway wall remodeling to functional and clinical changes has been emphasized *(2,3)*. Although the methods of sampling of bronchial tissue were previously limited, being obtained mostly from autopsic or surgical specimens, they have improved recently.

The safety and usefulness of bronchial biopsies obtained by bronchoscopic procedures have now been established. The analysis of inflammatory and structural airway changes has significantly contributed to our understanding of asthma pathophysiology *(4–7)*. This mode of sampling bronchial tissue has provided new means of obtaining materials for cell culture *(8)*.

One of the key cells involved in airway structural changes is the fibroblast *(9)*. For example, the typical subepithelial collagen deposition seen in asthma has been attributed to myofibroblasts, and the number of these cells found in the subepithelial area of the airways correlates with the basement membrane thickness *(10)*. The myofibroblast is probably involved in changes of the contractile properties of the airways following the repair process induced by the inflammatory insult. Furthermore, this cell has been involved in the modulation of the inflammatory process *(11,12)*.

Phenotypic cell changes may occur under the influence of the asthmatic inflammatory process. Cytokines produced by inflammatory cells can modulate fibroblast functions and extracellular matrix deposition. Among those, transform-

From: *Methods in Molecular Medicine, vol. 44: Asthma: Mechanisms and Protocols*
Edited by: K. F. Chung and I. Adcock © Humana Press Inc., Totowa, NJ

ing growth factor-β and platelet-derived growth factor are probably the most potent cytokines affecting ECM component synthesis, fibroblast proliferation, and structural cell phenotypes *(12)*.

The isolation and culture of fibroblastic cells from bronchial biopsies may therefore contribute to elucidating the influence of the inflammatory process on structural cells such as the fibroblast, and vice versa. There are, however, inherent difficulties, in order to maximize the chances of obtaining appropriate cell cultures from those techniques. These are discussed in the following subheadings.

2. Materials

2.1. Subjects: Selection and Evaluation

In published studies *(13)*, most bronchial biopsies have been obtained from mildly asthmatic subjects whose diagnosis of asthma corresponded to the American Thoracic Society criteria. More severe asthmatics have also been subjected to those techniques, which should always be performed very carefully. The reader is referred to published guidelines *(14,15)* on how to perform bronchoscopies and biopsies in asthmatic subjects. Ideally, asthma should be stable, subjects must be nonsmokers, without evidence of recent respiratory infection. Inhaled or systemic corticosteroid-free subjects have been considered ideal for those techniques, because of the possible effect of these agents on structural cells.

As a safety measure, most airflow obstruction is measured by spirometry before the bronchoscopy, according to standardized procedures *(16)*. Methacholine responsiveness is often determined, to measure severity of asthma, and to establish correlations between physiological and histopathological markers *(17)*.

2.2. Biopsy Sampling

In humans, bronchial fibroblasts have been isolated from bronchial biopsies or surgical specimens. Before the bronchoscopy, a 200-μg dose of salbutamol was given, usually using a metered-dose inhaler. All subjects received oxygen (e.g., 5 L/min by nasal catheter) during bronchoscopy. After local anesthesia of the throat, larynx, and bronchi with 2 and 4% xylocaine, the flexible bronchoscope was introduced into the bronchial tree, and up to 12 bronchial biopsies were taken from the carinae of the right upper and middle lobes and the segmental bronchi of the upper and lower lobes on both sides, using conventional or alligator forceps *(18)*. Vital signs, electrocardiograph, and oximetry were recorded throughout the procedure.

For a more detailed method for fiberoptic bronchoscopy, *see* Chapters 3 and 5.

2.3. Cell Culture Medium

Dulbecco's Modified Eagle's Medium (DMEM) (Gibco-BRL, Grand Island, NY) containing 10% fetal calf serum (FCS) (Gibco-BRL). Add stock antibiotic and fungicides to give a working concentration of 100 IU penicillin, 25 µg/mL gentamycin, and 2.5 µg/mL Fungizone (an antifungal agent, Sigma) (*see* **Note 1**).

2.4. Fibroblast Isolation

1. Collagenase solution: 0.1% (0.2 U/mL) collagenase H (Boehringer-Mannheim, Montreal, Canada) prepared in DMEM culture containing 10 m*M* $CaCl_2$, without any supplement.
2. Cell passage: trypsin–ethylenediamine tetraacetic acid (EDTA) solution (0.1% trypsin [Sigma] and 1 m*M* EDTA [Sigma] in DMEM).
3. Freezing media: 15% dimethylsulfoxide (DMSO; Sigma) in FCS.

2.5. Light Microscopy

1. 10% formalin buffer (4% formaldehyde): 100 mL 40% formaldehyde in 1000 mL.
2. Masson's trichrome: 0.5% acid fushsin in 0.5% acetic acid, 1% phosphomolybdic acid, and 2% methyl blue in 2.5% acetic acid.
3. Weigert's hematoxylin stain: 1% hematoxylin in ethanol (*see* **Note 2**) and 1.2% anhydrous ferric chloride containing 1% hydrochloric acid (HCl). Mix equal volumes just prior to use (solution should be a violet-black color).

2.6. Electron Microscopy

1. Karnovsky's fluid: Dissolve 2 g paraformaldehyde in 25 mL distilled water by heating to 60°C, with continuous stirring in a covered beaker. Add 1 *M* sodium hydroxide (NaOH) dropwise, until the solution clears.
2. Cacodylate buffer: 25 mL 0.2 *M* Na cacodylate plus 1.4 mL 0.2 *M* HCl in 100 mL, pH 7.4. Add 10 mL 25% glutaraldehyde to 25 mL Karnovsky's fluid. Make up to 50 mL with cacaodylate buffer. The final solution is 5% glutaraldehyde and 4% paraformaldehyde in 0.1 *M* cacodylate buffer, pH 7.2. It should be used when fresh.
3. 1% Osmium tetroxide: Add 41.5 mL 2.26% Na dihydrogen orthophosphate to 8.5 mL 2.52% NaOH. Add 5 mL 5.4% glucose to 45 mL of phosphate buffer, and finally add 0.5 g osmium tetroxide.
4. Epon embedding mixture: 13 mL Epon 812, 8 mL Hardener dodecenyl succinic anhydride (DDSA), 7.5 mL Hardener MNA and 0.42 mL Acclerator dimethyl aminomethyl-phenol (DMP/30).
5. Lead citrate: Add 1.3 g lead nitrate and 1.76 g Na citrate to 30 mL water, and shake vigorously for 1 min. A heavy white precipitate will form (*see* **Note 3**). Add 8 mL 1 *N* NaOH with agitation, and dilute to 50 mL (*see* **Note 4**).

2.7. Immunoflourescence

Mounting medium (phosphate-buffered saline [PBS]/glycerol: 30% glycerol, 70% PBS 1X, 2 g/100 mL gelatin, heated and adjusted to pH 7.6).

2.8. Collagen Gel Contraction Buffer

Stock solution of bovine type I collagen (dissolving 4.22 mg/mL of the powder overnight at 4°C in sterile 0.017 *M* acetic acid).

3. Methods

3.1. Bronchial Biopsy Processing and Bronchial Cell Culture (see Note 5)

Herein is described the method currently used in this laboratory.

1. Immediately upon sampling, biopsies were kept in supplemented DMEM–FCS kept at 4°C on ice (*see* **Note 6**).
2. Bronchial biopsies were digested in collagenase H overnight at 4°C.
3. Homogenates were centrifuged for 10 min at 300*g* at 4°C.
4. Cell pellets resuspended in supplemented DMEM–10% FCS in 35-mm Petri dishes (Falcon; Becton Dickinson, Oxnard, CA), and kept in an 8% CO_2 atmosphere at 37°C *(8)*.

A summary of the procedure can be found on **Fig. 1**. Culture medium was changed every 2 d. After 2 wk in culture, bronchial fibroblasts usually reach approx 85% confluency, and were ready to be subcultured or stored (*see* **Note 7**). For experimental use, cultured fibroblasts could be amplified by increasing their number and by extending their life-span (*see* **Note 8**). Continued cell growth could be maintained by passing the cells to larger surface area plates *(8)*.

3.1.1. Passaging

1. Aspirate medium and rinse cells with DMEM without FCS.
2. Add trypsin–EDTA just enough to cover all cells.
3. Incubate at 37°C 2–3 min, until cell detachment.
4. Add an equal volume of trypsin-inhibitor soybean (trypsin inhibitor [Sigma] 1 mg/mL in DMEM).
5. Collect and pellet cells 10 min at 500*g*.
6. Resuspend the cells in complete DMEM.

3.1.2. Cryopreservation

Primary cultures of fibroblasts can be frozen and stored for years by addition of cryopreservation products that inhibit the formation of ice crystals. The following protocols produce thawed cells with 90% viability.

3.1.3. Freezing

1. Trypsinize cells and suspend them in culture medium at a density of 1×10^6/mL.
2. Pellet cells 5 min at 500*g*.
3. Resuspend cells gently in freezing solutions (15% DMSO in FCS).
4. Aliquot 1 mL (1×10^6 cells) to previously labeled cryovials.

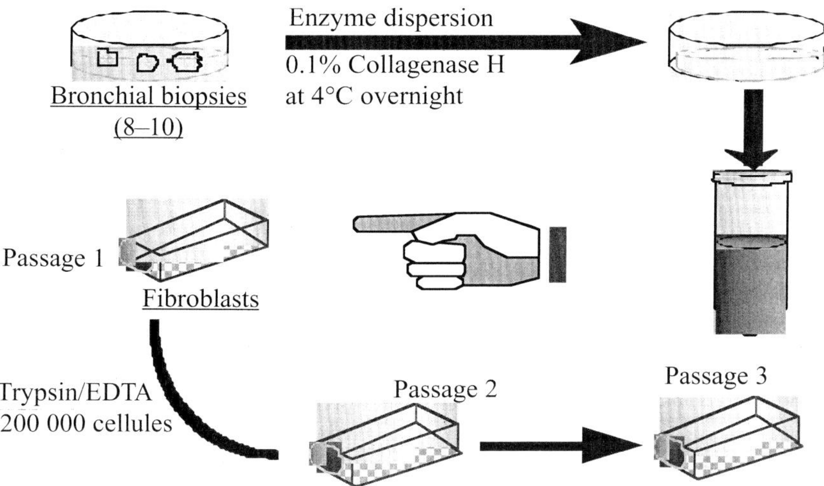

Fig. 1. Schematic illustration of the procedure for the isolation of bronchial fibroblasts from bronchial biopsies of normal and asthmatic subjects.

5. Put vials in styrofoam box and place in a –70°C freezer overnight.
6. Transfer vials to a liquid nitrogen storage tank.

3.1.4. Thawing

1. Remove the vial from liquid nitrogen and thaw in warm water (37°C).
2. Add prewarmed culture medium to the cryovial and gently transfer the cells to a 50 mL tube containing prewarmed culture medium.
3. Pellet cells 5 min at 500*g*.
4. Resuspend in medium supplemented with 10% FCS.
5. Count cells and assess viability by trypan blue (0.1% in PBS).

3.2. Cell Identification on Bronchial Biopsies

Two biopsies harvested from each subject were used for bronchial fibroblast identification by light and electron microscopy (**Fig. 2**).

3.2.1. Light Microscopy

1. Biopsies were fixed in 10% formalin buffer overnight.
2. The biopsy was dehydrated through increasing percentages of alcohol (70, 90, 100%) for 90 min each solution.
3. Dehydrate overnight in absolute alcohol.
4. Clear biopsy by 2 × 2 h washes in trichloroethane.
5. Embed in paraffin wax. Several changes in hot wax are required to remove all trichloroethane before cooling and trimming block.
6. Cut 4–5-µm sections using a microtome, and position adjoining sections onto slides. Dry slides in an oven for 45 min.

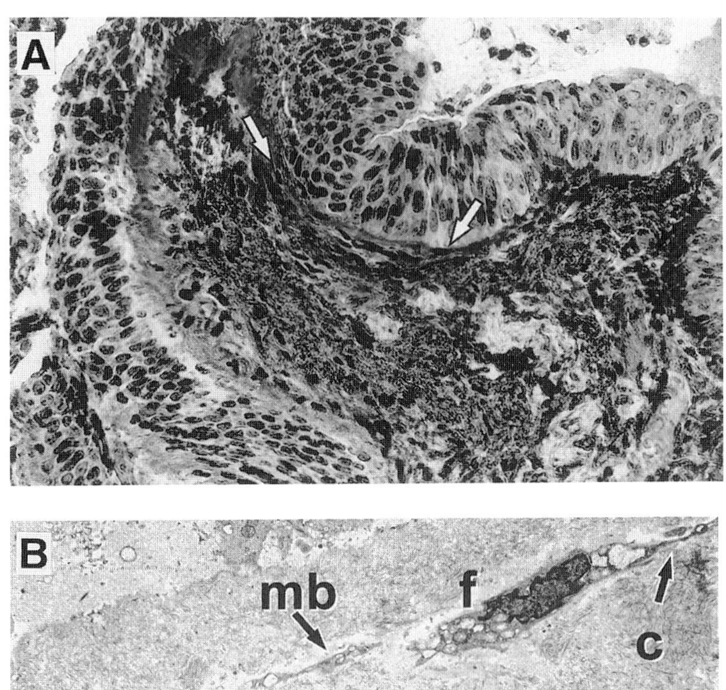

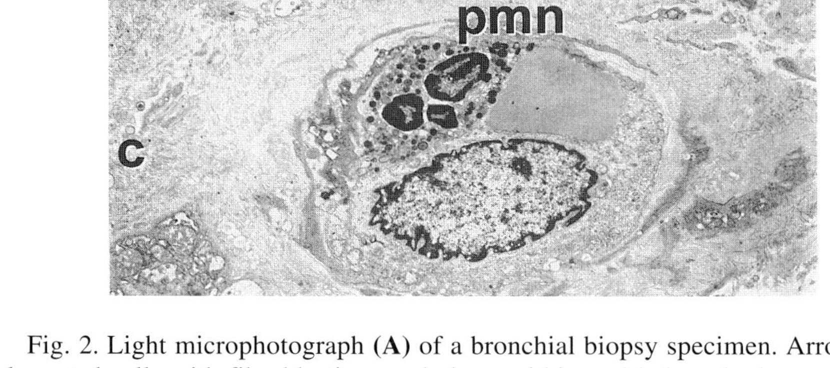

Fig. 2. Light microphotograph **(A)** of a bronchial biopsy specimen. Arrows show elongated cells with fibroblastic morphology within and below the basement membrane (original magnification ×400). **(B)** Electromicrograph of a bronchial biopsy specimen from an asthmatic subject, showing a fibroblast (f and arrow) within the basement membrane (bm) (original magnification ×2700).

3.2.1.1. Staining Sections with Masson's Trichrome and Weigert's Stain

1. Dewax sections and bring to water.
2. Wash in tap water.
3. Stain nuclei for 15–30 min with Weigert's stain.
4. Differentiate with 1% acid alcohol.

5. Wash well in tap water.
6. Stain in acid fuchsin solution (A), 5 min.
7. Rinse in distilled water.
8. Treat with phosphomolybdic acid solution (B) 5 min.
9. Drain.
10. Stain with methyl blue solution (C) for 2–5 min.
11. Rinse in distilled water.
12. Treat with 1% acetic acid 2 min (*see* **Note 9**).
13. Dehydrate through alcohols.
14. Clear in xylene, mount in EUKITT (Kuelab).

3.2.2. Electron Microscopy Analysis

1. Biopsies are fixed by immersion in Karnovsky's fixative for 15 min.
2. Rinse 3 × 1 min in 0.1 *M* cacodylate buffer, pH 7.4.
3. Postfix in 1% osmium tetroxide for 10 min.
4. Rinse 3 × 1 minute in 0.1 *M* cacodylate buffer, pH 7.4.
5. Dehydrate in 70% ethanol; two changes over 3 min.
6. Dehydrate in 85% ethanol; two changes over 3 min.
7. Dehydrate in 95% ethanol; three changes over 8 min.
8. Dehydrate in absolute ethanol; three changes over 8 min.
9. Dehydrate in absolute acetone; three changes over 8 min.
10. Infiltrate with absolute acetone–Epon mixture (1:1) for 10 min.
11. Remove from infiltrate, blot off excess mixture, and transfer to Epon embedding mixture for 10 min.
12. Remove from embedding mixture and blot off excess. Embed in rubber moulds in Epon embedding mixture.
13. Polymerize for 1 h at 100°C.
14. Cool rapidly at –20°C for 5 min, and section.
15. Stain grid sections in saturated uranyl acetate, pH 3.3 (in 50% ethanol), for 10 min in the dark.
16. Remove from dark, and wash rapidly in 50% ethanol, followed by two changes of distilled water.
17. Remove excess fluid, and stain with lead citrate for 5–10 min.
18. Wash in 0.02 *N* NaOH, followed by two washes in distilled water.
19. Electron microscopic studies evaluated the presence of fibroblasts in the basement membrane area.

3.2.3. Fibroblast Identification in Cell Culture

Cultured fibroblasts were identified and characterized by immunofluorescence and flow cytometry (FCM) using antivimentin and a mouse monoclonal antihuman fibroblast antibody (Ab), a fibroblast antigen Ab-1 from Calbiochem (San Diego, CA), which shows no cross-reactions with epithelial cells, endothelial cells, smooth muscle cells, and many other cell types (***19***; **Fig. 3**).

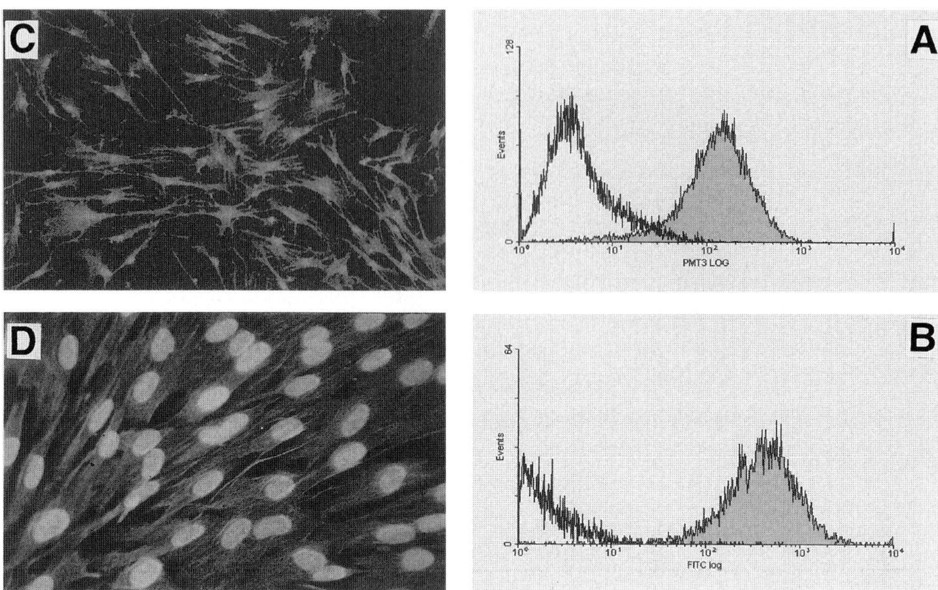

Fig. 3. Characterization of bronchial fibroblasts by FCM and immunofluorescence. (**A**, **B**) Typical fluorescence histogram obtained by flow cytometry. The X-axis of the scattergram shows the intensity of fluorescence and the Y-axis the number of cells. The white peak (left) represents the isotype control and the dark peak (right) the fluorescence associated with the Ab-1 and vimentin Abs. (**C**, **D**) Immunostaining of bronchial fibroblasts by anti-Ab-1 and antivimentin.

3.2.3.1. Protocol for Indirect Immunofluorescence

1. Fix confluent cell layers grown on glass slides 10 min in methanol at –20°C.
2. Wash with PBS.
3. Incubate with antivimentin or anti-Ab-1 Abs diluted with PBS 1% bovine serum albumin (BSA) for 45 min at room temperature.
4. Rinse 3× with PBS.
5. Overlay with the corresponding fluorescein-conjugated Ab for 30 min.
6. Wash with PBS.
7. Stain cell nuclei with Hoechst 33258 dye (Sigma) diluted 1/1000 in water for 5 min.
8. Mount slides in mounting medium (PBS–glycerol: 30% glycerol, 70% PBS 1X, 2 g/100 mL of gelatin, heated and adjusted to pH 7.6).

For negative controls, the primary Ab is omitted. The slides were analyzed under a fluorescence microscope, and positively labeled cells of each population (minimum of 500 cells) were counted.

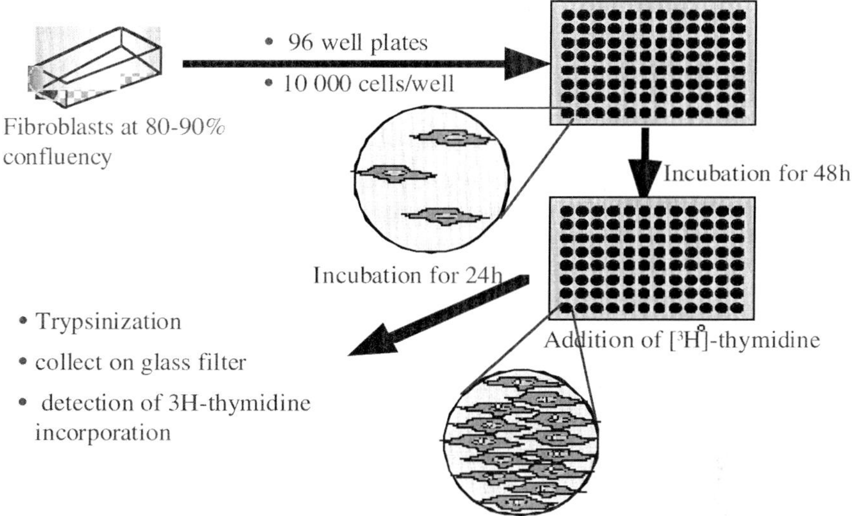

Fig. 4. Schematic illustration of the procedure for bronchial fibroblast DNA synthesis.

3.2.3.2. Protocol for FCM

1. Incubate 5×10^5 cells with 0.6 μg mouse vimentin and antihuman Ab-1 Abs for 30 min at 4°C.
2. Wash cells twice with PBS–1% BSA.
3. Resuspend cells in 100 μL containing 1 μg goat $F(ab')_2$ antimouse immunoglobulin G (H+L) Ab label with fluorescein isothiocyanate.
4. Incubate cells in the dark at 4°C for another 30 min.
5. Wash with PBS/1% BSA, then analyze by FCM (*see* Chapter 5).

3.2.3.3. Proliferative Phenotype of Bronchial Fibroblasts

DNA synthesis measurements by ^{3}H-thymidine incorporation were used to measure bronchial fibroblast proliferation (**Fig. 4**):

1. Culture normal and asthmatic bronchial fibroblasts to 80–90% confluence.
2. Trypsinize and wash in DMEM containing 10% FCS, antifungal agent, and gentamycin.
3. Seed 1×10^4 cells/well in flat-bottomed 96-well plates.
4. Incubate for 48 h at 37°C, 5% CO_2.
5. Add ^{3}H-thymidine (1 μCi/well) to the culture medium, and incubate for 24 h.
6. Remove medium and wash cells twice with PBS.
7. Trypsinize cells and collect on a glass filter with a cell harvester.
8. Detect ^{3}H-thymidine incorporation on a β-counter.

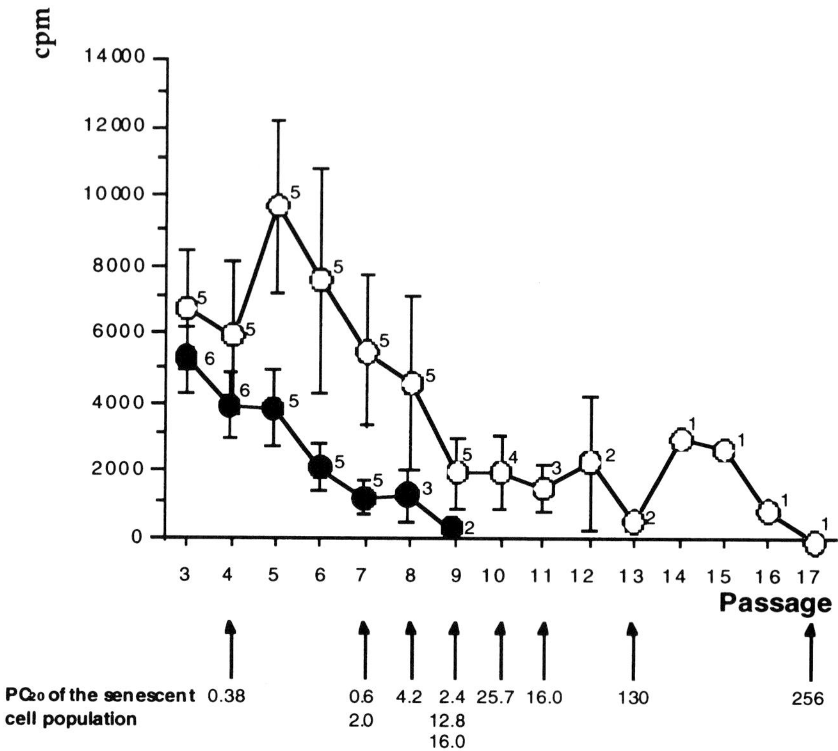

Fig. 5. Mean ^{3}H-thymidine uptake in relation to cell passage. The peak ^{3}H-thymidine uptake of the normal fibroblasts was 1.9× higher than the maximum average uptake rate reached by asthmatic fibroblasts. Bronchial fibroblasts of the most hyperreactive subjects stopped proliferating at an earlier passage than the least hyperreactive *(20)*.

For all subjects, results were expressed as mean ^{3}H-thymidine incorporation ± SEM of four replicate wells at each passage. Each cell population was passed serially, until DNA synthesis decreases below 500 cpm, at which time cells were considered to be senescent. At this stage, increases in cell size associated with senescence could be observed by microscopy. Senescence occurred at different passages for different subjects, ranging from passage 4 to 17 ***(20)***. The fibroblast in vitro life-span was calculated as the number of passages before cells reach senescence (**Fig. 5**).

3.2.3.4. Collagen Gel Contraction

The ability of bronchial fibroblasts to contract collagen fibrils in floating gels was tested according to the following protocol ***(8)***:

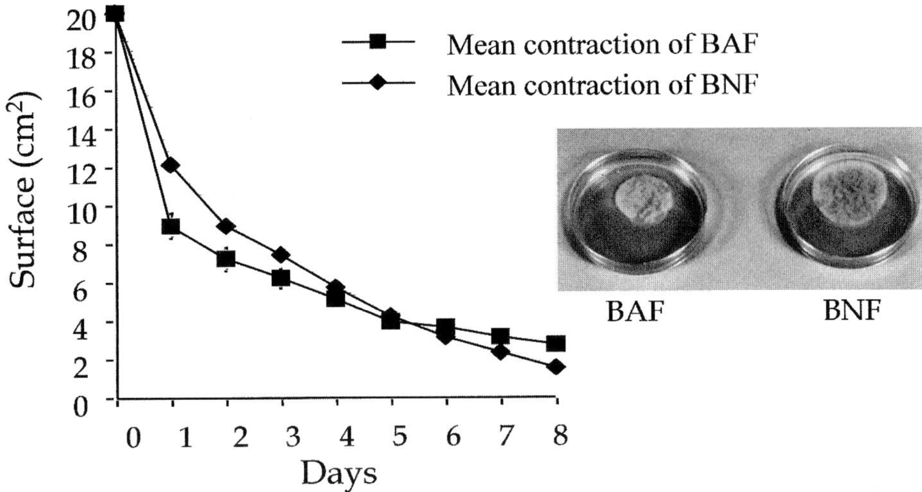

Fig. 6. Collagen gel contraction of bronchial fibroblasts. Asthmatic fibroblasts contract floating gel more than normal fibroblasts.

1. Prepare a stock solution of bovine type I collagen by dissolving 4.22 mg/mL of the powder overnight at 4°C in sterile 0.017 *M* acetic acid.
2. Prepare a solution of DMEM 2.7X containing 200 IU/mL penicillin G and 50 mg/mL gentamycin, pH 8.0.
3. Mix a solution of 5.6 mL DMEM 2.7X + 3.7 mL FCS, 9.5 mL stock collagen solution, 0.2 mL NaOH 0.7 *N*, and 1 mL fibroblast suspension (2.5×10^5 cells/mL).
4. Distribute quickly in 60-mm bacteriological Petri dishes (5 mL/dish).
5. Allow collagen polymerization for 2 h at 37°C.
6. Cover the gels with 2 mL DMEM supplemented with 10% FCS, 100 IU/mL penicillin G, and 25 mg/mL gentamicin.

The diameter of each collagen gel is directly measured daily over a period of 9 days or more (**Fig. 6**). The total surface area of each gel is determined using the following formula: P (D^2)/4, where P is a constant (3.1416) and *D* corresponds to the gel diameter ***(8)***.

4. Notes

1. Because xylocaine reduces cell viability, the culture medium must be changed twice. Culture contamination can occur. All materials used for bronchoscopy and cell culture must be sterilized, and antibiotics and antifungal agents must be added to culture media.
2. The hematoxylin solution should be allowed to ripen naturally for 4 wk before use.
3. Shake the solution every 5 min over a 30-min period to facilitate conversion of lead nitrate to lead citrate.

4. The stain is ready for use and will keep for 6 mo at room temperature. With age, a white precipitate will form, but this can be removed by filtration prior to use.
5. The technique described here was optimized for isolation of bronchial mesenchymal cells. The authors chose enzymatic digestion instead of explant technique in which cells are selected on their ability to migrate, and the resulting cells are possibly clones that are not necessarily representative of the total tissue cell population *(8)*.
6. The processing should be performed rapidly following the bronchoscopy (1–2 h).
7. The chief problem encountered in establishing primary bronchial fibroblasts are the number of bronchial biopsies. 10–12 biopsies are often required to establish cell population.
8. The phenotypic properties expressed by bronchial fibroblasts are dependent on the number of passages. All experiments must be done on passage 2–4 for asthmatic fibroblasts and no more than passage 5 for normal fibroblasts ***(20)***.
9. Nuclei are blue-black, cytoplasm, muscle, and erythrocytes are red and collagen is blue.

References

1. Lask, B. (1993) International consensus report on diagnosis and treatment of asthma. *Clin. Exp. Allergy* **23,** 155–157.
2. Bousquet, J., Chanez, P., Lacoste, J. Y., Barnéon, G., Ghavanian, N., Enander, I., et al. (1990) Eosinophilic inflammation in asthma. *N. Engl. J. Med.* **323,** 1033–1039.
3. Boulet, L. P., Chakir, J., Dubé, J., Laprise, C., Boutet, M., and Laviolette, M. (1998) Airway inflammation and structural changes in airway hyper-responsiveness and asthma: an overview. *Can. Respir. J.* **5,** 16–21.
4. Jeffery, P. K., Wardlaw, A. J., Nelson, F. C., Collins, J. V., and Kay A. B. (1989) Bronchial biopsies in asthma. An ultrastructural, quantitative study and correlation with hyperreactivity. *Am. Rev. Respir. Dis.* **140,** 1745–1753.
5. Djukanovic, R., Roche, W. R., Wilson, J. W., Beasley, C. R. W., Twentyman, O. P., Howarth, P. H., and Holgate, S. T. (1990) Mucosal inflammation in asthma. *Am. Rev. Respir. Dis.* **142,** 434–457.
6. Boulet, L. P., Laviolette, M., Turcotte, H., Milot, J., Cartier, A., Dugas, M., Malo, J. L., and Boutet, M. (1997) Bronchial subepithelial fibrosis correlates with airway responsiveness to methacholine. *Chest* **112,** 45–52.
7. Chakir, J., Laviolette, M., Boutet, M., Laliberté, R., Dubé, J., and Boulet, L. P. (1996) Lower airways remodeling in nonasthmatic subjects with allergic rhinitis. *Lab. Invest.* **75,** 735–744.
8. Goulet, F., Boulet, L. P., Chakir, J., Tremblay, N., Dubé, J., Laviolette, M., et al. (1996) Morphologic and functional properties of bronchial cells isolated from normal and asthmatic subjects. *Am. J. Respir. Cell Mol. Biol.* **15,** 312–318.
9. Roche, W. R. (1991) Fibroblasts and asthma. *Clin. Exp. Allergy* **5,** 56–58.
10. Brewster, C. E., Howarth, P., Djukanovic, R., Wilson, J., and Holgate, S. T. (1990) Myofibroblasts and subepithelial fibrosis in bronchial asthma. *Am. J. Respir. Cell Mol. Biol.* **3,** 507–511.

11. Gauldie, J., Jordana, M., and Cox, G. (1993) Cytokines and pulmonary fibrosis. *Thorax* **48,** 931–935.
12. Sime, P. J., Tremblay, G. M., Xing, Z., Sarnstrand, B. O., and Gauldie, J. (1997) Interstitial and bronchial fibroblasts, in *Asthma* (Barnes, P. J., Grunstein, M. M., Leff, A. R., and Woolcock, A. J., eds.), Lippincott-Raven, Philadelphia, pp. 475–489.
13. American Thoracic Society Board of Directors (1987) Standards for the diagnosis of patients with COPD and asthma. *Am. Rev. Respir. Dis.* **136,** 225–244.
14. Anonymous (1992) Investigative use of bronchoscopy, lavage and bronchial biopsies in asthma and other airways diseases. *Eur. Respir. J.* **5,** 115–121.
15. Anonymous (1991) Workshop summary and guidelines: investigative use of bronchoscopy, lavage, and bronchial biopsies in asthma and other airway diseases. *J. Allergy Clin. Immunol.* **88,** 808–814.
16. American Thoracic Society (1995) Standardization of spirometry, 1994 update. *Am. J. Respir. Crit. Care Med.* **152,** 1107–1136.
17. Juniper, E., Cockcroft, D. W., and Hargreave, F. E. (1992) Histamine and methacholine inhalation tests: tidal breathing method. Laboratory procedure and standardization. Canadian Thoracic Society. AB Draco, Lund, Sweden.
18. Laviolette, M., Carreau, M., and Coulombe, R. (1988) Bronchoalveolar lavage cell differentia*l*tial on microscope glass cover. *Am. Rev. Respir. Dis.* **138,** 451–457.
19. Saalbach, A., Anderegg, U., Bruns, M., Schnabel, E., Herrmann, K., and Haustein, U. F. (1996) Novel fibroblast-specific monoclonal antibodies: properties and specificities. *J. Invest. Dermatol.* **106,** 1314–1319.
20. Dubé, J., Chakir, J., Laviolette, M., Saint-Martin, S., Boutet, M., Desrochers, C., Auger, F., and Boulet, L. P. (1998) In vitro procollagen synthesis and proliferative phenotype of bronchial fibroblasts from normal and asthmatic subjects. *Lab. Invest.* **78,** 297–307.

5

Flow Cytometric Analysis of Blood Monocytes and Alveolar Macrophages

Marcia L. Taylor and Bruce S. Bochner

1. Introduction

Pulmonary monocytes and macrophages are believed to function in a wide range of biological roles, including host defense against foreign organisms, maintenance of immunological homeostasis in the lung, presentation of antigen to lymphocytes, and migration to sites of tissue injury and inflammation *(1)*. There is also mounting evidence that recruited blood monocytes and resident alveolar macrophages (AM) in lung disease express an activated phenotype, suggesting that they may play important roles in chronic respiratory diseases, including asthma and interstitial lung diseases *(2–6)*.

The hallmarks of chronic inflammation and tissue fibrosis are the influx of inflammatory cells, resultant accumulation of inflammatory mediators, an expansion of the mesenchymal cell population, and increased deposition of extracellular matrix components *(7)*. AMs are believed to orchestrate this inflammatory and fibrotic process through the release of a variety of mediators, including proinflammatory cytokines (interleukin-1 [IL-1], interferon-γ, tumor necrosis factor-α and macrophage inhibitory protein-1β) ***(8)***; reactive oxygen species ***(9)***; proteases such as plasminogen activator ***(10)***; chemokines, including IL-8, MIP-1α, macrophage chemotactic protein-1, and regulated on activation normal T-cell expressed and secreted RANTES ***(11–16)***, mitogens for mesenchymal cells (platelet-derived growth factor, fibroblast growth factor, insulin-growth factor) ***(2,3,17)***; and mediators that are directly fibrogenic (transforming growth factor-β).

The function of monocytes and AM may also be regulated by cell–cell interactions and interactions with soluble proinflammatory and anti-inflammatory factors, which are in turn mediated through multiple receptors located on their

From: *Methods in Molecular Medicine, vol. 44: Asthma: Mechanisms and Protocols*
Edited by: K. F. Chung and I. Adcock © Humana Press Inc., Totowa, NJ

surface. This is supported by evidence that these cells have the ability to change their phenotypic pattern ***(18)*** and functional properties ***(10)*** in response to exogenous stimuli and/or pathological processes in the lung ***(19,20)***. Therefore, knowledge of monocyte and AM surface molecule expression is important in examining the potential roles of these cells in the lung. A variety of approaches, discussed below, provide quantitative measures of cell surface phenotype, which, along with confirmatory functional studies, yield insight into their biological roles in pulmonary homeostasis and disease.

2. Materials

2.1. Isolation of Peripheral Blood Mononuclear Cells

1. Percoll (Phamacia, Uppsala, Sweden).
2. 10X concentrated piperazine-N, *N'*-bis-2-ethanesulfonic acid (PIPES) buffer (Sigma, St. Louis, MO): 250 m*M* PIPES, 100 m*M* NaCl, 60 m*M* KCl, 400 m*M* NaOH, pH 7.4, kept at 4°C.
3. PIPES (1:10 dilution of the 10X PIPES).
4. 0.9% NaCl (Abbott, N. Chicago, IL).
5. 90% Percoll (nine parts Percoll and one part 10X PIPES).
6. Percoll at a density of 1.080 g/L (80 mL 90% Percoll and 40 mL PIPES).
7. 0.1 *M* ethylenediamine tetraacetic acid (EDTA) (Sigma).

2.2. Collection of AMs by Bronchoalveolar Lavage

1. Phosphate-buffered saline (PB)–0.1% bovine serum albumin (BSA): 100 mL Dulbecco's PBS (Biofluids, Rockville, MD) containing 100 mg BSA (Sigma).
2. PIPES/albumin/glucose buffer: PIPES buffer containing 0.003% human serum albumin and 0.1% glucose.

2.3. Culturing of Monocyte/Macrophage Cell Lines

1. THP-1 cells: Human acute monocytic leukemia cell line (American Type Culture Collection [ATCC] no. 45502 or 45503) (*see* **Note 1**).
2. THP-1 culture media: RPMI 1640 medium with 2 m*M* L-glutamine, adjusted to contain 1.5 g/L Na bicarbonate, 4.5 g/L glucose, 10 m*M* HEPES, and 1 m*M* Na pyruvate, and supplemented with 10% fetal bovine serum (FBS) and 0.05 m*M* 2-mercaptoethanol.
3. U937 cells: Human monocyte-like, histiocytic lymphoma (ATCC no. CRL 1593).
4. U937 culture media: RPMI-1640 with 25 m*M* HEPES buffer, 1% penicillin–streptomycin, 1% L-glutamine, 5% FBS.

2.4. Indirect Immunofluorescent Labeling of Cells

1. PBS–0.2% BSA: 100 mL Dulbecco's PBS (Biofluids) containing 200 mg BSA (Sigma).
2. Human immunoglobulin G (IgG) (Sigma), used to reduce nonspecific binding of antibodies (Abs) via Fcγ receptors: To make a working 12 mg/mL stock from a

main 100 mg/mL stock, combine 120 µL human IgG (100 mg) and 880 µL PBS–0.2% BSA.
3. Tricolor (R-phycoerythrin [R-PE]-cyanine dye [Cy]5 fluorochrome)-conjugated, FITC-conjugated, or R-PE-conjugated polyclonal $F(ab')_2$ goat antimouse IgG (Caltag, Burlingame, South San Francisco, CA) used at a saturating concentration (typically a 1:5 dilution).
4. 1% paraformaldehyde, used as a fixative to sterilize the sample and preserve it for analysis: 0.6 g paraformaldehyde (Sigma) dissolved in 60 mL Dulbecco's PBS. Place in a 100-mL glass bottle, and stir on a hot plate, using moderate heat until the solution is clear. Filter and refrigerate to 4°C before use.

3. Methods

Immunofluorescence and flow cytometric methods are typically combined with light microscopic analysis of stained cells to count monocytes and AM, and provide an estimate of percentages in the starting cell suspensions to aid and corroborate information obtained by flow cytometry. Examples of the latter include the Diff-Quik stain (Dade Diagnostics, Aguada, PR), a modification of the Wright stain, in which blood smears or cytocentrifugation preparations are fixed using a methanolic fixative solution to stabilize cellular components. Two aqueous solutions are then applied individually to the fixed smear to differentially stain specific cellular components. Solution 1 is a buffered solution of eosin Y (an anionic dye); solution 2 is a buffered solution of thiazine dyes (cationic dyes) consisting of methylene blue and Azure A ***(21)***. Another example is staining for nonspecific esterase (α-naphthyl acetate esterase [ANAE] with fluoride inhibition kit (Sigma) (*see* **Note 2**).

3.1. Isolation of Peripheral Blood Mononuclear Cells by Density Gradient Centrifugation

Density gradient centrifugation is the most common and useful method for initial blood monocyte enrichment. Reagents such as Percoll, diluted to a specific gravity (1.080 g/L with buffer), are used to separate cells of lower density (lymphocytes, monocytes, and basophils) from cells of higher density (neutrophils, eosinophils, and erythrocytes, specific gravity >1.080 g/L) following centrifugation.

1. Peripheral venous blood is drawn and anticoagulated with EDTA (0.01 *M* final concentration, i.e., 1 mL of 0.1 *M* EDTA/10 mL blood).
2. Each 10 mL chelated blood is diluted with 25 mL 0.9% NaCl at room temperature (RT), and layered on 10 mL Percoll solution, with a density of 1.080 g/L. The blood is then centrifuged for 15 min at 400*g* at RT.
3. Carefully collect the cells above the interface, and wash twice in PBS–0.1% BSA at 4°C.

4. The total cell count and viability of recovered cells is determined.
5. The purity of the monocyte population is determined from cytocentrifugation preparations (Cytospin 2, Shandon, Pittsburgh, PA) stained with Diff-Quik or nonspecific esterase, using an ANAE kit.

3.2. Collection of Alveolar Macrophages by Bronchoalveolar Lavage

Bronchoscopy should be performed only by experienced pulmonologists under guidelines established by various panels of experts and workshops, and with informed consent ***(22,23)***.

3.2.1. Bronchoalveolar Lavage Procedure and Collection of Cells

1. Premedicate subjects with atropine (0.6 mg iv) and fentanyl (0.1 mg iv). Local anesthesia is achieved with administration of 4% nebulized and 2% instilled lidocaine into the lower airways ***(24)***.
2. Bronchoalveolar Lavage (BAL) is performed using five 20-mL aliquots of normal saline prewarmed to 37°C. The saline is instilled and suctioned sequentially from three sites (right middle lobe, right lower lobe, and lingula), and the pooled BAL fluids are immediately placed on ice.
3. Collect the cells by centrifugation at 500*g* for 6 min at 4°C.
4. Wash the cells twice in PBS–0.1% BSA at 4°C.
5. Resuspend cells in PAG buffer for a cell count (typical yield: total count $2–10 \times 10^7$ cells, >80% macrophages).
6. Determine the total cell count and viability in a hemocytometer by light microscopy and erythrocin B dye exclusion, as above.
7. Perform cell differentials by counting 100 cells on cytocentrifuge slides stained with Diff-Quik and ANAE (*see* **Subheading 3.1., step 5**).
8. Pellet and resuspend cells in PBS–0.2% BSA (used to minimize sticking of anticell surface antigen monoclonal antibodies [MAbs] to the plastic tubes), so that there will be a minimum of $0.3–1 \times 10^5$ BAL cells/tube or condition before addition of Abs for labeling.

3.3. Culturing and Maintenance of Monocyte/Macrophage Cell Lines

3.3.1. Growing Cells from Frozen Aliquots

1. Thaw cells at RT.
2. Add thawed cells to media with 30% FBS (7 mL RPMI + 3 mL FBS).
3. Centrifuge cells at 500*g* for 6 min, aspirate supernatant, and resuspend cells in media with 20% FBS (8 mL RPMI + 2 mL FBS).
4. Centrifuge cells at 500*g* for 6 min at RT, aspirate supernatant, and resuspend cells in appropriate media with FBS concentration in 1 mL, if culturing in a T75 flask, or 0.5 mL, if culturing in a T25 flask.
5. Start cultures at 10^5 cells/mL and maintain between $10^5–10^6$ cells/mL.

3.3.2. Cell Culturing, Feeding, and Subculturing

1. The monocytic cell lines U937 and THP-1 are cultured in their respective media (*see* **Subheading 2.3.**).
2. Add 1 mL resuspended cells to 9 mL media in a T75 flask, or 0.5 mL resuspended cells in 4.5 mL media in a T25 flask, maintaining the appropriate concentrations of cells.
3. The cells are incubated in a fully humidified air atmosphere containing 5% CO_2 at 37°C.
4. For feeding, transfer cells in media, and centrifuge at 500*g* for 6 min.
5. Aspirate the supernatant and resuspend the cells in an appropriate volume of media, depending on size of flask (*see* **step 2**).
6. Dispense cells into new flasks, and supplement with the appropriate amount of fresh media.
7. Media is replaced at least twice a week, depending on the growth rate (*see* **Note 4**).
8. For subculturing, remove cells and media from the flask, and centrifuge at 500*g* for 6 min.
9. Aspirate the supernatant, and resuspend cells in twice the appropriate volume of media.
10. Split cells between two flasks, and supplement with the appropriate volume of media.

3.4. Indirect Immunofluorescent Labeling of Cells

The combination of two approaches, immunofluorescence and flow cytometry (FCM), allows both quantitative and specific cell surface analysis. This requires a cell suspension and at least 30,000 cells (ideally, 1 million cells) per analysis. Previously, a major limiting factor of AM flow cytometry was interference by autofluorescence, emitted in the absence of any exogenous fluorochrome ***(25–27)***. Fortunately, because blood monocytes, like other leukocytes, lack this magnitude of autofluorescence, fluorescein isothiocyanate (FITC) or R-PE can be used for their analysis. In human AM, this intense autofluorescence (even more intense in AM from smokers) is emitted when cells are excited by light from 488 nm lasers, the excitation wavelength of the most commonly used air-cooled argon lasers. Because this intense autofluorescence occurs at a peak of 540 nm, with a range spanning the emission spectrum for both FITC and R-PE (480–580 and 540–640 nm, respectively ***[26,28,29]***), it essentially obscures fluorescence from these fluorochromes, making their use impractical. One potential solution to the problem of autofluorescence is to use fluorescent reagents whose excitation and/or emission spectra are distinct from that of AM autofluorescence. One such reagent, allophycocyanin (APC), is a fluorescent reagent that is excited at a wavelength of >600 nm and emits at 660 nm, beyond the range of AM autofluorescence ***(30–32)***. Although this reagent can be employed for AM phenotyping, it requires access to a significantly more expensive and sophisticated dual or tunable laser flow cytometer. As an alternative, a two-color FCM method using a single 488-nm laser, allowing the identification and quantitative phenotypic analysis of AM, has been developed *(33)*. This method employs a fluorescent tandem phycobiliprotein conjugate for indirect immunofluorescence, and is similar to another conjugate initially developed as a combination of PE and APC *(34)*. With the original conjugate, 90% of emitted energy from R-PE (excited by the 488-nm laser, emitted at a peak of 590 nm) is absorbed by, and excites, the APC, which then emits at a peak of 660 nm, coming almost entirely from APC itself. Following the development of the R-PE–APC conjugate, a new family of Cy reagents was developed *(35)*, and one of the Cy fluorochromes, with peak emission at 670 nm, was used, linked to R-PE as a second fluorochrome in the tandem dye, replacing APC. The fluorochrome found to be optimal for use as the secondary reagent with a tandem dye termed "tricolor" consisting of R-PE linked to Cy5, conjugated to a polyclonal F(ab')$_2$ preparation of goat antimouse IgG.

1. Add 10 µL 12 mg/mL human block IgG (this will reach 4 mg/mL final concentration in a total final volume of 30 µL), to reduce nonspecific binding of the primary murine MAb to Fcγ receptors or other surface structures.
2. Add the primary AB, using a saturating concentration of an antihuman MAb (typically mouse) recognizing a specific surface molecule. An irrelevant isotype-matched MAb at an identical concentration (typically about 10 µg/mL) is used as a control (*see* **Note 5**).
3. Incubate for 30 min at 4°C.
4. After 30 min, spin down and pellet the cells in a refrigerated microcentrifuge (4°C) for 20 s at 10,000*g*.
5. Remove the supernatant and resuspend pellets in 100 µL cold PBS–0.2% BSA, and centrifuge again in the refrigerated microcentrifuge.
6. Remove the supernatant, then resuspend the pellet in 20 µL prediluted secondary Ab (e.g., 1:5 dilution of tricolor-conjugated polyclonal F(ab')$_2$ goat antimouse IgG for AM and monocytes, or FITC or R-PE-conjugated polyclonal F(ab')$_2$ goat antimouse IgG for monocytes or cell lines) and incubate the cells on ice in the dark for 30 min.
7. Pellet the cells as above, wash once (100 µL cold PBS–0.2% BSA), pellet, and resuspend the cells in PBS–0.2% BSA (1×10^6 cells/mL PBS).
8. If cells cannot be analyzed the day that they are labeled, they can be fixed by resuspending them in fresh 1% paraformaldehyde, instead of the PBS suggested in **step 7**, and kept for up to 1 wk at 4°C, in the dark, until analyzed.

3.5. Flow Cytometry

1. Alveolar macrophages are identified by gating on cells with high autofluoresence in the FITC channel with typical forward- and side-scatter characteristics (*see* **Figs. 1** and **2**).

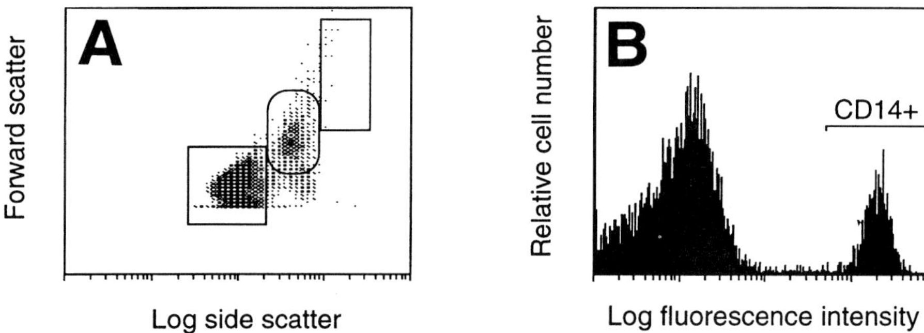

Fig. 1. FCM analysis of blood monocytes. **(A)** An example of scatter characteristics and **(B)** CD14 expression using mononuclear cells obtained by Percoll separation (*see* **Subheading 3.1.**). In **(A)**, the square represents lymphocytes, the oval represents monocytes, and the rectangle is the region where eosinophils and neutrophils would have been located. Basophils, which stay with the mononuclear cells (not the other granulocytes), are found in the region where the square and oval touch (i.e., they have light-scatter characteristics between the lymphocyte and monocyte populations). In **(B)**, an example of bright FITC–CD14 staining of monocytes in an ungated, mixed mononuclear cell preparation is shown.

2. To eliminate any light of wavelength <630 nm, including AM autofluorescence, a 630-nm long-pass filter is substituted for the standard long-pass filter used to analyze R-PE, allowing the collection of tricolor signals emitted beyond 630 nm (***33***; *see* **Note 6**).
3. Fluorescence histograms are generated using a four-log scale, and are expressed in units of net mean fluorescence, with IgG control values subtracted (net mean fluorescence intensity). Ideally, at least 5000 cells are analyzed to generate each histogram. Using these approaches, an extensive analysis of blood monocyte and AM phenotype has been generated, and can now be compared to that observed for monocyte and macrophage cell lines, such as THP-1 and U937 (*see* **Table 1**).

4. Notes

1. The ATCC web site for ordering the cell lines mentioned is *www.atcc.org*.
2. Although cellular esterases are ubiquitous in nature, ANAE is found primarily in cells of monocytic lineage. Blood, bone marrow films, or tissue preparations are incubated with α-naphthyl acetate in the presence of freshly formed diazonium salt. Enzymatic hydrolysis of ester linkages liberates free naphthol compounds, and these couple with the diazonium salt, forming highly colored deposits at sites of enzyme activity. It should be noted, however, that megakaryocytes and erythroid precursors are positive for this enzyme ***(36)***, and lymphocytes and some mature granulocytes can show occasional positivity ***(37)***. To differentiate these cells conclusively from monocytes, sodium fluoride is

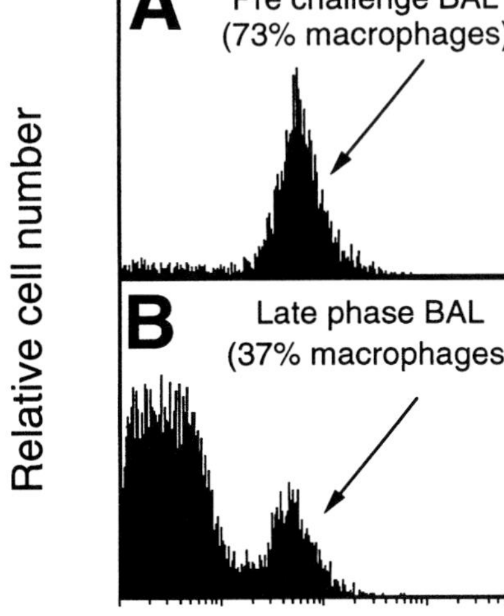

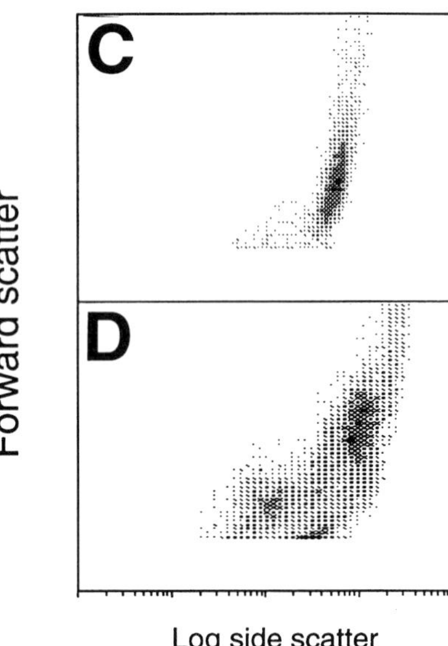

Fig. 2. FCM analysis of AMs. Examples of autofluorescence (monitored in the FITC channel, **A** and **B**) and typical scatter characteristics (**C** and **D**) for resident BAL cells obtained before allergen challenge (**A** and **C**), and approx 18 h after segmental allergen challenge of an allergic subject (**B** and **D**) *(24)*. Note that the bright autofluorescent staining (**A** and **B**) makes it easy to gate on the macrophages, which can then be specifically analyzed for indirect immunofluorescent tricolor staining for a specific marker (not shown). Also note that BAL macrophage scatter characteristics are broad and overlap with many leucocyte subpopulations. It is therefore recommended that autofluorescence analysis be performed first, so that AM can be gated away from other BAL cells for further analysis. In this particular example, the prechallenge BAL contained 73% macrophages, 25% lymphocytes, 1% neutrophils, and 1% eosinophils; the late phase BAL contained 37% macrophages, 20% lymphocytes, 16% neutrophils, and 27% eosinophils.

incorporated into the incubation system, resulting in the inactivation of the monocyte enzyme. Staining with α-naphthyl butyrate esterase (Sigma) will also demonstrate nonspecific esterase activity in monocytes and macrophages, but the α-naphthyl butyrate esterase assay is less sensitive than the ANAE procedure *(38)*.

3. If the Percoll density reading is greater than the required density, adjust by adding more PIPES buffer; if it is lower than the required density, add more 90% Percoll.
4. Usually, when cell lines are initially passaged, media is replaced twice a week (slower growing, fewer cells), but, as the cells become more confluent, the media is replaced 3–4×/wk.

Table 1
Expression of CD Cell Surface Markers on Human Blood Monocytes, Alveolar Macrophages, and the Monocyte/Macrophage Cell Lines THP-1 and U937

CD Number	Monocytes	AM	THP-1 cells	U937 cells
4	+	+	++++	++++
9	++++	+	++	+
11a	++++	++++	++++	++++
11b	++++	++	++++	++
11c	++++	++	++++	++
12	++++	not done	++++	+
13	++++	+	++++	++++
14	++++	+	++++	+
15	++++	+	++++	++++
15s	++++	not done	++++	++++
16	++	+++	++++	+
17	+++	+	++++	+
18	++++	++++	++++	++++
23	+	+	+	++++
24	+	+	++	+
29	++++	++	++++	++++
31	++++	+	++++	++++
32	++++	+++	++++	++++
33	++++	++	++++	++++
35	++++	++	+++	++++
36	++++	+	++++	++++
37	++++	+	+	++++
38	++++	+	++++	++++
39	++++	+	+++	+++
40	+++	+	++++	+
41	++++	+	+	+
42a	++++	+	+	+
42b	++++	+	++++	++++
42d	++++	+	not done	not done
43	++++	+	++++	++++
44	++++	++++	++++	++++
45	++++	++	++++	++++
45RA	+++	not done	++	++++
45RB	++++	not done	++++	++++
45RO	++++	not done	++++	+
46	++++	+	++++	++++
47	++++	++	++++	++++
48	++++	+	+	++++
49a	++	+	+	+
49b	++++	+	+	+
49c	++	+	++	++
49d	++++	+	++++	++++
49e	++++	+	++++	++++
49f	++++	+	++++	++++
50	++++	+	++++	++++
51	++	+	++	+
52	++++	++	++	+
53	++++	++	++++	+
54	++++	+	++++	++++
55	++++	+	++++	++++
58	++++	+	++++	++++
59	++	+	++++	+
61	++++	+	++	+

CD number	Monocyte	AM	THP-1	U937
62L	++++	+	+	+
63	++++	++++	++++	++++
64	++++	++++	++++	++++
w65	+	+	+++	++++
66acde	+	+	++++	++++
68	+	+	++	+
69	++	+	+++	++++
70	+	+	++++	+
71	+	++++	++++	++++
74	+++	not done	+	+
81	++++	++	++++	+
82	++++	+	++++	++++
w84	++++	not done	+++	+
85	++++	+	++	++++
86	++++	+	++	+
87	++++	++	++++	++++
88	++++	not done	++++	+
89	++++	+	++++	++++
90	+	+	++	+
91	++++	++	++++	+
w92	++++	+	++++	++++
93	++++	+	++++	++++
95	++++	not done	+	+
97	++++	+	++++	++++
98	++++	+	++++	++++
99	++++	+	++++	++++
99R	++++	not done	++++	++++
100	++++	+	+	++++
101	++++	+	++	+
102	++++	+	++++	++++
105	++++	+	++++	++++
107a	+	+	++	++
107b	+	+	+++	++++
109	++++	+	++++	+
115	++++	+	+	+
w116	++++	+	++	++++
w119	++++	+	++	++++
120a	++++	+	+	++
120b	++++	+	+	+++
121b	+	+	+	+++
126	++++	+	+	+
w128	+++	+	+	+
w130	+	+	+	+++
139	+++	not done	+	+++
141	+	not done	++++	+++
142	+	not done	+	++
147	++++	not done	++++	++++
148	++++	not done	++++	++++
149	++++	not done	++++	++++
151	++++	not done	++++	++++
154	++++	not done	++++	++++
155	++	not done	++++	++
157	+++	not done	+	++++
164	+	not done	+++	+++
165	+++	not done	+	+

5. It is useful to include CD14 (high on monocytes, low on AM) and CD71 (low on monocytes, high on AM) to help distinguish these cells in BAL fluids ***(51)***.
6. The filter substitution mentioned above for analysis of tricolor signals was necessary for older two-color flow cytometry machines (like the original Coulter EPICS Profile and Becton Dickinson FACScan). The appropriate filter sets are usually standard as part of the optics for newer machines equipped to perform three or more color analyses, such as the Coulter EPICS Profile 11, and the Becton Dickinson FACSCalibar.

References

1. Bilyk, N. and Holt, P. G. (1993) Inhibition of the immunosuppressive activity of resident pulmonary alveolar macrophages by granulocyte/macrophage colony-stimulating factor. *J. Exp. Med.* **177,** 1773–1777.
2. Martinet, Y., Rom, W. N., Grotendorst, G. R., Martin, G. R., and Crystal, R. G. (1987) Exaggerated spontaneous release of platelet-derived growth factor by alveolar macrophages from patients with idiopathic pulmonary fibrosis. *N. Engl. J. Med.* **317,** 202–209.
3. Rom, W. N. (1988) Alveolar macrophages release an insulin-like growth factor 1-type molecule. *J. Clin. Invest.* **82,** 1685–1693.
4. Kuhn, C. (1993) Pathogenesis of pulmonary fibrosis. *Monogr. Pathol.* **36,** 78–92.
5. Viksman, M. Y., Liu, M. C., Bickel, C. A., Schleimer, R. P., and Bochner, B. S. (1997) Phenotypic analysis of alveolar macrophages and monocytes in allergic airway inflammation. 1. Evidence for activation of alveolar macrophages, but not peripheral blood monocytes, in subjects with allergic rhinitis and asthma. *Am. J. Respir. Crit. Care Med.* **155,** 858–863.
6. Taylor, M. L., Noble, P. W., White, B., Wise, R., Liu, M. C., and Bochner, B. S. (2000) Extensive surface phenotyping of alveolar macrophages in interstitial lung disease. *Clin. Immunol.* **94,** 33–41.
7. Panos, R. J., Mortenson, R. L., Niccoli, S. A., and King, T. E. (1990) Clinical deterioration in patients with idiopathic pulmonary fibrosis: causes and assessment. *Am. J. Med.* **88,** 396–404.
8. Ziegenhagen, M. W., Schrum, S., Zissel, G., Zipfel, P. F., Schlaak, M., and Muller-Quernheim, J. (1998) Increased expression of proinflammatory chemokines in bronchoalveolar lavage cells of patients with progressing idiopathic pulmonary fibrosis and sarcoidosis. *J. Invest. Med.* **46,** 223–231.

Data for monocytes, and THP-1 and U937 cells are from published information from blind panel analyses performed as part of the Fifth and Sixth International Leukocyte Typing Workshops ***(39,40)***, and from web sites, including the one for the Sixth International Leukocyte Typing Workshop (mol.genes.nig.ac.jp/hlda/) and the CD Index (www.ncbi.nlm.nih.gov/prow/); data on AM are from both published ***(5,6)*** and unpublished observations, including experiments using the blind panel MAbs from the Sixth International Leukocyte Typing Workshop. Scales: + 0–25% positive; ++ 25–50%; +++. 50–75%; ++++ 75–100%. To conserve space, CD markers considered negative on all four cell types were excluded from the table.

9. Kiemle-Kallee, J. H., Kreipe, H., Radzun, H. J., Parwaresch, M. R., Auerswald, U., Magnussen, H., and Barth, J. (1991) Alveolar macrophages in idiopathic pulmonary fibrosis display a more monocyte-like immunophenotype and an increased release of free oxygen radicals. *Eur. Resp. J.* **4,** 400–406.
10. Crystal, R. G. (1991) *Alveolar Macrophages.* Raven, New York.
11. Carre, P. R., Mortenson, R., King, T., Noble, P., Sable, C., and Riches, D. (1991) Increased expression of the interleukin-5 gene by alveolar macrophages in idiopathic pulmonary fibrosis. A potential mechanism for recruitment and activation of neutrophils in lung fibrosis. *J. Clin. Invest.* **88,** 1802–1810.
12. Standiford, T., Rolfe, M., Kunkel, S., Lynch, J. D., Burdick, M., Gilbert, A., et al. (1993) Macrophage inflammatory protein-1 alpha expression in interstitial lung disease. *J. Immunol.* **151,** 2852–2863.
13. Iyonaga, K., Takeya, M., Saita, N., Sakamoto, O., Yoshimura, T., Ando, M., and Takahashi, K. (1994) Monocyte chemoattractant protein-1 in idiopathic pulmonary fibrosis and other interstitial lung diseases. *Hum. Pathol.* **25,** 455–463.
14. Smith, R. E., Strieter, R. M., Zhang, K., Phan, S. H., Standiford, T. J., Lukacs, N. W., and Kunkel, S. L. (1995) Role for C-C chemokines in fibrotic lung disease. *J. Leukoc. Biol.* **57,** 782–787.
15. Petrek, M., Pantelidis, P., Southcott, A. M., Lympany, P., Safranek, P., Black, C. M., et al. (1997) Source and role of RANTES in interstitial lung disease. *Eur. Respir. J.* **10,** 1207–1216.
16. Kodama, N., Yamaguchi, E., Hizawa, N., Furuya, K., Kojima, J., Oguri, M., Takahashi, T., and Kawakami, Y. (1998) Expression of RANTES by bronchoalveolar lavage cells in nonsmoking patients with interstitial lung diseases. *Am. J. Respir. Cell Mol. Biol.* **18,** 526–531.
17. Khalil, N., O'Connor, R. N., Flanders, K. C., and Unruh, H. (1996) TGF-beta 1, not TGF-beta 2 or TGF-beta 3, is differentially present in epithelial cells of advanced pulmonary fibrosis: an immunohistochemical study. *Am. J. Resp. Cell Mol. Biol.* **14,** 131–138.
18. Spiteri, M. A., Clarke, S. W., and Polter, L. W. (1992) Isolation of phenotypically and functionally distinct macrophage subpopulations from human bronchoalveolar lavage. *Eur. Respir. J.* **5,** 717–726.
19. Striz, I., Wang, Y.-M., Kalaycioglu, O., and Costabel, U. (1992) Expression of alveolar macrophage adhesion molecules in pulmonary sarcoidosis. *Chest* **102,** 882–886.
20. Barbosa, I. L., Gant, V. A., and Hamblin, A. S. (1991) Alveolar macrophages from patients with bronchogenic carcinoma and sarcoidosis similarly express monocyte antigens. *Clin. Exp. Immunol.* **86,** 173–178.
21. Thompson, S. W. and Hunt, R. D. (1996) Methods for the microscopic demonstration of morphologic components of animal tissue, in *Selected Histochemical Methods.* Charles C. Thomas, Springfield, IL.
22. (1991) Workshop summary and guidelines: investigative use of bronchoscopy, lavage, and bronchial biopsies in asthma and other airway diseases. *J. Allergy Clin. Immunol.* **88,** 808–814.

23. Rennard, S., Aalbers, R., Bleecker, E., Klech, H., Rosenwasser, L., Olivieri, D., and Sibille, Y. (1998) Bronchoalveolar lavage: performance, sampling procedure, processing and assessment. *Eur. Respir. J.* **26(Suppl.),** 13S–15S.
24. Liu, M. C., Hubbard, W. C., Proud, D., Stealey, B., Galli, S., Kagey-Sobotka, A., Bleecker, E. R., and Lichtenstein, L. M. (1991) Immediate and late inflammatory responses to ragweed antigen challenge of the peripheral airways in asthmatics: cellular, mediator, and permeability changes. *Am. Rev. Respir. Dis.* **144,** 51–58.
25. Edelson, J., Klein, M., Gallagher, B., Liu, F., Hornstein, A., Braude, A. C., and Rebuck, A. S. (1984) Bronchoalveolar lavage cells autofluoresce. *Am. Rev. Respir. Dis.* **4,** A164.
26. Edelson, J. D., MacFadden, D. K., Klein, M., and Rebuck, A. S. (1985) Autofluorescence of alveolar macrophages: problems and potential solutions. *Med. Hypotheses* **17,** 403–408.
27. Rossman, M. D., and Douglas, S. D. (1988) Alveolar macrophage: receptors and effector cell function, in *Immunology and Immunologic Diseases of the Lung* (Daniele, R. P., ed.), Blackwell, Chicago, pp. 167–183.
28. Crissman, H. A. and Steinkamp, J. A. (1990) Cytochemical techniques for multivariate analysis of DNA and other cellular constituents, in *Flow Cytometry and Sorting* (Melamed, M. R., Lindmo, T., and Mendelsohn, M. L., eds.), Wiley-Liss, New York, pp. 227–247.
29. Shapiro, H. (1988) Parameters and probes, in *Practical Flow Cytometry* (Shapiro, H., ed.), Liss, New York, pp. 115–198.
30. Fuchs, H. J., McDowell, J., and Shellito, J. E. (1988) Use of allophycocyanin allows quantitative description by flow cytometry of alveolar macrophage surface antigens present in low numbers of cells. *Am. Rev. Respir. Dis.* **138,** 1124–1128.
31. Loken, M. R., Keji, J. F., and Kelley, K. A. (1987) Comparison of helium-neon and dye lasers for the excitation of allophycocyanin. *Cytometry* **8,** 96–100.
32. Williams, D. H., Jeffery, L. H., and Murray, E. J. (1992) Aurothioglucose inhibits induced NF-κB and AP-1 activity by acting as an IL-1 functional antagonist. *Biochem. Biophys. Acta* **1180,** 9–14.
33. Viksman, M. Y., Liu, M. C., Schleimer, R. P., and Bochner, B. S. (1994) Application of a flow cytometric method using autofluorescence and a tandem dye to analyze human alveolar macrophage surface markers. *J. Immunol. Methods* **172,** 17–24.
34. Glazer, A. N. and Stryer, L. (1983) Fluorescent tandem phycobiliprotein conjugates. Emission wavelength shifting by energy transfer. *Biophys. J.* **43,** 383–386.
35. Ernst, L. A., Gupta, R. K., Mujumdar, R. B., and Waggoner, A. S. (1989) Cyanine dye labeling reagents for sulfhydryl groups. *Cytometry* **10,** 3–10.
36. Hayhoe, F. G. J. and Flemans, R. J. (1982) *Color Atlas of Hematological Cytology.* Wiley, New York, pp. 34–38.
37. Yam, L. T., Li, C. Y., Wolfe, N. J., and Moy, P. W. (1971) Cytochemical examination of monocytes and granulocytes. *Am. J. Clin. Pathol.* **55,** 283–287.
38. Basso, G., Cocito, M. G., Semenzato, G., and Pezzutto, A. (1980) Cytochemical study of thymocytes and T lymphocytes. *Br. J. Haematol.* **44,** 577–580.

39. Shaw, S., Luce, G. G., Gilks, W. R., Anderson, K., Ault, K., Bochner, B. S., et al. (1995) Leukoeyte differentiation antigen database, in *Leukocyte Typing V: White Cell Differentiation Antigens* (Schlossman, S., Boumsell, L., Gilks, W., Harlan, J., Kishimoto, T., Morimoto, C., eds.), Oxford University Press, New York, pp. 16–198.
40. Miyazaki, S., Sugawara, H., Tamura, T., Okayama, T., Ishii, J., Shimura, J., et al. (1997) Cross-lineage (blind panel) study and human leucocyte differentiation antigen database, in *Leucocyte Typing VI: White Cell Differentiation Antigens* (Kishimoto, T., Kikutani, H., von dem Borne, A. E. G. K., Goyert, S. M., Mason, D. Y., Miyasaka, M., eds.), Garland, New York, pp. 3–20.

6

Expression of Interleukin-10 and Granulocyte-Macrophage Colony-Stimulating Factor on Blood Monocytes and Alveolar Macrophages

Matthias John and Sam Lim

1. Introduction

Peripheral blood monocytes (PBMs) and alveolar macrophages (AMs) are widely recognized as cells that play a central role in the regulation of immune and inflammatory activities, as well as in tissue remodeling. The fulfillment of these activities is mediated by complex and multifactorial processes involving products derived from macrophages and monocytes *(1)*. Monocytes are an important source of cytokines that are released in asthma and are likely precursor cells to AMs. Macrophages usually elaborate powerful suppressive signals to limit the proliferative potential of T-cells, thus maintaining local immunologic homeostasis *(2)*. In asthma, macrophages and monocytes may be stimulated by specific allergens to augment T-cell proliferation *(3)*, which may result from a different profile of cytokines released from these cells. For example, increased release of granulocyte-macrophage colony-stimulating factor (GM-CSF) may inhibit the immunosuppressive effect of macrophages *(4)*. Indeed, macrophages and monocytes from asthmatic subjects release increased amounts of proinflammatory cytokines, such as interleukin-1β (IL-1), tumor necrosis factor-α, Interferon-γ (IFN-γ), IL-6, and GM-CSF *(5–8)*. Inhaled steroids used for the treatment of asthma reduce the number of infiltrating eosinophils, T-cells, macrophages, and mast cells in the airway submucosa *(9)*. Suppression of proinflammatory cytokine release, such as GM-CSF, IL-4, IL-5, and regulated upon activation, normal T-cell expressed and secreted (RANTES), from many inflammatory and resident airway cells, is a likely mechanism of steroid action *(10–12)*. Proinflammatory cytokine expression

From: *Methods in Molecular Medicine, vol. 44: Asthma: Mechanisms and Protocols*
Edited by: K. F. Chung and I. Adcock © Humana Press Inc., Totowa, NJ

by macrophages may also be inhibited, such as the release of GM-CSF, IL-6, and macrophage inflammatory protein (MIP-1α) as has been demonstrated in vitro ***(13,14)***.

IL-10 has numerous anti-inflammatory effects that would be beneficial in suppressing inflammatory mechanisms associated with asthma. In addition to inhibiting the production of IFN-γ and IL-2 by T-helper type-1 (Th1) lymphocytes ***(15)***, IL-10 also inhibits proinflammatory cytokine production (such as IL-1β, IL-6, IL-8, MIP-1α) by mononuclear phagocytes ***(16–20)*** at the level of cytokine gene transcription ***(21)***, and IL-4 and IL-5 production by Th2 T-cells ***(22)***. GM-CSF is a pleiotropic cytokine that can stimulate the proliferation, maturation, and function of hematopoietic cells, and has priming effects on inflammatory cells, such as neutrophils and eosinophils. There is evidence for increased expression of GM-CSF in the epithelial cells and PBMs from asthmatic patients ***(23,24)***.

The authors have shown ***(8)*** that chronic inhaled corticosteroid therapy alters the balance of pro- and anti-inflammatory cytokine expression and release from AMs in asthma by decreasing the production of the proinflammatory cytokines MIP-1α, GM-CSF, and IFN-γ. Corticosteroids convert the cytokine response of the AM of the asthmatic subject into the range found in normal subjects, and this may underlie the improved functional effects observed, such as the attenuation of bronchial hyperresponsiveness. A previous study by the authors demonstrated that PBMs of mildly asthmatic patients, with a dual early and late response following allergen challenge, express and release significantly greater amounts of IL-10. Asthmatic subjects who demonstrated only an early response released significantly less IL-10 and MIP-1α from their monocytes at baseline and following stimulation by exogenous stimuli, such as lipopolysaccharide and IL-1β. In addition, single responders express a lesser amount of IL-10 mRNA, indicating that the difference in IL-10 release results from a reduction in IL-10 transcription (**Fig. 1**). For all these reasons, IL-10 may be a key cytokine for the regulation of the inflammatory response in the airways. The potential role of IL-10 in asthma remains to be determined.

Molecular techniques that are commonly employed to describe the regulation of cytokines, such as IL-10 and GM-CSF in AMs and PBM, include reverse transcription-polymerase chain reaction (RT-PCR) for the mRNA quantification, and enzyme-linked immunosorbent assays (ELISA) for protein measurement.

2. Materials

2.1. Cell Isolation

1. Hank's balanced salt solution (HBSS) (Sigma).
2. RPMI-1640 culture medium (Sigma).

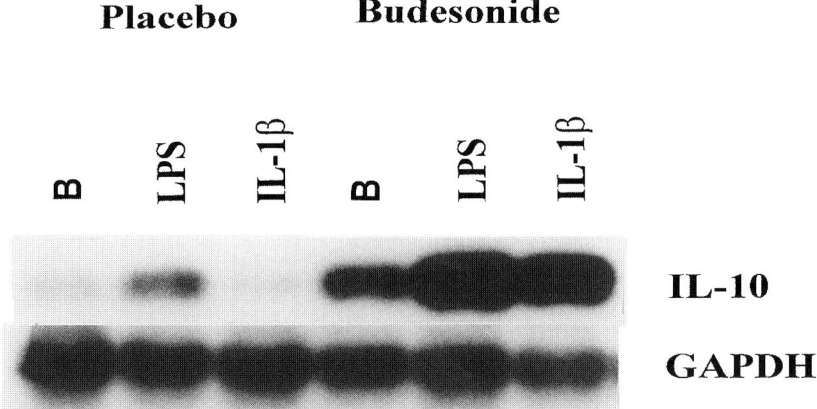

Fig. 1. Effect of inhaled corticosteroid, budesonide, given over 1 mo on IL-10 expression in AMs at baseline (baseline B) and after 24 h of stimulation with lipopolysaccharide (LPS, 1 µg/mL) and IL-1β (10 ng/mL). The upper panel shows representative Southern blot of IL-10 and GAPDH cDNA expression from the same asthmatic patient treated with placebo, and following 4-wk treatment with budesonide. The lower panel shows IL-10 protein concentration in the cell culture supernatants from AMs of 11 untreated (open bar) asthmatics, and following 4 wk of budesonide treatment (solid bar). Data shown as mean ± SEM. $*p < 0.05$, $**p < 0.01$, compared between the groups.

3. Dextran (Sigma).
4. Ficoll-Hypaque (Pharmacia).
5. 1.5 g citric acid, 2.5 g sodium citrate, 2.0 g D-glucose (ACD) (all from Sigma) in 100 mL distilled water).
6. Fetal calf serum (FCS) (Sigma).
7. Penicillin, streptomycin (Sigma).
8. L-Glutamin (Sigma).

2.2. RNA Extraction

1. Solution D: Add 586 mL distilled sterile water to 500 g guanidium isothiocyanate (Sigma). Add 35.2 mL 0.75 *M* sterile sodium citrate solution, pH 7.0, and 52.4 mL 10% *N*-lauroyl-sarcosine sodium salt solution (Sigma). This stock is stable for several months. To 50 mL stock, add 360 µL mercaptoethanol just before use. This solution D is stable for 3 d.
2. Isopropanol (BDH).
3. Phenol (Rathburne).
4. Chloroform (BDH).

2.3. Reverse Transcription Reaction

1. Hexamer primer (Promega).

2. Deoxynucleotide triphosphates (dNTPs): 10 m*M* each deoxyadenosine triphosphate (dATP), deoxyguanosine triphosphate (dGTP), deoxycytidine triphosphate (dCTP), deoxythymidine triphosphate (dTTP) (Promega).
3. Avian myeloblastosis virus (AMV) buffer (5X) (Promega).
4. RNase inhibitor (Promega).
5. AMV reverse transcript (Promega).
6. Nuclease-free water (Sigma).

2.4. PCR for IL-10

1. 10X: PCR buffer (50 m*M* KCl, 10 m*M* Tris-HCl (pH 8.4), 1.5 m*M* $MgCl_2$).
2. dNTPs: 10 m*M* each of dATP, dGTP, dCTP, dTTP (Promega).
3. *Taq* polymerase (Promega).
4. Mineral oil (Sigma).

2.5. ELISA for IL-10 and GM-CSF

1. Quantikine ELISA Kit (R&D, Abingdon, UK).
2. GM-CSF rat monoclonal antibody (mAb) (Cambridge Bioscience).
3. Biotynilated rat antihuman GM-CSF mAb (Cambridge Bioscience).
4. Avidin-peroxidase (Sigma).
5. 2.2'-Azino-*bis*(3-ethylbenzthiazoline-6-sulfonic acid) (ABTS) (Sigma).
6. Human recombinant GM-CSF (Genzyme).

3. Methods

3.1. Isolation of AMs

1. Filter the lavage fluid through sterile gauze into 50-mL Falcon tubes.
2. Centrifuge 10 min at 4°C at 1700 rpm, and remove the supernatant, which may kept for further analysis at –70°C.
3. Resuspend the cell pellet with 50 mL HBSS, and centrifuge 10 min at 4°C at 1700 RPM. Repeat this washing step once.
4. Resuspend the cell pellet in 2 m cell culture medium RPMI-1640, supplemented with 10% FCS, 1% L-glutamin, and 1% penicillin–streptomycin.
5. Determine total cell and macrophage count using a Neubauer chamber, and determine the cell viability with trypan blue exclusion.
6. Plate the cells in complete media (as described above) at a concentration of 1×10^6/mL in a 24-well plate.
7. Incubate the cells at 37°C with 5% CO_2 for 2 h, then change the medium to remove the nonadherent cells, such as lymphocytes, in order to obtain a pure population of macrophages, which have adhered to the bottom of the plate. Stimulate the cells with cytokines and incubate the plates again.

3.2. Isolation of PBMs

The principle of the isolation of PBMs from venous blood is the separation from other blood cells, using a density gradient centrifugation.

1. Mix venous blood with ACD in a proportion of 6:1, to prevent clotting. Add 6% dextran solution (1:5), and mix gently to accelerate red blood cell separation.
2. Leave the tube for 40–50 min at room temperature, until the red cells are separated from the leukocytes.
3. Remove the buffy coat, and transfer it into a new 50-mL Falcon tube. Centrifuge 10 min at 18°C at 1700 rpm. The cell pellet contains monocytes and other leucocytes.
4. Pipet the plasma off, leaving 5 mL in the tube. Resuspend the pellet with the remaining plasma.
5. Fill a 15-mL Falcon tube with 8 mL Ficoll-Hypaque. Pipet the resuspended cells very carefully on the surface of the Ficoll Hypaque. Centrifuge for 30 min at 18°C at 1600 rpm. At the end of this step, the mononuclear cells will remain in a layer on the Ficoll surface.
6. Remove the monocyte layer from the Ficoll surface with a one way pipet, and transfer it to a new 50-mL Falcon tube. Add 50 mL HBSS, and centrifuge 10 min at 18°C at 1700 rpm. Repeat this washing step twice.
7. After the second washing step, remove the HBSS completely, and resuspend the cell pellet in 3 mL cell culture medium RPMI-1640, supplemented with 10% FCS, 1% L-glutamin, and 1% penicillin–streptomycin.
8. Cell counting and viability testing should be performed as described in subheading XX for AMs.
9. Plate the cells in complete media at a concentration of 1×10^6 /mL in a 24-well plate.
10. Incubate the cells at 37°C with 5% CO_2 for 2 h, then change the medium, to remove nonadherent cells. Stimulate the cells with cytokines, and incubate the plates again.

3.3. RNA Extraction from AMs and Blood Monocytes

In order to describe the regulation of cytokine gene expression in monocytes or macrophages, the cells need to be lysed and the RNA extracted. The method of RNA extraction uses phenol–chloroform, as described by Chomczynski and Sacchi *(25)*.

1. After removing the cell culture supernatant, add 800 μL solution D to each culture well, and rinse the bottom carefully, to lyse the cells. Transfer the solution into a 2-mL Eppendorf tube.
2. Add 90 μL Na acetate (2 *M*, pH 4.0), and vortex the tube.
3. Add 800 μL phenol, and vortex the tube.
4. Add 160 μL chloroform–isoamyl alcohol, and vortex the tube again.
5. Put the tube on ice for 15 min, and spin it for 15 min at 200*g* (4°C).
6. Very carefully remove the upper aqueous-phase supernatant, which contains the RNA, and transfer it into a fresh 1.5-mL Eppendorf tube. Avoid aspirating fluid from the lower organic phase that contains DNA.
7. Add isopropanol in an equal volume to the supernatant, and store the assay overnight at –20°C.

Table 1
Amount for One Reverse Transcription Reaction

	μL
Hexamer primer 0.2 μg/μL	1
dNTPs (10 m*M*)	2
AMV buffer (5X)	4
RNase inhibitor	0.75
AMV reverse transcription	0.75
Final reaction volume	8.5

8. Spin the tube for 30 min at 200*g* (4°C), and pour off the supernatant.
9. For RNA washing, add 250 μL solution D, vortex, and add 1 mL 100% ethanol, and vortex again. Keep the assay on dry ice or, alternatively, in a –70°C freezer for 1 h.
10. Spin the tube for 30 min at 200*g* (4°C), and pour off the supernatant. Add 1 mL 75% ethanol, vortex, and spin 10 min at 200*g* (4°C). Pour out the supernatant, and freeze-dry for 15 min. The pellet contains the extracted RNA. Before putting the tube in the freeze-dryer, occlude the apperture with foil, and puncture it with a needle. Following freeze-drying, there is a tiny pellet containing RNA at the bottom of the Eppendorf tube.

3.4. Reverse Transcription Reaction

1. Resuspend the RNA pellet in 18 μL nuclease-free water, and spin the tube for 30 s. Transfer the RNA solution into a 0.5-mL Eppendorf tube. Measure the amount of yielded RNA, using a spectrophotometer.
2. Take a volume of RNA solution that is equal to 1 μg RNA, and add nuclease-free water to a final volume of 11.5 μL.
3. Incubate the assay for 5 min at 70°C, using a thermal cycler in order to denature the double-stranded RNA.
4. Prepare a master mix of nucleotides, enzymes, and buffer. Calculate the master mix resulting from the amount of samples that you will transcribe. A master mix volume of 8.5 μL is required for one sample (**Table 1**).
5. Place the tubes in a thermal cycler, and incubate 1 h at 42°C and 4 min at 90°C, then add 80 μL water. Aliquot samples (0.5 μL) in a PCR plate, and store it at –70°C.

3.5. PCR for IL-10

PCR is a valuable method for investigating the nucleic acid synthesis. A particular sequence of DNA can be replicated specifically. Only small amounts of DNA are required for PCR analysis; therefore, the method is useful for cell

Table 2
Amount for One PCR

	μL
PCR buffer with $MgCl_2$	2.5
dNTPs (10 m*M*)	0.5
Oligonucleotide primer (forward)	0.25
Oligonucleotide primer (reverse)	0.25
distilled water	16.4
Taq-polymerase	0.1
Final reaction volume	25

culture with limited amounts of cells. The preparation of pure DNA is important for a successful amplification.

1. Prepare DNA samples from stimulated macrophages or monocytes, as described above.
2. Carry out PCR reaction in a 96 well PCR plate. The basic procedure for PCR amplification is as in **Table 2**.
3. Add 20 μL PCR reaction mix to 5 μL IL-10 DNA template, and mix gently by pipeting. Add two drops of mineral oil to prevent sample evaporation.
4. Place the plate on a thermal cycler, and perform amplification. The cycling profile will vary, depending on individual PCR experiments.
5. The products can be distinguished by electrophoresis on a 1.5% agarose, ethidium bromide-stained gel, and then visualized using ultraviolet luminescence.

3.6. ELISAs for IL-10 and GM-CSF

IL-10 and GM-CSF were assayed using a quantitative sandwich-enzyme immunoassay technique.

3.6.1. IL-10

For IL-10, a commercially available kit was used (Quantikine, R&D). An anti-IL-10 mAb was coated onto a microtiter plate, to which standards and samples were added. An enzyme-linked polyclonal Ab specific for IL-10 was added to the wells, to sandwich-immobilized IL-10. Addition of a stabilized chromogen and hydrogen peroxide allowed a color development in proportion to the amount of IL-10 assayed by measurement of optical density using a spectrophotometer set to 450 nm. The lower limit of detection was 1.5 pg/mL for IL-10. Every sample should be assayed in duplicate. A sample volume of 200 μL is required for each measurement.

3.6.2. GM-CSF

1. Coat round-bottomed plates overnight with a rat antihuman GM-CSF mAb (50 µL 2 µg/mL) at 4°C.
2. Wash the plates two times with phosphate-buffered saline (PBS)–Tween pH 7.4.
3. Add 200 µL PBS–10% FCS in order to block the Ab, and incubate the assay for 2 h at 4°C.
4. Wash the plates again with PBS–Tween, and add 200 µL GM-CSF standard and samples to the wells, and incubate the plate overnight at 4°C.
5. Wash the plate 4× with PBS–Tween.
6. Add the secondary biotinylated anti-GM-CSF Ab (100 µL 2 µg/mL in PBS–10% FCS), and incubate for 45 min at room temperature, and wash with PBS–Tween again. Then add 100 µL 1:400 avidin–peroxidase solution, and incubate for 30 min at room temperature.
7. Wash the plates again, and add for development 100 µL ABTS substrate solution.
8. Measure GM-CSF colometrically, using a spectrophotometer set at 405 nm. The cytokine concentration was quantified by interpolation from a standard curve. The lower limit of detection was 16 µg/mL.

4. Notes

1. The viability of AMs and PBMs should be >85%, to obtain reproducible data.
2. For Northern blot analysis, a cell density of 5×10^6/mL in a 6-well plate is required.
3. Add the enzymes for the reverse transcription reaction and PCR at last to the mastermix, in order to prevent a denaturation of the enzyme proteins.
4. PCR cycling temperatures normally used for IL-10 gene amplification are as follows: denaturation of the DNA strands at 94°C for 30 s; annealing of primers to templates, 58°C; and extension of primers at 72°C for 30 s. Primers for IL-10 were 5' ATGCCCCAAGCTGAGAACCAAGACCCA and 3'TCTC AAGGGGCTGGGTCAGCTATCCCA, giving a product of 351 bp. The number of cycles was set to 29, which was chosen after determination of the linear phase of the product amplification curve from serial sampling, with increasing cycles of amplification.
5. The quantification of IL-10 gene expression can be performed either by Southern blot analysis or densitometric evaluation of the negative of the gel photogaph. For both methods, it is necessary to calculate the ratio of IL-10 to a standard gene, which is expressed independent of any stimulation. The authors have used the glyceraldehyde-phosphate dehydrogenase (GAPDH) gene. The GAPDH primers are: 5' TCTAGACGGCAGGCTAGGTCCACC and 3'CCACCCATGG CAAATTCCATGGCA, giving a product of 598 bp. The annealing temperature is 58°C. All other conditions are the same as for IL-10 PCR. Alternatively, it is also possible to use β-actin as the standard gene.

References

1. Nathan, C. F. (1987) Secretory products of macrophages. *J. Clin. Invest.* **79,** 319–326.
2. Holt, P. G. (1985) Downregulation of immune responses in the lower respiratory tract: role of alveolar macrophages. *Clin. Exp. Immunol.* **63,** 261–270.
3. Spiteri, M., Knight, R. A., Jeremy, J. Y., Barnes, P. J., and Chung, K. F. (1994) Alveolar macrophage-induced suppression of T-cell hyperresponsiveness in bronchial asthma is reversed by allergen exposure. *Eur. Respir. J.* **7,** 1431–1438.
4. Bilyk, N. and Holt, P. G. (1993) Inhibition of the immunosuppressive activity of resident pulmonary alveolar macrophages by granulocyte/macrophage colony-stimulating factor. *J. Exp. Med.* **177,** 1773–1777.
5. Spiteri, M. A., Prior, C., Herold, M., Knight, R. A., Clarke, S. W., and Chung, K. F. (1992) Spontaneous release of IL-1, IL-6, TNF-α and GM-CSF by alveolar macrophages (AM) in bronchial asthma. *Am. Rev. Respir. Dis.* **145,** A239
6. Hallsworth, M. P., Soh, C. P. C., Lane, S. J., Arm, J. P., and Lee, T. H. (1994) Selective enhancement of GM-CSF, TNF-α, IL-1β and IL-8 production by monocytes and macrophages of asthmatic subjects. *Eur. Respir. J* **7,** 1096–1102.
7. Cembrzynska-Norvak, M., Szklarz, E., Inglot, A. D., and Teodorczyk-Injeyan, J. A. (1993) Elevated release of TNF-α and interferon-gamma by bronchoalveolar leukocytes from patients with bronchial asthma. *Am. Rev. Respir. Dis.* **147,** 291–295.
8. John, M., Lim, S., Seybold, J., Jose, P. J., Robichaud, A., O' Connor, B., Barnes, P. J., and Fan Chung, K. (1998) Inhaled corticosteroids increase IL-10 but reduce MIP-1α, GM-CSF and IFNγ release from alveolar macrophages in asthma. *Am. J. Respir. Crit. Care Med.* **157,** 256–262
9. Djukanovic, R., Wilson, J. W., Britten, K. M., Wilson, S. J., Walls, A. F., Roche, W. R., Howarth, P. H., and Holgate, S. T. (1992) The effect of an inhaled corticosteroid on airway inflammation and symptoms in asthma. *Am. Rev. Respir. Dis.* **145,** 669–674.
10. Robinson, D. S., Hamid, Q., Ying, S., Bentley, A. M., Assoufi, B., North, J., Qui, M., Durham, S. R., and Kay, A. B. (1993) Prednisolone treatment in asthma is associated with modulation of bronchoalveolar lavage cell IL-4, IL-5 and IFN-γ cytokine gene expression. *Am. Rev. Respir. Dis.* **148,** 401–406.
11. Wang, J. H., Trigg, C. J., Devalia, J. L., Jordan, S., and Davies, R. J. (1994) Effect of inhaled beclomethasone dipropionate on expression of proinflammatory cytokines and activated eosinophils in the bronchial epithelium of patients with mild asthma. *J. Allergy Clin. Immunol.* **94,** 1025–1034.
12. Davies, R. J., Wang, J. H., Trigg, C. J., and Devalia, J. L. (1995) Expression of granulocyte/macrophage-colony-stimulating factor, interleukin-8 and RANTES in the bronchial epithelium of mild asthmatics is down-regulated by inhaled beclomethasone dipropionate. *Int. Arch. Allergy Immunol.* **107,** 428–429.

13. Berkman, N., Jose, P., Williams, T., Barnes, P. J., and Chung, K. F. (1995) Corticosteroid inhibition of macrophage inflammatory protein-1α expression in human monocytes and alveolar macrophages. *Am. J. Physiol.* **269,** L443–L452.
14. Linden, M. and Brattsand, R. (1994) Effects of a corticosteroid, budesonide, on alveolar macrophage and blood monocyte secretion of cytokines: differential sensitivity of GM-CSF, IL-1β and IL-6. *Pulm. Pharmacol.* **7,** 43–47.
15. Fiorentino, D. F., Bond, M. W., and Mosmann, T. R. (1989) Two types of mouse helper T cells. IV. Th 2 clones secrete a factor that inhibits cytokine production by Th 1 clones. *J. Exp. Med.* **170,** 2081–2090.
16. de Waal Malefyt, R., Abrams, J., Bennett, B., Figdor, C. G., and De Vries, J. E. (1991) Interleukin 10 (IL-10) inhibits cytokine synthesis by human monocytes: an autoregulatory role of IL-10 produced by monocytes. *J. Exp. Med.* **179,** 1209–1220.
17. Bogdan, C., Vodovotz, Y., and Nathan, C. (1991) Macrophage deactivation by interleukin 10. *J. Exp. Med.* **174,** 1549–1555.
18. Fiorentino, D. F., Zlotnik, A., Mossmann, T. R., Howard, M., and O'Garra, A. (1991) IL-10 inhibits cytokine production by activated macrophages. *J. Immunol.* **147,** 3815–3822.
19. Oswald, I. P., Wynn, T. A., Sher, A., and James, S. L. (1992) Interleukin 10 inhibits macrophage microbicidal activity by blocking the endogenous production of tumor necrosis factor alpha required as a costimulatory factor for interferon gamma-induced activation. *Proc. Natl. Acad. Sci. USA* **89,** 8676–8680.
20. Berkman, N., John, M., Roesems, G., Jose, P. J., Barnes, P. J., and Chung, K. F. (1995) Inhibition of macrophage inflammatory protein-1α by interleukin-10: differential sensitivities in human blood monocytes and alveolar macrophages. *J. Immunol.* **155,** 4412–4418.
21. Wang, P., Wu, P., Siegel, M. I., Egan, R. W., and Billah, M. M. (1994) IL-10 inhibits transcription of cytokine genes in human peripheral blood mononuclear cells. *J. Immunol.* **153,** 811–816.
22. Moore, K. W., O'Garra, A., de Waal Malefyt, R., Vieira, P., and Mosmann, T. R. (1993) Interleukin-10. *Annu. Rev. Immunol.* **11,** 165–190.
23. Gelder, C. M., Morrison, J. F. J., Southcot, A. M., Adcock, I. M., Kidney, J., Peters, M., et al. (1993) Cytokine mRNA profiles in asthmatic endobronchial biopsies. *Am. Rev. Respir. Dis.* **147,** A786
24. Nakamura, Y., Ozaki, T., Kamgi, T., Kawaji, K., Banno, K., Miki, S., et al. (1993) Increased GM-CSF production by mononuclear cells from peripheral blood of patients with bropnchial asthma. *Am. Rev. Respir. Dis.* **147,** 87–91.
25. Chomczynski, P. and Sacchi, N. (1987) Single step method of RNA isolation by acid guanidinium thiocyanate-phenol-chloroform extraction. *Anal. Biochem.* **162,** 156–160.

7

Mitogen-Activated Protein Kinase Activation in Eosinophils

Patricia M. de Souza, Hannu Kankaanranta, Mark A. Giembycz, and Mark A. Lindsay

1. Introduction

The mitogen-activated protein kinases (MAPK) are an expanding family of proline-directed serine/threonine kinases that are activated, following their dual phosphorylation at conserved threonine and tyrosine residues, by a family of MAPK kinases (MEK). Presently, the MAPK family can be divided into three groups: the extracellular signal-regulated kinases (ERK), composed of ERK-1/2/3/4/5, the c-jun N-terminal kinases (JNK)-46/54; and the p38 MAP kinase (p38 MAPK) composed of p38/p38β/p38γ/p38δ *(1)*. Of these enzymes, the authors have detected ERK-1/2/3/5, JNK-46/54, and p38 in guinea pig peritoneal eosinophils by Western analysis: ERK-4 and p38β were apparently absent.

A number of physiological stimuli have been demonstrated to induce the activation of the ERK kinases in eosinophils. In human cells, interleukin-5 (IL-5) and granulocyte-macrophage colony-stimulating factor (GM-CSF) transiently activate (15–60 min) members of the ERK family, although, at present, there are contradictory reports regarding whether it is the ERK-1 or ERK-2 isoform *(2–6)*. The upstream events linking ERK activation to the IL-5 receptor are presently unknown. Antisense studies have implicated a role for Src homology protein tyrosine phosphatase 2 in ERK-2 activation *(7)*; inhibitor studies have shown that both IL-5- and GM-CSF-induced ERK-1 activation could be inhibited by wortmannin, thereby implicating a role for phosphatidylinositol 3-kinase *(5)*. Studies in guinea pig peritoneal eosinophils have demonstrated the rapid and transient activation of ERK-1 and ERK-2 after exposure to the G-protein-linked agonist, leukotriene B_4 (LTB_4)

From: *Methods in Molecular Medicine, vol. 44: Asthma: Mechanisms and Protocols*
Edited by: K. F. Chung and I. Adcock

(8). PD098059, at concentrations that completely attenuated ERK-1/2 activation, was found to have no significant affect on either LTB_4-induced H_2O_2 generation by the NADPH nor phospholipase A_2 catalyzed [^{3}H]arachidonic acid release *(8)*.

In contrast to ERK, IL-5 and LTB_4 failed to activate JNK or p38 MAPK. However, incubation of human eosinophils in the absence of cytokines, which is associated with apoptosis, induced the activation of p38 MAPK. The selective p38 MAPK inhibitor, SB203580, was found to increase the rate of apoptosis suggesting that p38 MAPK activation was required for eosinophil survival *(9)*.

2. Materials

2.1. Cell Lysis

RIPA buffer: 10 m*M* Tris-HCl, pH 7.2, 150 m*M* sodium chloride (NaCl), 1 m*M* ethylenediamine tetraacetic acid (EDTA), 1% (v/v) Triton X-100, 0.5% (w/v) Na deoxycholate, 0.1% (w/v) Na dodecyl sulfate (SDS), 1 m*M* phenylmethylsulfonyl fluoride (PMSF), 2 m*M* Na orthovanadate, 10 μg/mL leupeptin, 25 μg/mL aprotinin, 10 μg/mL pepstatin, 1.25 m*M* sodium fluoride, 1 m*M* sodium pyrophosphate (*see* **Note 1**).

2.2. Immunoprecipitation

1. Washing buffer: 10 m*M* Tris-HCl, pH 7.2 (0.605 g), 150 m*M* NaCl (4.383 g), 1 m*M* ethyleneglycol-*bis*(β-amonoethylether)-*N,N,N',N'*-tetra-acetic acid (EGTA) (add 5 mL form 100 m*M* stock) made up in 500 mL distilled water.
2. Protein A/G Plus-agarose (Santa Cruz).

2.3. Western Blotting

1. 1.5 *M* Tris-HCl, pH 8.8 (45.4 g/250 mL).
2. 0.5 *M* Tris-HCl, pH 6.8 (6.05 g/100 mL).
3. 10% SDS (1 g/10 mL).
4. 10% ammonium persulfate (APS) (100 mg/mL): Make up fresh each day.
5. Running buffer (10X solution): 25 m*M* Tris-HCl (15 g), 192 m*M* glycine (72 g), 0.1% (w/v) SDS (5 g) in 500 mL distilled water (do not pH solution).
6. Transfer buffer (10X solution): 20 m*M* Tris-HCl (12.1 g), 192 m*M* glycine (72 g), 0.1% (w/v) SDS (5 g) in 500 mL distilled water (do not pH solution).
7. Tris-buffered saline–Tween (TBS–T) (10X solution): 20 m*M* Tris-HCl, pH 7.6 (12.1 g), 150 m*M* NaCl (43.8 g), 0.1% (v/v) Tween-20 (5 mL) in 500 mL distilled water.
8. Sample buffer: glycerol (1 mL), 2-mercaptoethanol (2-ME) (0.5 mL), 10% SDS (3 mL), 0.5 *M* Tris-HCl, pH 6.8 (2.5 mL), 1 mg bromophenol blue.

2.4. In-Gel Renaturation Assay (Two Gels)

2.4.1. Stock Solutions

1. Myelin basic protein (MBP): Reconstitute 5 mg protein (derived from bovine brain) in 1 mL water.
2. Tris stock solution (TSS): 1 *M* Tris-HCl, pH 8.0: 242.2 g Tris-HCl in 2000 mL, adjusted to pH 8.0.
3. Denaturation buffer stock (DBS): 6 *M* guanidine-HCl, 50 m*M* Tris-HCl (pH 8.0): 573.2 g guanidine-HCl + 50 mL TSS in 1000 mL water (*see* **Note 2**).
4. Re-equilibration buffer stock (RBS): 40 m*M* HEPES (pH 8.0), 10 m*M* $MgCl_2 \cdot 6H_2O$: 10.41 g HEPES + 2.03 g $MgCl_2 \cdot 6H_2O$ in 1000 mL water, adjusted to pH 8.0.
5. Kinase assay buffer stock (KABS): 40 m*M* HEPES pH 8.0, 10 m*M* $MgCl_2 \cdot 6H_2O$, 0.5 m*M* EGTA: 2.08 g HEPES + 0.406 g $MgCl_2 \cdot 6H_2O$ + 0.038 g EGTA in 200 mL water. Then adjust to pH 8.0. Store as 10-mL aliquots at –20°C.
6. Cold adenosine triphosphate (ATP): Prepare a 55-m*M* ATP (0.30 g in 10 mL water, adjusted to pH 7.4). Store 9.5 mL as 0.5-mL aliquots at –20°C. Dilute remaining 0.5 mL to give 0.55-m*M* ATP (1:100 dilution). 0.55-m*M* ATP is to be used for in-gel assays, and can be stored as 1-mL aliquots at –20°C.
7. Protein kinase inhibitor (PKI): Prepare 20 m*M* PKI (45 mg/mL) and store as 10-μL aliquots at –20°C. Dilute 1:100 just before use, to give 200 μ*M* PKI.
8. Trichloroacetic acid (TCA): Prepare 100% solution (500 g in 500 mL water).

2.4.2. Ready-to-Use Buffers

1. Buffer A: 50 m*M* Tris-HCl (pH 8.0), 20% (v/v) isopropanol: 15 mL TSS + 60 mL isopropanol + 225 mL water.
2. Buffer B: 50 m*M* Tris-HCl (pH 8.0), 5 m*M* 2-ME: 15 mL TSS + 105 μL 2-ME + 285 mL water.
3. Buffer C: 6 *M* guanidine-HCl, 50 m*M* Tris-HCl (pH 8.0), 5 m*M* 2-ME: 200 mL DBS + 70 μL 2-ME.
4. Buffer D: 50 m*M* Tris-HCl (pH 8.0), 5 m*M* 2-ME, 0.04% Tween-40: 25 mL TSS + 475 mL water + 200 μL Tween-40+ 175 μL 2-ME.
5. Buffer E: 40 m*M* HEPES (pH 8.0), 10 m*M* $MgCl_2$, 2 m*M* dithioreitol (DTT): 200 mL RBS + 0.0617 g DTT.
6. TCA wash (2000 mL): 5% (w/v) TCA, 1% (w/v) Na pyrophosphate: To 2000 mL water, add 25 g Na pyrophosphate and 125 mL 100% TCA (in this order).

3. Methods

3.1. Cell Preparation

Following cell separation (*see* Chapter 00), human eosinophils are aliquoted on 12-well plates at 1×10^6/well in 0.5 mL RPMI-1640 + 10% fetal calf serum (FCS). These plates had been treated with FCS for 60 min, to coat the plates and prevent cellular adhesion. Cells are treated with stimuli and incubated at 37°C in O_2–CO_2 (95–5%). At the specified times, eosinophils are carefully pipeted into a 1-mL Eppendorf, the plates washed with an additional 0.5 mL RPMI-1640–FCS, and the cells pelleted by a 5-min spin at 18,000*g*. Cells are resuspended in 50 μL ice-cold Hank's balanced salt solution (HBSS) buffer is followed by 50 μL 2X lysis buffer (*see* **Note 1**), vortexed, and left to stand on ice for 20 min. The lysate is centrifuged at 18,000*g* at 4°C for 10 min, and the supernatant removed (the pellet is discarded). The supernatant is then boiled in 20 μL sample buffer ready for use in measuring ERK-1/2, JNK-46/54, or p38 MAPK. When using immunoprecipitation studies for measurement of other MAPK family members cells are initially resuspended in 250 μL HBSS buffer and 250 μL RIPA buffer (2X).

3.2. Measurement of ERK-1/2, JNK-46/54, and p38 MAPK Activation

The recent commercial availability of antibodies (Abs) (e.g., New England Biolabs, Santa Cruz, CA) that recognize the dual phosphorylation (tyrosine/threonine) and activated form of ERK-1/2, JNK-46/54, and p38 MAPK, means that this can be readily measured by Western blot analysis (*see* **Note 3**).

Samples are initially separated on a Bio-Rad mini-gel system (Bio-Rad) by SDS-polyacrylamide gel electrophoresis (SDS-PAGE). The gel is composed of a 10% resolving gel (bottom) and 3% stacking gel (top), and is made from the following solution (sufficient for two gels) using the manufacturers instructions (*see* **Subheading 2.3.**):

1. Resolving gel: acrylamide–*bis*-acrylamide solution (40:2%) (2.5 mL), distilled water (4.8 mL), 1.5 *M* Tris-HCl, pH 8.8 (2.5 mL), 10% SDS (100 μL), 10% APS (75 μL), *N',N',N',N'*-tetramethylethylenediamine (TEMED) (8 μL).
2. Stacking gel: acrylamide–*bis*-acrylamide solution (40:2%) (1 mL), distilled water (6.3 mL), 0.5 *M* Tris-HCl, pH 6.8 (2.5 mL), 10% SDS (100 μL), 10% APS (80 μL), TEMED (14 μL).
3. Following sample separation, proteins are transblotted (Bio-Rad Mini-Gel Transblotter) to nitrocellulose (Hybond-ECL, Amersham) for 2 h at 1000 mA in transblotting buffer.
4. The nitrocellulose is incubated for 1 h in TBS-T + 5% nonfat milk to block non-specific Ab binding, and incubated overnight in TBS-T containing 5% bovine serum albumin and the relevant phospho-Ab.
5. Membranes are washed with TBS-T (5 × 5 min), and incubated with either HRPO-linked antirabbit immunoglobulin G (IgG) (diluted 1:2000) or HRPO-linked antigoat IgG (diluted 1:1000) in TBS-T + 5% nonfat dry milk for 1 h at room temperature (RT).
6. The nitrocellulose is then washed in TBS-T (5 × 5 min) and antibody-labeled proteins are detected by enhanced chemiluminescence (ECL), using HyperFilm ECL (Amersham) (*see* **Fig. 1**). The intensity of the relevant bands is quantified by laser-scanning densitometry.

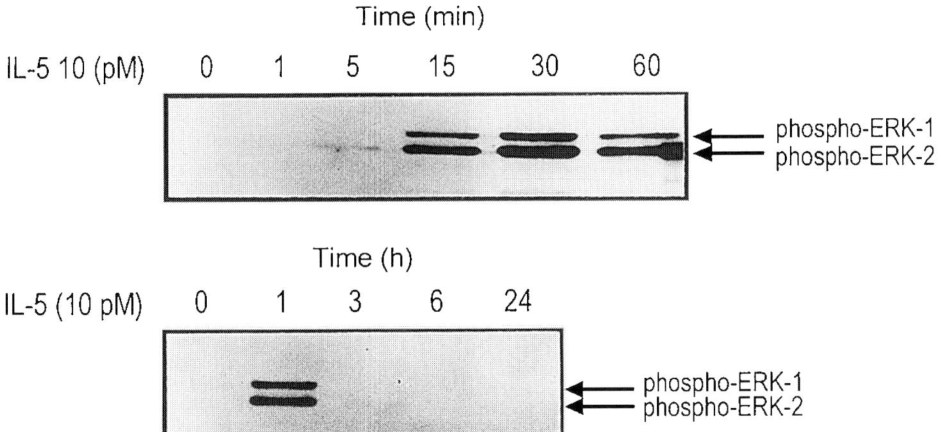

Fig. 1. Time-course of IL-5-induced (10 p*M*) ERK-1 and ERK-2 activation in human eosinophil, measured by immunoblotting with Abs raised to the dual phosphorylated enzyme (*see* **ref. *9***).

3.3. Measurement of MAPK Activity Using In-Gel Renaturation Assay

For those MAPKs that cannot be detected by Western blot analysis (i.e., ERK-3/4/5 and p38β/γ/δ), activation can be detected by immunoprecipitation of the individual enzyme and measurement of activity using an in-gel renaturation assay.

3.3.1. Immunoprecipitation

For immunoprecipitation, eosinophil samples were prepared as described in **Subheading 3.1.**, with the exception that the lysate supernatant was made up to 500 µL with lysis buffer (i.e., with 500 µL lysis buffer [1X]), and not boiled in Laemmli buffer. Immunoprecipitation was then performed as follows:

1. Samples are clarified by incubation (end-over-end) for 60 min at 4°C in the presence of 1 µg of a nonspecific control IgG Ab (i.e., if employing rabbit primary Ab for immunoprecipitation, use rabbit IgG) and 5 µL protein A/G-Plus agarose (Santa Cruz), pelleted by centrifugation (16,000*g* for 3 min), and the supernatant removed for **step 2**.
2. Supernatant is incubated overnight (end-over-end) at 4°C with 1 µg of the relevant MAPK Ab. Samples were then incubated for 120 min (end-over-end) at 4°C, following the addition of 20 µL protein A/G-Plus agarose.
3. Immunoprecipitated protein is then pelleted by centrifugation (18,000*g* for 3 min) (*see* **Note 3**) and washed 3× with 1 mL immunoprecipitation wash buffer (*see* **Subheading 3.2.**). Following the last wash, the pellet is resuspended in 100

μL immunprecipitation wash buffer, boiled with 20 μL Laemmli buffer, and stored at –20°C.

3.3.2. In-Gel Assay (Two Gels)

The in-gel renaturation assay initially involves the separation of immunoprecipitated sample upon a 10% SDS-PAGE, into which MBP, a substrate for ERK-3/4/5 and p38β/γ/δ, has been incorporated. The MAPKs are then renaturated and their activity determined by autoradiography, following the addition of a [^{32}P]ATP, which is incorporated into MBP. The details are as follows (please refer to **Subheading 2.4.** for preparation of stock buffers and reagents and ready-to-use buffers):

1. Gels are prepared as in **Subheading 3.2.** However, when making the resolving gel, add 400 μL MBP (MAPK substrate) to the resolving gel solution. Mix well, before addition of APS and TEMED.
2. Immunoprecipitated protein samples are then separated on SDS-PAGE.
3. Following electrophoresis, SDS is removed from gel with 3 × 20 min (50 mL per gel) washes at RT in buffer A (TSS + 20% [v/v] isopropanol).
4. Isopropanol is removed from gel with 3 × 20 min (50 mL/gel) washes at room temperature in buffer B (TSS + 5 m*M* 2-ME).
5. Gel protein is denatured with 2 × 30 min (50 mL/gel) washes at RT in buffer C (TSS + 5 m*M* 2-ME + 6 *M* guanidine-HCl). Remember, after each wash, to return the used denaturation buffer C to the stock bottle of DBS (*see* **Note 2**).
6. Gel protein is renatured with five washes (50 mL/gel) at RT in buffer D (TSS + 5 m*M* 2-ME + 0.04% Tween-40) as follows: 1 × 30 min, 2 × 60 min, overnight, 1 × 60 min.
7. Gels are then re-equilibrated with two washes (50 mL/gel) at RT in buffer E (RBS + 2 m*M* DTT).
8. In-gel kinase assay: For two gels, add 0.55 m*M* ATP (1 mL) and 200 μ*M* PKI (5 μL) to 10 mL KABS. Then add 25 μCi [^{32}P]ATP (>5000 Ci/mmol). Place the two gels in containers with flat surfaces, and gently layer assay solution on the gels, ensuring that the whole surface is covered. Leave for 3 h, returning occasionally to ensure that the gel surfaces are covered evenly.
9. Wash unlabeled [^{32}P]ATP from gels with nine washes (50 mL/gel) at 4°C with TCA wash solution, as follows: 3 × 5 min, 3 × 10 min, and, with rocking, 2 × 30 min, overnight, 1 × 60 min.
10. Place gels (face down) on cling film or Saran Wrap (Dow Chemical Co., Middlesex, UK), then lay Whatman blotting paper (Whatman, Kent, UK) on them. Dry gels using Savant (Stratech Scientific, Luton, UK) gel dryer, and expose to Kodak, Biomax-MS film (Amersham, Buckinghamshire, UK) (1–20 d at –70°C) to detect radiolabeled MBP (**Fig. 2**).

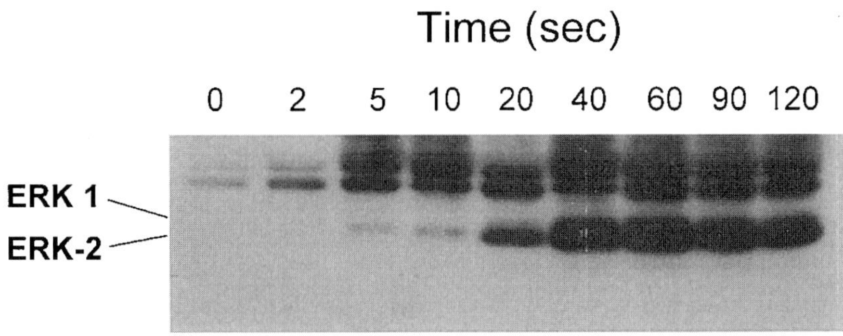

Fig. 2. Time-course of LTB_4-induced (1 μ*M*) ERK-1 and ERK-2 activity in guinea pig peritoneal eosinophils measured by in-gel renaturation assay (*see* **ref. *8***).

4. Notes

1. Prepare 150 mL of a 2.66X concentrated solution of RIPA buffer: Tris-HCl, pH 7.2 (0.48 g), NaCl (3.5 g), EDTA (149 mg), Triton X-100 (4 mL), sodium deoxycholate (2 g), SDS (0.4 g), and store at 4°C. Initially dissolve Tris-HCl and NaCl in 120 mL, then add, in order (waiting until each is dissolved, which can take from 5–30 min), sodium deoxycholate, EDTA, SDS, Triton X-100, and then pH solution to 7.4 with HCl.

   Prepare stock aliquots of the inhibitors, as follows (these may be stored for 4–6 mo):

   a. PMSF (34.8 mg/mL in isopropanol), store at 4°C (50-μL aliquots).
   b. Na_3VO_4 (36.8 mg/mL in H_2O), store at –20°C (50-μL aliquots).
   c. Leupeptin (4 mg/mL in H_2O), store at –20°C (50-μL aliquots).
   d. Aprotinin (10 mg/mL in H_2OHH), store at –20°C (50-μL aliquots).
   e. Pepstatin (4 mg/mL in methanol), store at –20°C (50-μL aliquots).
   f. NaF (4.2 mg/mL in H_2O), store at –20°C (0.5-mL aliquots).
   g. Sodium pyrophosphate (8.9 mg/mL in H_2O), store at –20°C (0.5-mL aliquots).

   Take 7.5 mL RIPA buffer (2.67X), add one aliquot of each inhibitor and then make up the volume to 10 mL (2X RIPA solution) or 20 mL (1X lysis solution) with ice-cold distilled water. PMSF may require a vigorous vortex to resuspend, and should be added just prior to lysis, because this compound is unstable in water.
2. 1000 mL DBS may be reused for up to 30 gels, only if the used buffer is returned to the stock bottle after each wash. Remember to keep a record of how many gels DBS has been used on.
3. Use Abs that recognize dual phosphorylation of both tyrosine and threonine, since Abs that detect tyrosine phosphorylation alone may not reflect enzyme activation. These antibodies can be obtained from an increasing number of companies, including New England Biologicals and Santa Cruz.

References

1. Widmann, C., Gibson, S., Jarpe, M. B., and Johnson, G. L. (1999) Mitogen-activated protein kinase: conservation of a three-kinase module from yeast to human. *Physiol. Rev.* **79,** 143–180.
2. Alam, R., Pazdrak, K., Stafford, S., and Forsythe, P. (1995) The interleukin-5/ receptor interaction activates Lyn and Jak2 tyrosine kinases and propagates signals via the Ras-Raf-1–MAP kinase and the Jak-STAT pathways in eosinophils. *Int. Arch. Allergy Immunol.* **107,** 226–227.
3. Pazdrak, K., Schreiber, D., Forsythe, P., Justement, L., and Alam, R. (1995) The intracellular signal transduction mechanism of interleukin 5 in eosinophils: the involvement of lyn tyrosine kinase and the Ras-Raf-1-MEK-microtubule-associated protein kinase pathway. *J. Exp. Med.* **181,** 1827–1834.
4. Bates, M. E., Bertics, P. J., and Busse, W. W. (1996) IL-5 activates a 45–kilodalton mitogen-activated protein (MAP) kinase and Jak-2 tyrosine kinase in human eosinophils. *J. Immunol.* **156,** 711–718.
5. Hiraguri, M., Miike, S., Sano, H., Kurasawa, K., Saito, Y., and Iwamoto, I. (1997) Granulocyte-macrophage colony-stimulating factor and IL-5 activate mitogen-activated protein kinase through Jak2 kinase and phosphatidylinositol 3-kinase in human eosinophils. *J. Allergy Clin. Immunol.* **100,** S45–51.
6. Coffer, P. J., Schweizer, R. C., Dubois, G. R., Maikoe, T., Lammers, J. W., and Koenderman, L. (1998) Analysis of signal transduction pathways in human eosinophils activated by chemoattractants and the T-helper 2-derived cytokines interleukin-4 and interleukin-5. *Blood* **91,** 2547–2557.
7. Pazdrak, K., Adachi, T., and Alam, R. (1997) Src homology 2 protein tyrosine phosphatase (SHPTP2)/Src homology 2 phosphatase 2 (SHP2) tyrosine phosphatase is a positive regulator of the interleukin 5 receptor signal transduction pathways leading to the prolongation of eosinophil survival. *J. Exp. Med.* **186,** 561–568.
8. Lindsay, M. A., Hadded, E.-L., Rousell, J., Teixiera, M. M., Hellewell, P. G., Barnes, P. J., and Giembycz, M. A. (1998) Role of mitogen-activated protein kinases and tyrosine kinases during leukotriene B_4 induced eosinophil activation. *J. Leuc. Biol.* **64,** 555–562.
9. Kankannranta, H., de Souza, P. M., Salmon, M., Barnes, P. J., Giembycz, M. A., and Lindsay, M. A. (1999) SB203580, an inhibitor of p38 mitogen-activated protein kinase, enhances constitutive apoptosis of cytokine deprived human eosinophils. *J. Pharmacol. Exp. Ther.* **290,** 621–628.

8

Human Eosinophil Isolation and the Measurement of Apoptosis

Hannu Kankaanranta, Patricia M. de Souza, Mark A. Giembycz, and Mark A. Lindsay

1. Introduction

Eosinophils have been implicated in allergic diseases, such as bronchial asthma, which is characterized by elevated eosinophil numbers in the bronchoalveolar lavage fluid and peripheral blood. Their accumulation and activation within the airway mucosa is thought to cause tissue injury, contraction of airway smooth muscle, and increased bronchial responsiveness ***(1–3)***. The balance between cell maturation and death is of great importance in determining the number of eosinophils in the blood and tissues ***(4–6)***. Following in vitro culture in the absence of cytokines, eosinophils undergo apoptosis, or programmed cell death ***(7,8)***, a process that can be inhibited by cytokines such as interleukin-3 and -5 and granulocyte-macrophage colony-stimulating factor (GM-CSF), and accelerated by such factors as corticosteroids and Fas ***(7–11)***.

Although eosinophils are believed to play a pivotal role in the development of a number of inflammatory lung diseases, until relatively recently, the study of human eosinophil biology has been fraught with methodological difficulties. A primary obstacle was obtaining cells in sufficient numbers and purity for detailed functional and biochemical experiment. Recently, the development of CD16-negative selection methodology, to isolate eosinophils ***(12)***, offered a solution to the problem of the purity of the eosinophil population. However, the number of cells isolated from human blood still remains a major obstacle in studying human eosinophil biology. The methods described below not only allow isolation of a pure eosinophil population, which are only present in low numbers in human peripheral blood, but they also enable the experimenter to

From: *Methods in Molecular Medicine, vol. 44: Asthma: Mechanisms and Protocols*
Edited by: K. F. Chung and I. Adcock © Humana Press Inc., Totowa, NJ

detect the critical hallmarks of cell death. In addition, these methods allow for the distinction between cells undergoing apoptosis or primary necrosis, as well as determination of the percentage of apoptotic cells in a given cell population.

Apoptosis is characterized by specific morphological and biochemical changes, including cell shrinkage, surface blebbing, chromatin condensation, and endonuclease-catalyzed DNA breakdown. This is then followed by fragmentation of the eosinophil into discrete apoptotic bodies, which are recognized and engulfed by phagocytic cells without inducing inflammatory reaction. Because the plasma membrane of the apoptotic cell remains relatively intact until the later phases of apoptosis (i.e., late apoptotic secondary necrosis), the cytotoxic cellular contents remain within the cell ***(13–15)***, thus averting induction of an immune response. This process is distinct from cell necrosis, which is characterized by cell lysis and the uncontrolled release of cellular contents, which may be harmful to surrounding tissues, and result in an inflammatory response.

Assessment of plasma membrane integrity/permeability serves as a starting point in determining whether the cells are dying via primary necrosis or apoptosis. When accompanied by more specific measurements of morphological changes and DNA fragmentation, conclusions concerning the mode of cell death can be drawn. However, assessment of apoptosis with only the classical DNA-laddering gel electrophoresis may lead to wrong conclusions, because DNA fragmentation may occur also during primary necrosis of DNA ***(15)***. The same applies to the flow cytometry (FCM) measurements of relative DNA content and other methods measuring DNA breakdown. Generally, to distinguish whether the cells die via apoptosis or primary necrosis, the use of at least three different methods that assess various aspects of cell death is recommended: measurement of membrane permeability and cell viability, assessment of the morphological changes, and biochemical changes.

2. Materials

2.1. Eosinophil Separation

1. Aqueous solution of 0.277 *M* D-glucose and 0.16 *M* $Na_2HC_6H_5O_7 \cdot 1.5H_2O$ (ACD) (may be prepared in larger quantities, filter sterilized, and stored in aliquots at –20°C).
2. 10% ACD: aqueous solution of 27.7 m*M* D-glucose, 16 m*M* ACD, and 154 m*M* NaCl (may be prepared in larger quantities, filter-sterilized, and stored in aliquots at –20°C).
3. Hydroxyethyl starch (60 mg/mL) solution ([HAES]-sterile Fresenius AG, Bad Hamburg, Germany).
4. Ficoll-Paque (Pharmacia Biotech, Uppsala, Sweden).
5. Hank's balanced salt solution (HBSS) without phenol red (Gibco-BRL, Paisley, UK).

6. RPMI-1640A (without phenol red and L-glutamine) (Gibco-BRL) with 5 m*M* ethylenediamine tetraacetic acid (EDTA) and 2% fetal calf serum (FCS).
7. RPMI-1640B (Dutch Modification; Gibco-BRL) with penicillin (50 IU/mL), streptomycin (50 μg/mL), L-glutamine (2 m*M*) and 10% FCS.
8. Magnetic cell sorting (MACS) CD16 magnetic microbeads (Miltenyi Biotech, Bergisch Gladbach, Germany).
9. VarioMACS magnetic cell separation system (Miltenyi Biotech).
10. CS negative selection columns (Miltenyi Biotech).
11. FCS (low endotoxin) (Gibco-BRL) (*see* **Note 1**).
12. Aqueous solution of 1.8% NaCl.

2.2. Flow Cytometry

1. Propidium iodide (PI) (Sigma, St. Louis, MO) in hypotonic solution: aqueous solution of 0.1% Triton X-100 (w/v), 3.8 m*M* ACD and 50 μg/mL PI, filter-sterilize (stable for some days in the dark at +4°C).
2. PI in isotonic solution: 1 mg/mL in HBSS.
3. Fluorescein diacetate (FDA) (Sigma): 1 mg/mL in acetone.

2.3. Light Microscopy

1. May-Grünwald solution (Sigma).
2. Giemsa solution (BDH, Poole, UK).
3. Xylene, methanol, and ethanol (Merck, Darmstadt, Germany).
4. Mountex (Histolab, Göteborg, Sweden).

2.4. DNA Fragmentation Assay

1. DNA extraction buffer: aqueous solution of 100 m*M* NaCl, 10 m*M* Tris-HCl. pH 8.0, 25 m*M* EDTA, 0.5% sodium dodecyl sulfate, and 0.2 mg/mL proteinase K.
2. Aqua Phenol (highly toxic; Appligene-Oncor, Durham, UK), chloroform (Merck), isoamyl alcohol (Sigma).
3. 7.5 *M* ammonium acetate.
4. Ethidium bromide (Sigma).
5. Agarose (Promega, Madison, WI).
6. Electrophoresis running buffer: aqueous solution of 40 m*M* Tris-base, pH 8.0, 1.1 m*M* glacial acetic acid, 1 m*M* EDTA, pH 8.0, and 0.5 mg/L ethidium bromide.
7. (TE)-buffer: aqueous solution of 10 m*M* Tris-HCl, pH 8.0, and 5 m*M* EDTA.
8. Orange G solution: aqueous solution of 8.8 m*M* Orange G, 1 mM EDTA, and glycerol (50%; v/v).

3. Methods

3.1. Eosinophil Isolation and Culture

The number of eosinophils isolated from human blood remains a limiting factor in studying human eosinophil biology. With the isolation method described subsequently, 1–10 × 10^6 eosinophils can be isolated from 50 mL human blood, with a purity of ≥99%. However, because the proportion of contaminating cells tends to increase along with the decreasing yield, it is inadvisable to continue the isolation process if the number of eosinophils in the first cell count is very low (<3–4 × 10^6). Moreover, only cell preparations of high purity should be used, because contaminating cells may secrete cytokines, which affect eosinophil survival.

1. Collect 50 mL blood into 10 mL ACD solution.
2. Gently add the blood–ACD mix (2 × 30 mL) to two 50-mL tubes containing 20 mL eloHAES and 5 mL 10% ACD, invert tubes to mix, and leave to stand at room temperature (RT) for 40–60 min, while red blood cells settle.
3. Remove supernatant with a Pasteur pipet (containing eosinophils and leucocytes) and centrifuge at 320*g* for 5 min to obtain a cell pellet.
4. Discard supernatant, resuspend pellet in 5 mL HBSS, and layer on 7 mL Ficoll-Paque. Centrifuge at 700*g* for 30 min at 20°C.
5. Carefully remove monocyte pellet (see **Note 2**), then resuspend, and wash phagocyte pellet twice with 50 mL ice-cold HBSS. Resuspend final pellet in 5 mL HBSS.
6. Lyse remaining red blood cells with 25 mL ice-cold distilled water for 30 s, then add 25 mL 1.8% NaCl solution. Centrifuge at 320*g* for 5 min at 4°C.
7. Wash twice with 50 mL ice-cold HBSS. Resuspend pellet in 2 mL ice-cold RPMI-1640A. Remove a small aliquot for cell count. Count the total number of cells, to determine how much CD16 conjugated magnetic microbeads is to be added to the cells. Wash remaining cells with 50 mL ice-cold RPMI-1640A solution. Then resuspend in 300 μL RPMI-1640A. Add CD16 magnetic microbeads (1 μL/2 × 10^6 cells), and incubate on ice for 40 min, with occasional shaking.
8. Prepare the CS-negative selection column by washing through twice with RPMI-1640A. Resuspend cell pellet in 6 mL RPMI-1640A, and add the suspension to top of the column. Flush sample through with 40 mL RPMI-1640A (*see* **Note 3**).
9. Centrifuge at 320*g* for 10 min. Wash sample in RPMI-1640B.
10. Resuspend the sample in 1 mL RPMI-1640B, and count the cells.

Eosinophils adhere to plastic surfaces, which may affect the survival of these cells. Therefore, plates are precoated with FCS to prevent eosinophil adhesion.

1. Coat the wells with FCS by adding 1.5 mL (for 12-well plate) and 200 μL FCS (for 96-well plate) for 60 min at 37°C. Remove FCS by washing twice with HBSS.
2. Suspend isolated eosinophils at 1–2 × 10^6/mL in RPMI-1640B. Add 100–200 μL/well to the 96-well plate (for measurements of viability and apoptosis by FCM or light microscopy) or 1–2 mL/well to the 12-well plates (for determination of DNA fragmentation by gel electrophoresis). The density of cells seeded in the 96 well plates must equal that of those seeded in 12-well plates, to ensure that results can be compared.

3. Incubate cells at 37°C with 5% CO_2 for the desired time.
4. At the desired time-point, detach the cells by mixing with pipet, and transfer to a centrifuge tube. For FCM and DNA fragmentation assays, centrifuge the cells down at 320*g* for 8 min at 4°C, and remove supernatant. For morphological analysis, cells may be used directly from the plates in their current medium.

3.2. Measurement of Cell Viability and Necrosis by FCM

A feature of viable, metabolically functioning cells is an intact plasma membrane. In contrast, when cells die, the cell membrane is disrupted, rendering the cell permeable to their external environments. Over the years, a number of dyes have been employed in the assessment of cell viability and necrosis, which include FDA and PI. FDA is a nonpolar, nonfluorescent fatty acid ester, which is able to penetrate viable cells through their intact plasma membranes. Once inside the cell, FDA can be hydrolyzed by esterases to produce free fluorescein, which is highly fluorescent. Because of its polar nature, fluorescein becomes trapped within the cell, emitting a green fluorescence, which can be detected by FCM.

On the other hand, PI is a charged dye that stains DNA. Since PI is unable to penetrate intact plasma membranes, it only stains the DNA of cells with disrupted cell membranes resulting from primary or secondary necrosis. Thus, incubation of cells with FDA and PI for short time periods permits the experimenter to assess cell viability and necrosis, because viable cells, possessing intact outer membranes, will exhibit green fluorescence resulting from fluorescein; dead cells with disrupted membranes display red fluorescence caused by PI staining of DNA. However, low cellular red fluorescence (usually indicative of viability) does not exclude apoptotic death, since DNA fragmentation leads to reduced DNA binding by PI (*see* **Subheading 3.3.**). Typical FCM patterns of cytokine-deprived and interleukin-5 treated eosinophils are shown in **Fig. 1**.

1. Prepare FCM apparatus (refer to your instruction manual for the general settings of your flow cytometer).
2. At the desired time-point, detach cultured cells from wells of 96-well plates, with pipet, transfer to fluorescence-activated cell sorter (FACS) tubes, and centrifuge the cells at 320*g* for 5 min. Resuspend the cell pellet in 250 μL HBSS. Prepare all the samples to be tested in this way, before proceeding to the next step.
3. Add 0.5 μL FDA solution to each tube, and incubate for 15 min at 37°C, then add 5 μL PI in isotonic solution. Incubate cells at RT for 5 min.
4. Register green fluorescence from fluorescein at 530 ± 20 nm and red fluorescence from PI at >630 nm (excitation at 488 nm of the argon ion laser). Usually, a compensatory adjustment, because of an overlap in green and red fluorescence, is needed (refer to your operating manual).

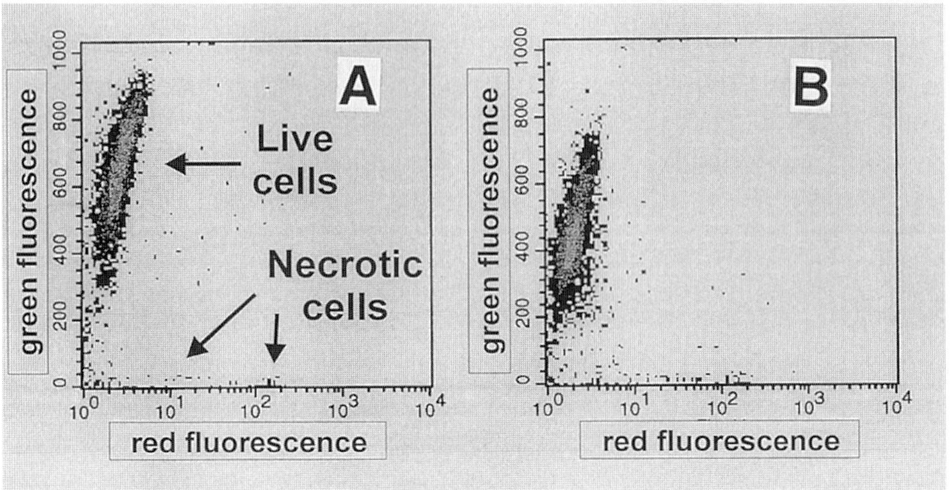

Fig. 1. Staining of eosinophils cultured with **(A)** and without **(B)** 10 p*M* IL-5 for 48 h with FDA and PI. Live cells show high green fluorescence, and necrotic cells show high red fluorescence. In B, the group of cells show lower green fluorescence than in A, and low red fluorescence probably reflects a population of apoptotic cells. However, this analysis can only be used to discriminate between live and necrotic cells, but not between apoptotic and nonapoptotic cells.

3.3. Measurement of Apoptosis by FCM

Apoptosis is characterized by DNA fragmentation following endonuclease nicking at the internucleosomal linker regions. As stated earlier, PI penetrates the perforated membranes of dead cells (PI is unable to enter live or apoptosing cells), where it intercalates into intact and, to a much lesser degree, fragmented DNA, to produce a red fluorescent signal. However, the addition of PI in a hypotonic solution containing detergent, allows the permeabilization of the membranes of apoptotic and viable cells. Because fragmented DNA is a feature of apoptotic cells, less DNA is stained, compared with viable cells.

The reduced DNA content of apoptotic nuclei results in a hypodiploid DNA peak, which can usually be discriminated from the narrow peak of cells with normal diploid DNA (G_0/G_1 peak) content in the red fluorescence channels ***(19)***. This method allows quantitative assessment of the degree of apoptosis in a given sample, and can be performed with relatively low numbers of cells. Results obtained by this method correlate well with the appearance of morphological characteristics of eosinophil apoptosis ($r = 0.95$; $P < 0.0001$) ***(16,17)***. To further validate the method, apoptosis of a pure eosinophil population in culture was measured twice over a period of 11–35 wk when between-day coefficient of variation of 8.1% was obtained ***(17)***.

Many authors uncritically consider all cells showing decreased relative DNA content as cells undergoing apoptosis. Generally, the mean fluorescence channel of apoptotic cells is considered to lie approximately one-half to one-third below the fluorescence channel of the peak of cells containing normal diploid DNA (**Fig. 1**; ***20***). However, the authors have observed that eosinophils appearing at a much lower fluorescence channel are late apoptotic eosinophils, which have lost most of their chromatin, and appear as ghosts by morphological analysis. Occasionally, morphologically apoptotic eosinophils may only appear at a slightly lower fluorescence than the nonapoptotic cells. It must be noted that assessment of apoptosis using PI in a hypotonic solution only allows the discrimination between apoptotic and nonapoptotic, and not between apoptotic and live or necrotic cells.

1. At the desired time, detach cultured cells from 96-well plates with pipet, transfer to a FC tube, and centrifuge at 320*g* for 5 min. Remove supernatant and resuspend the pellet in 200–400 µL of hypotonic PI solution.
2. Store the samples at +4°C in the dark, from 1 to 24 h before reading them by FACS.
3. Set up the FCM apparatus (refer to your instruction manual for the general settings of your flow cytometer).
4. Measure red fluorescence at >620 nm (excitation at 488 nm of the argon ion laser) to give the relative DNA content of the cells.
5. Analyze the number of cells showing decreased relative DNA content (apoptotic cells) and cells having normal diploid DNA content (considered as nonapoptotic cells), as shown in **Fig. 2** (*see* **Note 4**).

3.4. Morphological Determination of Apoptosis

Apoptosis was originally distinguished from necrosis on the basis of its ultrastructural changes. Electron microscopy still provides the most reliable method for recognizing these two death processes, although, with respect to eosinophils, apoptotic and necrotic cells can be also be identified using light microscopy. Another advantage of using morphological analysis for identifying cell death is the independent recognition of apoptosis and necrosis in situations in which these processes occur simultaneously ***(21)***. The earliest morphological feature of the onset of apoptosis is the condensation of chromatin. In eosinophils, it can be seen as disappearance of normal bilobular nucleus (**Fig. 3A**) and formation of intensely stained rounded nucleus (**Fig. 3B**). Other features include shrinkage of the cell and overall condensation of the cytoplasmic material. Membrane blebs may be formed, which finally leads to formation of apoptotic bodies of varying size and composition. Late apoptotic secondary necrotic cells (termed "ghosts") will appear as rounded and shrunken cells, possibly containing granules, although an intact nucleus may be absent (**Fig. 3C**). In contrast to apoptosis, primary necrotic cells will appear as swollen cells, typically having broken plasma membrane and bursting nucleus.

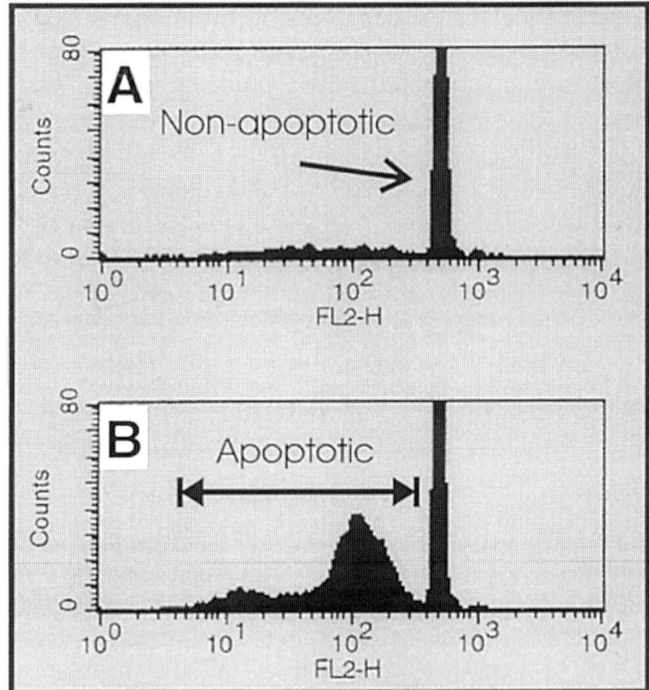

Fig. 2. Assessment of percentages of apoptotic (hypodiploid DNA content) and nonapoptotic (normal diploid DNA) cells in eosinophil cultures with **(B)** and without **(A)** 1 μ*M* dexamethasone. Apoptotic cells are seen as appearance of a hypodiploid peak at approx one-third of the fluorescence channel of that of G_0/G_1 peak of normal diploid cells.

1. At the desired time, detach cultured cells from 96-well plates with pipet, and transfer to the cytospin centrifuge chamber.
2. Centrifuge the cells, as recommended.
3. Air-dry the cytospin slides at RT for at least 30 min (samples must be run without any delay, because apoptosis is progressing while cells are in culture medium).
4. Fix the cytospin slides for 15 min in methanol, stain with routine May-Grünwald-Giemsa-staining, dehydrate, mount with DPX, and insert cover glass.
5. Analyze the cytospin slides by light microscopy with magnification of ×400–1000 for the appearance of normal, apoptotic, late apoptotic secondary necrotic, and primary necrotic cells.

3.5. DNA Fragmentation Assay by Agarose Gel Electrophoresis

The classical biochemical feature of apoptosis is the appearance of oligonucleosome-sized fragments of DNA. First, the genome is cleaved into large DNA fragments that vary from 300 to 50 kb in size, and finally into 180 bp

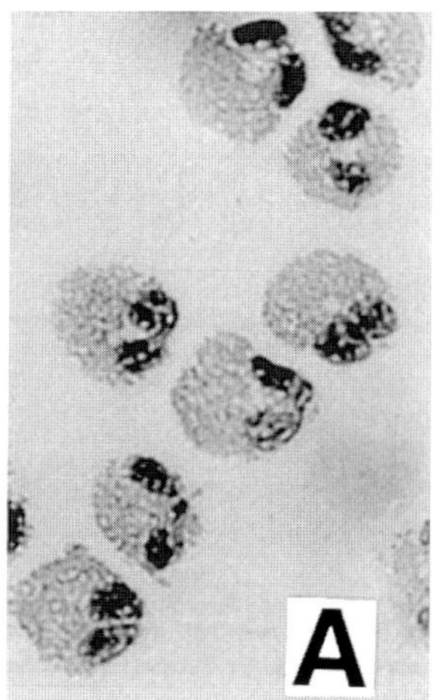

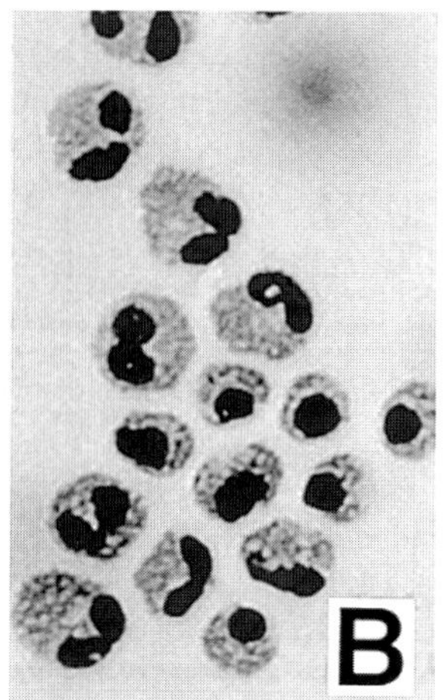

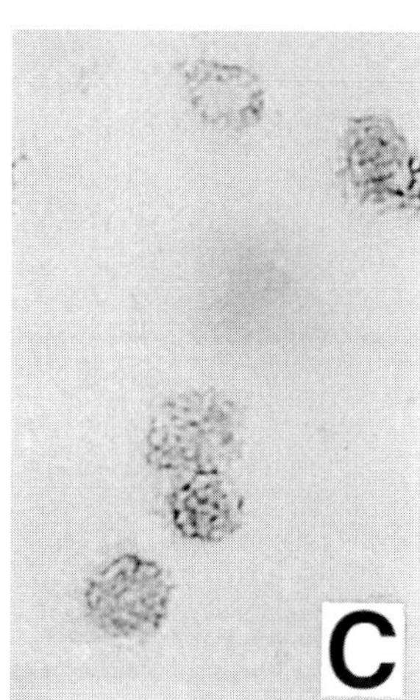

Fig. 3. **(A)** Freshly isolated eosinophils showing normal morphology. **(B)** Eosinophils cultured for 24 h, showing typical apoptotic morphology, such as chromatin condensation and cell shrinkage. **(C)** Eosinophils cultured for 48 h, showing typical morphology of late apoptotic secondary necrotic cells. Magnification ×400.

multiples. When run on agarose gel, they produce ladders, as shown in **Fig. 4**. Current scientific literature includes many cases in which DNA fragmentation (by agarose gel analysis) has been misinterpreted as a sign of apoptosis, because, in several forms of cell death, including necrosis, DNA becomes degraded at some point. DNA fragmentation during necrosis is random, and, indeed, forms a smear, on agarose gel analysis ***(15)***. Thus, to obtain evidence for the occurrence of apoptotic cell death, only results showing a clear ladder pattern should be accepted (**Fig. 4**). The 180-bp periodicity of the DNA fragments visible on agarose gels, together with typical morphological changes, is an indicator of apoptotic cell death ***(15–18)***.

1. Stop the incubation, at the desired time-point, by removing cells from the plate with a pipet, transfer cells to a centrifuge tube, and centrifuge at 320*g* for 8 min at 4°C. Carefully remove the supernatant, and add 0.5 mL of DNA-extraction buffer.
2. Incubate at +50°C for 12 h.
3. Extract once with 0.5 mL phenol:chloroform:isoamyl alcohol (25:24:1; v/v/v).
4. Extract twice with 0.5 mL chloroform:isoamyl alcohol (24:1; v/v).
5. Add 133 µL ammonium acetate to a final concentration of 2.5 *M* to precipitate the DNA and add 1.1 mL 100% ethanol. Vortex, and place tubes at –20°C for >2 h.
6. Pellet DNA by centrifugation (12,000*g* for 30 min) at RT.
7. Pour the supernatant off, add 0.5 mL ethanol:water (75:25; v/v), and repeat centrifugation.

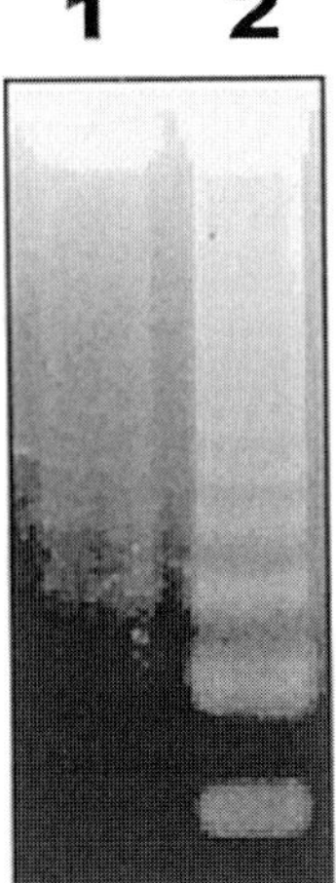

Fig. 4. Induction of apoptosis and DNA fragmentation by Fas antibody CH-11 in human eosinophils after culture for 18 h. **(A)** Cells cultured with control antibody (IgM); **(B)** with CH-11 (10 ng/mL). DNA was extracted and subjected to agarose gel electrophoresis.

8. Pour the supernatant off, and freeze-dry the sample for 2–4 min.
9. Dissolve DNA pellet in 30 μL TE buffer; take an aliquot for spectrophotometric readings at 260 nm and 280 nm. Add 3 μL Orange G solution per sample.
10. Load samples to agarose gel, and run at 25 V for 4–6 h.
11. Visualize the gel on a ultraviolet illuminator box, and observe the samples for the 180-bp multiples (**Fig. 4**).
12. The appearance of bands composed of approx 180-bp fragments, and its multimers (i.e., ladder formation), indicates that at least some of the cells in the population underwent apoptosis.

4. Notes

1. The authors recommend the use of FCS with very low endotoxin content (1 ng/mL) because endotoxin/lipopolysaccharide, at concentrations as low as 1 ng/mL, may affect eosinophil survival.
2. The mononuclear cells (MNCs) are found within the upper layer (at the interface between HBSS and Ficoll-Paque); the neutrophil/eosinophil are found within the pellet. It is essential to prevent contamination of the pellet with MNCs through the use of thin-tipped plastic pasteur pipets to remove the MNC layer and sterile cotton sticks to remove MNCs attached to the inner surface of centrifuge tubes.
3. Neutrophil contamination of the eosinophil preparation may result from a high column flow rate, and can be prevented by using a lower-bore needle (at the bottom of the CS column).

4. Eosinophils isolated from most healthy and asthmatic donors showed 20–50% apoptotic cell death after culture for 48 h. However, the authors were able to identify donors (most of whom were asthmatics) whose cells spontaneously survived in culture up to 4–5 d without any added cytokine ***(16,17)***.

References

1. Barnes, P. J. (1996) Pathophysiology of asthma. *Br. J. Clin. Pharmacol.* **42,** 3–10.
2. Seminario, M.-C. and Gleich, G. J. (1994) Role of eosinophils in the pathogenesis of asthma. *Curr. Opin. Immunol.* **6,** 860–864.
3. Desreumaux, P. and Capron, M. (1996) Eosinophils in allergic reactions. *Curr. Opin. Immunol.* **8,** 790–795.
4. Simon, H.-U. and Blaser, K. (1995) Inhibition of programmed eosinophil death: a key pathogenic event for eosinophilia? *Immunol. Today* **16,** 53–55.
5. Simon, H.-U., Yousefi, S., Schranz, C., Schapowal, A., Bachert, C., and Blaser, K. (1997) Direct demonstration of delayed eosinophil apoptosis as a mechanism causing tissue eosinophilia. *J. Immunol.* **158,** 3902–3908.
6. Walsh, G. M. (1997) Mechanisms of human eosinophil survival and apoptosis. *Clin. Exp. Allergy* **27,** 482–487.
7. Yamaguchi, Y., Suda, T., Ohta, S., Tominaga, K., Miura, Y., and Kasahara, T. (1991) Analysis of the survival of mature human eosinophils: interleukin-5 prevents apoptosis in mature human eosinophils. *Blood* **78,** 2542–2547.
8. Stern, M., Meagher, L., Savill, J., and Haslett, C. (1992) Apoptosis in human eosinophils. *J. Immunol.* **148,** 3543–3549.
9. Tai, P. C., Sun, L., and Spry, C. J. F. (1991) Effects of IL-5, granulocyte/macrophage colony-stimulating factor (GM-CSF) and IL-3 on the survival of human blood eosinophils in vitro. *Clin. Exp. Immunol.* **85,** 312–316.
10. Meagher, L. C., Cousin, J. M., Seckl, J. R., and Haslett, C. (1996) Opposing effects of glucocorticoids on the rate of apoptosis in neutrophilic and eosinophilic granulocytes. *J. Immunol.* **156,** 4422–4428.
11. Matsumoto, K., Schleimer, R. P., Saito, H., Iikura, Y., and Bocher, B. S. (1995) Induction of apoptosis in human eosinophils by anti-Fas antibody treatment in vitro. *Blood* **86,** 1437–1443.
12. Hansel, T. T., Pound, J. D., Pilling, D., Kitas, G. D., Salmon, M., Gentle, T. A., Lee, S. S., and Thompson, R. A. (1989) Purification of human blood eosinophils by negative selection using immunomagnetic beads. *J. Immunol. Methods* **122,** 97–103.
13. Anderson, G. P. (1996) Resolution of chronic inflammation by therapeutic induction of apoptosis. *Trends Pharmacol. Sci.* **17,** 438–442.
14. Darzynkiewicz, Z., Li, X., and Gong, J. (1994) Assays of cell viability: discrimination of cells dying by apoptosis in *Methods in Cell Biology,* vol. 41 (Darzynkiewicz, Z., Robinson, J. P., and Crissman, H. A., eds.), Academic, San Diego, pp. 15–79.
15. Ramachandra, S. and Studzinski, G. P. (1995) Morphological and biochemical criteria of apoptosis, in *Cell Growth and Apoptosis* (Studzinski, G. P., ed.), IRL, Oxford University Press, Oxford, UK, pp. 119–142.

16. Kankaanranta, H., De Souza, P. M., Salmon, M., Barnes, P. J., Giembycz, M. A., and Lindsay, M. A. (1999) SB 203**580,** an inhibitor of p38 mitogen-activated protein kinase, enhances constitutive apoptosis of cytokine-deprived human eosinophils. *J. Pharm. Exp. Ther.* **290,** 621–628.
17. Kankaanranta, H., Lindsay, M. A., Giembycz, M. A., Moilanen, E., and Barnes, P. J. (1999) Delayed eosinophil apoptosis in asthma. *J. Allergy Clin. Immunol.,* in press.
18. Gschwind, M. and Huber, G. (1997) Detection of apoptotic or necrotic death in neuronal cells by morphological, biochemical and molecular analysis in *Neuromethods, vol. 29: Apoptosis Techniques and Protocols* (Poirier, J., ed.), Humana, Totowa, NJ, pp. 13–31.
19. Nicoletti, I., Migliorati, G., Pagliacci, M. C., Grignani, F., and Riccardi, C. (1991) Rapid and simple method for measuring thymocyte apoptosis by propidium iodide staining and flow cytometry. *J. Immunol. Methods,* **139,** 271–279.
20. Fraker, P. J., King, L. E., Lill-Elghanian, D., and Telford, W. G. (1995) Quantification of apoptotic events in pure and heterogeneous populations of cells using the flow cytometer, in *Methods in Cell Biology,* vol. 46 (Schwartz, L. M. and Osborne, B. A., eds.), Academic, San Diego, pp. 57–76.
21. Kerr, J. F. R., Gobe, G. C., Winterford, C. M., and Harmon, B. V. (1995) Anatomical methods in cell death, in *Methods in Cell Biology,* vol. 46 (Schwartz, L. M. and Osborne, B. A., eds.), Academic, San Diego, pp. 1–27.

9

Adhesion of T-Cells to Airway Smooth Muscle Cells

Aili L. Lazaar and Reynold A. Panettieri, Jr.

1. Introduction

Cell adhesion molecules (CAMs) have been implicated in many cellular functions, including development, tumor metastasis, leukocyte activation, homing, and transendothelial migration, and can also serve as viral receptors. The role of CAMs on leukocytes and endothelial cells, and the interactions between these cell types, have been extensively characterized. The current model of leukocyte recruitment and homing involves the expression and activation of a cascade of CAMs, as well as the local production of chemoattractants, leading to leukocyte adhesion and transmigration into lymph nodes and sites of inflammation *(1)*. Most studies have focused on the mechanisms that control leukocyte adhesion and transendothelial migration, yet the subsequent interactions of infiltrating leukocytes with other cell types in the submucosa, and with the extracellular matrix, may also be important for sustaining the inflammatory response.

Integrins, which are expressed at high levels on the surface of leukocytes, normally exist in a low-affinity state. Integrin activation can be upregulated by a variety of factors, including divalent cations, cytokines, and phorbol esters *(2)*. Crosslinking of these cell surface receptors, such as CD3, CD44, or CD28, can also increase integrin function and subsequent lymphocyte adhesion. The rapid modulation of integrin affinity by T-cell receptor crosslinking or phorbol esters is transient, and probably results from both conformational changes within the molecule and interactions with the cytoskeleton. In contrast, intercellular adhesion molecules (ICAM-1) and vascular cell adhesion molecules (VCAM-1), members of the immunoglobulin gene superfamily, are constitutively avid. ICAM-1 and VCAM-1 are normally expressed at low levels on the cell surface, but can be induced on a wide variety of cell types by inflammatory mediators, such as cytokines or lipopolysaccharides *(2)*.

From: *Methods in Molecular Medicine, vol. 44: Asthma: Mechanisms and Protocols*
Edited by: K. F. Chung and I. Adcock

Lymphocyte infiltration is prominent in many diseases characterized by smooth muscle cell (SMC) hyperplasia, including asthma and atherosclerosis. T-cell adhesion to airway smooth muscle (ASM) via integrins and CD44 has been described by Lazaar et al. *(3)*. This interaction leads to increased expression of major histocompatibility complex class II and ICAM-1 on ASM *(4)*, as well as to induction of SMC DNA synthesis *(3)*. These findings suggest that T-cells, either by direct cell–cell contact or through secretion of cytokines, induce changes in gene expression and cell growth in the target cell, and can have profound effects on parenchymal cells in areas of inflammation.

ASM may be considered an important participant in the airway inflammatory response, because it can both synthesize cytokines and support adhesion of activated T-lymphocytes. Lymphocyte binding to ASM cells can have effects on both lymphocyte activation and function, as well as on SMC growth and reactivity. Further studies of the interaction between T-cells and ASM cells may provide insight into the mechanisms that induce bronchial inflammation and the airway remodeling seen in asthma.

The techniques that are commonly used to measure CAM expression and cell adhesion include the isolation of pure populations of ASM and/or T-lymphocytes, adhesion assays, and fluorescene-activated cell sorting (FACS) analysis. Details necessary to carry out these procedures are described below.

2. Materials

2.1. Cell Separation: T-Cells

1. Hank's balanced salt solution (HBBS) (Gibco-BRL, Grand Island, NY).
2. RPMI-1640 (Gibco).
3. Ficoll-Paque (Pharmacia, Uppsala, Sweden).
4. Neuraminidase (N-6514, Sigma, St. Louis, MO).
5. Sheep red blood cells (SRBCs) in Alsever's solution (Rockland, Gilbertsville, PA).
6. Lysis buffer: 16 m*M* NH_4Cl, 1 m*M* $KHCO_3$ (should be freshly prepared and sterile-filtered before use).
7. Antibody (Ab)-coated magnetic beads and magnetic particle concentrator for cell separation (Dynal, Lake Success, NY).

2.2. Cell Separation: ASM

1. Media 199 (Gibco).
2. Ham's F12 (Gibco).
3. Collagenase (Boehringer-Mannheim, Indianapolis, IN).
4. Soybean trypsin inhibitor (Sigma).
5. Elastase (Worthington Biochemical, Freehold, NJ).
6. Fetal calf serum (FCS) (Hyclone, Logan, UT).
7. 0.25% trypsin/1 m*M* ethylenediamine tetraacetic acid (EDTA) (Gibco).
8. Polypropylene mesh 125 μm (Spectrum, Houston, TX).

2.3. Cell Culture

1. T-cells: Complete RPMI contains RPMI-1640 supplemented with 10% heat-inactivated FCS, 2 m*M* glutamine, 100 U/mL penicillin, 100 μg/mL streptomycin, 100 μg/mL gentamicin, and 2.5 μg/mL amphotericin.

   Note: To heat-inactivate fetal calf serum (FCS), heat it at 56°C for 30 min. Shake well and sterile-filter. The serum should be stored at 4°C.
2. ASM: Complete Ham's F12 contains Ham's F12 supplemented with 10% FCS (not heat-inactivated), 2 m*M* glutamine, 25 m*M* HEPES, 12 m*M* NaOH, 1.5 m*M* $CaCl_2$, 100 U/mL penicillin, 100 μg/mL streptomycin.

2.4. Adhesion Assay

1. Phorbol 12,13-dibutyrate (PDBU) (Sigma).
2. Ionomycin (Sigma).
3. [^{3}H]-thymidine (Amersham, Arlington Heights, IL).
4. Blocking monoclonal antibodies (Abs) to CAMs (if desired).
5. 1% Triton X-100 in phosphate-buffered saline (PBS).

3. Methods

Adhesion of cells to ASM can be performed using a purified population of T-cells, or even a subset of T-cells (such as CD4$^+$). Ficoll density centrifugation is widely used to prepare peripheral blood mononuclear cell (PBMC) fractions. T-lymphocytes may be further purified by rosetting with SRBCs; subpopulations of T-cells can be obtained using magnetic bead separation.

3.1. Peripheral Blood Cell Fractionation

3.1.1. Ficoll Separation of Mononuclear Cells

This preparation can be scaled up or down, depending on the number of cells needed for a particular application. In general, a yield of approx 1–1.5 × 10^6 PBMCs/mL whole blood can be expected. Approximately 50% of these will be obtained as purified T-cells.

1. Draw 60 mL blood into heparinized syringes, and divide into two sterile 50-mL conical tubes. Fill the tubes with HBSS at room temperature (RT).
2. Layer 25 mL diluted blood onto 10 mL Ficoll-Paque, using a wide-bore pipet. Centrifuge for 30 min at 400*g* at RT, with no brake.
3. Carefully remove the interface between the Ficoll and the serum, which contains the mononuclear cell fraction, and transfer to a sterile 50-mL conical tube (the interfaces of two tubes can be pooled into one tube). Avoid aspirating the upper layer, because this can contaminate the prep with platelets.
4. Fill tubes with HBSS and centrifuge at 400*g*, 10 min, at RT.
5. Remove supernatant by aspiration, resuspend cells in HBSS, and repeat **steps 4** and **5** two additional times.

6. After the third wash, resuspend, and combine pellet in final volume of 5 mL RPMI. Determine the cell concentration using a hemocytometer or automated cell counter.

3.1.2. T-Cell Separation

1. Adjust the concentration of PBMC to 10–20 × 10^6 cells/mL using RPMI. Add an equal volume of neuraminidase-treated sheep red blood cells (N-SRBC, *see* **Subheading 3.1.3.**), and mix once by pipeting up and down. Divide the mixture evenly, so there is no more than 20 mL/tube. Allow the tubes to sit for 5 min at RT. Centrifuge at 400*g* for 10 min at RT, without brake. Place the tubes at 4°C for 1 h, being careful not to disturb the red cell pellet.
2. Add HBSS to a final volume of 30 mL, and gently resuspend the pellet, using a wide-bore pipet. Underlay with 12.5 mL Ficoll-Paque, and centrifuge 30 min at 400*g* at RT with no brake.
3. Remove everything, except the red cell pellet, by aspiration. To each tube, add 30 mL lysis buffer, and gently resuspend the red cell pellet, using a wide-bore pipet. The solution should go from an opaque to a dark clear red, indicating RBC lysis.
4. Centrifuge 400*g* for 10 min, at RT. Repeat washes two additional times.
5. After the final wash, resuspend and combine the pellets in 5 mL RPMI, and determine the cell number. These purified T-cells contain both CD4- and CD8-positive cells, and can be cultured at 2 × 10^6 cells/mL in complete RPMI media (*see* **Subheading 2.3.**). To purify T-cell subsets, refer to **Subheading 3.2.**

3.1.3. Neuraminidase-Treated SRBC

1. Divide 50 mL SRBCs into two sterile 50-mL conical tubes. Fill each tube with HBSS, and mix by inversion.
2. Centrifuge for 15 min at 830*g* at RT with no brake. Remove the supernatant by careful aspiration.
3. Resuspend the pellets, using a wide-bore pipet and repeat **step 2** twice.
4. After the third wash, resuspend, and combine the pellets in a final volume of 100 mL RPMI-1640 containing 100 U/mL penicillin and 100 μg/mL streptomycin. Transfer the cells to a sterile T-75 tissue culture flask. Add 1 U neuraminidase, parafilm the top, and place the flask in a shaking water bath at 37°C. Incubate in the shaking bath for 45 min.
5. Divide the cells into two sterile 50-mL conicals, and centrifuge as in **step 2**. Wash 3× with cold RPMI, as in **steps 2** and **3**.
6. After the final wash, resuspend and combine the pellets in a final volume of 100 mL RPMI containing penicillin, streptomycin, and 10% FBS. Store the N-SRBC at 4°C. Before use, gently resuspend the RBCs, using gentle aspiration with a wide-bore pipet. The N-SRBCs will keep for several weeks; however, if the supernatant begins to turn dark red, this indicates RBC lysis, and the cells should be discarded.

3.1.4. Purification of T-Cell Subsets

Purification of T-cell subsets is a valuable tool, and can be performed easily using magnetic beads coated with Ab, which binds to specific receptors on the cell surface. These cells can then be removed using a magnet. Removal of cells from a population is referred to as "negative selection."

1. Incubate the T-cells with Abs specific for the cell types that are to be removed. For example, if a population of purified $CD4^+$ cells is desired, incubate the T-cells with Abs to CD8 and CD56 (a natural killers cell marker, since there will be some contaminating natural killer cells in the E-rosetted T-cell fraction). The optimal concentration of Ab to use should be determined individually, but, generally, 10–20 μg/mL is adequate. Make sure all the Abs are from the same species (i.e., mouse antihuman). Incubate the cells, with gentle mixing, for 30 min at 4°C (*see* **Note 1**).
2. Wash the cells twice with cold RPMI, to remove unbound Ab, and resuspend in a small volume of RPMI.
3. To calculate the number of magnetic beads needed, estimate the number of $CD8^+$ and $CD56^+$ cells in the population (approx 40–50% of the total T-cell number), and use at least four beads per cell. The final reaction volume should have a concentration of at least 2×10^7 beads/mL. Wash the beads 5–6× with RPMI before using, because they are stored in azide.
4. Incubate the beads and cells in a sterile conical tube for 20 min on a nutator platform at 4°C.
5. Transfer cells to a 15-mL polypropylene tube, and place on the magnetic particle separator to remove the $CD8^+$ and $CD56^+$ cells, which should now be bound to the Ab-coated magnetic beads.
6. While the tube is still on the magnet, use a plugged Pasteur pipet to transfer the remaining unbound cells to a new tube. Wash these cells once in HBSS, determine the cell number, and culture in complete RPMI at 2×10^6 cells/mL.

3.2. Human ASM Cell Culture

Human ASM can be obtained from the trachea of lung transplant donors, from segments of bronchus resected for peripheral carcinoma, or from postmortem specimens (*see* **Note 2**).

1. The muscle is dissected free under sterile conditions, minced, centrifuged, and resuspended in 10 mL Media 199 containing 1.7 m*M* ethyleneglycol-*bis*-(β-aminoethylether)-*N,N,N',N'*-tetraacetic acid, 640 U/mL collagenase, 10 mg/mL soybean trypsin inhibitor, and 10 U/mL elastase. Digest the tissue for 30–60 min in a shaking water bath at 37°C.
2. Filter the cell suspension through the sterile mesh, and wash the filtrate in an equal volume of cold Ham's F12 containing 10% FBS. Plate the cell suspension in a six-well plate at a density of 1×10^4 cells/cm^2, in complete Ham's F12 *(see* **Subheading 2.3.**) plus 2.5 μg/mL amphotericin. Media should be replaced every 72 h.

3. To passage the cells, remove the media and add one-half vol trypsin–EDTA. Incubate the cells for 7 min at 37°C. Remove the cells using a pipet, and add to an equal volume of complete Ham's F12 media (*see* **Subheading 2.3.**). Determine the cell number, and replate at the required density.

   Cells isolated in this manner represent a pure population of SMCs. These cells stain uniformly for SMC-specific actin (*see* Chapter 5 for methods) and retain their responsiveness to contractile agonists, as has been described by Panettieri et al. ***(5)***. Ideally, cells should be used between the third and sixth passage, in order to retain these characteristics.

3.3. Adhesion Assay

Adhesion assays can be useful as an in vitro measure of cell–cell interactions under resting or inflammatory conditions. The use of blocking mAbs to cell adhesion or other molecules can further define the role of particular receptors in mediating this interaction.

1. Mitogen-activated T-cells can be prepared by stimulating T-cells with 5 ng/mL PDBU and 250 n*M* ionomycin for 36–42 h (*see* **Note 3**).
2. Radiolabel the T-cells with 2 μCi/mL ^{3}H-thymidine for the final 16 h of incubation (*see* **Note 4**). Prior to use in the assay, wash the T-cells once with RPMI, to remove the unincorporated thymidine. Determine the cell number, because there will be cell death during the activation process.
3. SMCs are grown in 24-well tissue culture dishes in 1 mL of media. Confluent cells should be treated with inflammatory mediators for 24 h prior to the assay (though the cells can be stimulated for longer or shorter periods, as desired).
4. T-cells and/or ASM cells can be pretreated with blocking mAbs for 30 min at 4°C prior to performing the adhesion assay. Abs should not be washed out.
5. Add 6×10^5 T-cells/well and allow them to adhere for 1 h at 37°C. Each condition should be performed in triplicate. Nonadherent cells are removed by gentle washing 6× with warmed media. After removing the media, adherent cells are lysed by adding 300 μL 1% Triton X-100 in PBS to each well. Pipet up and down several times to ensure cell lysis.
6. Transfer the contents of each well to a scintillation vial and quantitate counts (*see* **Note 5**). Be sure to include a vial containing the same volume of cells (also lysed in 1% Triton) that was originally added to each well (input cells). Percent binding is calculated as counts recovered from adherent cells/total input counts × 100 (**Fig. 1**).

3.4. Fluorescence Activated Cell Sorting

FACS analysis is a powerful and relatively simple method for measuring the expression of cell surface receptors or intracellular proteins. FACS analysis can be used to determine the effects of inflammatory stimuli (such as cyto-

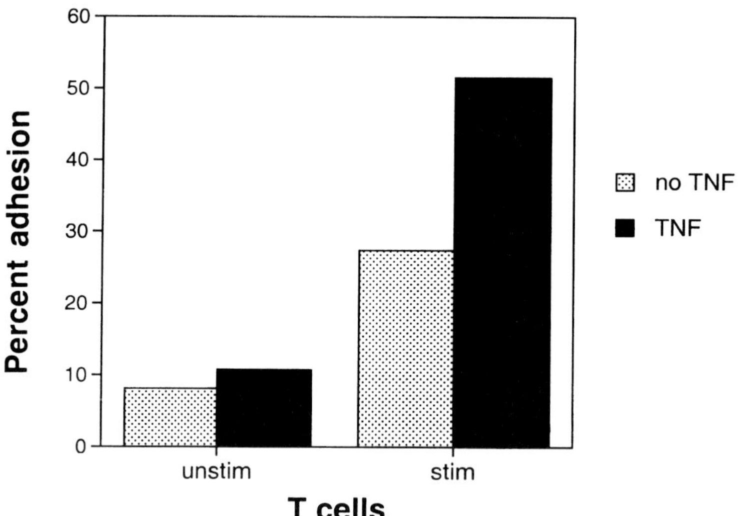

Fig. 1. Schematic illustration of T-cell adhesion to ASM. T-cells were either unstimulated (unstim) or were activated with PDBU and ionomycin (stim). ASM cells were incubated in control media (speckled bars) or in the presence of tumor necrosis factor-α (TNF-α) (gray bars) for 24 h.

kines) on SMC phenotype, including CAMs, growth factor receptors, and intracellular cytokines (**Fig. 2**). By gating on specific-sized cells, FACS can also be used to analyze mixed cell populations, such as T-cell-SMC cocultures.

The methods necessary for performing FACS analysis are detailed in Chapters 6 and 15, and can be applied to SMCs as well as to T-lymphocytes. The primary and secondary Abs used for detection will be determined by the receptor or protein of interest (*see* **Note 6**).

4. Notes

1. The beads referred to in this protocol are coated with secondary antibody (e.g., goat antimouse immunoglobulin G). Anti-CD8 and anti-CD4 Abs directly conjugated to magnetic beads are also available. This can simplify the procedure from two steps to one.
2. Bronchial SMCs are available commercially; however, these cells are highly passaged, and, therefore, may not retain all the characteristics of freshly isolated cells.
3. In this assay, T-cells are activated by mitogen. A more physiologic method of activation would involve plating the T-cells, in the presence of MAbs to CD28 on plates that had been previously coated with anti-CD3 (T-cell receptor) antibodies. The combination of immobilized CD3 with soluble CD28 more closely mimics in vivo T-cell activation.

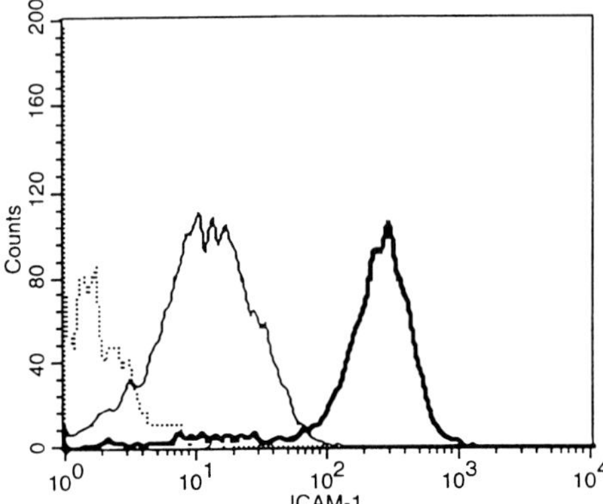

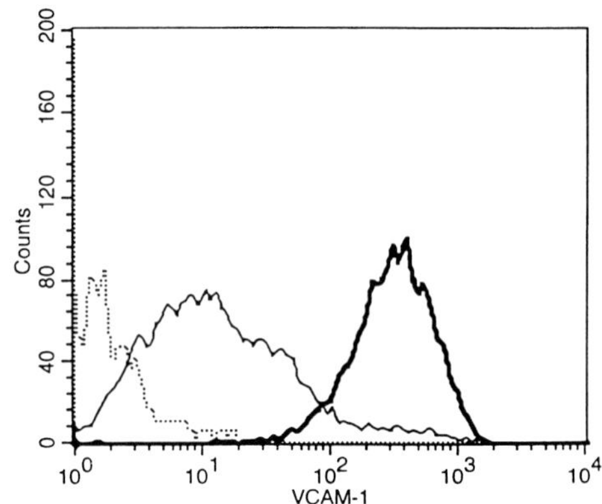

Fig. 2. FACS plot demonstrating the induction of ICAM-1 and VCAM-1 on ASM by TNF-α. Cells were stained with a control Ab (dotted line) or with Abs specific for ICAM-1 (left) or VCAM-1 (right), after being incubated in control media (thin line) or in the presence of TNF-α (thick line) for 24 h.

4. Alternately, cells can be labeled with ^{51}chromium for 1–2 h *(6)*.
5. The method outlined above utilizes radiolabeled cells. As an alternative, nonradioactive approach, cells could be labeled with a fluorescent dye *(7)*, and adherent cells then measured in a fluorimeter. Additionally, one could count the actual number of cells in a given number of high-power fields, and express the data as a percentage of number of cells added *(8)*.
6. Because ASM cells are adherent, it is necessary to remove them from the plate prior to staining for FACS. Usually, cells are removed using trypsin–EDTA; however, trypsin can cleave certain cell surface receptors, such as ICAM-1 (although this is more of a problem with murine, rather than human, cells). If there is a concern regarding the stability of the receptor in the presence of trypsin, ASM cells can be lifted by incubating them in 5 m*M* EDTA in calcium/magnesium-free PBS for 10 min at 37°C.

References

1. Dustin, M. L. and Springer, T. A. (1991) Role of lymphocyte adhesion receptors in transient interactions and cell locomotion. *Annu. Rev. Immunol.* **9,** 27–66.
2. Springer, T. A. (1990) Adhesion receptors of the immune system *Nature* **346,** 425–434.
3. Lazaar, A. L., Albelda, S. M., Pilewski, J. M., Brennan, B., Puré, E., and Panettieri, R. A. (1994) T-lymphocytes adhere to airway smooth muscle via integrins and CD44 and induce smooth muscle cell DNA synthesis. *J. Exp. Med.* **180,** 807–815.
4. Lazaar, A. L., Rietz, H. E., Panettieri, R. A., Peters, S. P., and Puré, E. (1997) Antigen receptor-stimulated peripheral blood and bronchoalveolar lavage-derived T-cells induce MHC class II and ICAM-1 expression on human airway smooth muscle. *Am. J. Resp. Cell Mol. Biol.* **16,** 38–45.

5. Panettieri, R. A., DePalo, L. R., Murray, R. K., Yadvish, P. A., and Kotlikoff, M. I. (1989) A human airway smooth muscle cell line that retains physiological responsiveness. *Am. J. Physiol. Cell* **256,** C329–C335.
6. Dustin, M. L., Singer, K. H., Tuck, D. T., and Springer, T. A. (1988) Adhesion of T-lymphoblasts to epidermal keratinocytes is regulated by interferon γ and is mediated by intercellular adhesion molecule 1 (ICAM-1). *J. Exp. Med.* **167,** 1323–1340.
7. Brenan, M. and Parish, C. R. (1984) Intracellular fluorescent labeling of cells for analysis of lymphocyte migration. *J. Immunol. Methods* **74,** 31–38.
8. Piela-Smith, T. H., Aneiro L., and Korn, J. H. (1991) Binding of human rhinovirus and T cells to intercellular adhesion molecule-1 on human fibroblasts. *J. Immunol.* **147,** 1831–1836.

10

Proliferation of Circulating T-Lymphocytes

Mark Larché

1. Introduction

Together with B-lymphocytes, T-lymphocytes (or T-cells) comprise the antigen (Ag)-specific arm of the immune response. The Ag receptors of both cell types are generated by recombination of multiple gene segments *(1)*, giving rise to a large repertoire of receptors of differing specificity. When a lymphocyte encounters Ag, cellular activation occurs via aggregation of cell surface Ag receptors *(2)*. The consequences of activation are numerous, but, in the case of the T-cell, include clonal expansion, via proliferation, and also secretion of soluble mediators and growth factors, such as interleukin-2 (for a review of the role of the T-lymphocyte in allergic disease, *see* **ref.** ***3***).

Proliferation and mediator release can be used as surrogate markers of T-cell activation, and in this sense may be useful in determining whether T-cells are being activated by a given stimulus (i.e., a qualitative outcome), and also the extent of the activation (i.e., a quantitative outcome). This chapter focuses on measurement of proliferation in cultures of circulating T-cells, although the principles and methods may be easily extended to the investigation of other T-cell populations, or other cell types.

In order to accurately assess proliferative responses, a number of considerations need to be taken into account, which will allow optimization of the assay system prior to its use in the laboratory. In general, the investigator will wish to examine the proliferative response of T-cells to an external stimulus, such as an Ag or a growth factor. Many variables, such as cell number, Ag or growth factor concentration, and duration of assay, will require definition. These parameters may be defined by simple titration of reagents and time-course studies. Thus, the first steps in designing an assay will be to initiate a number of cul-

From: *Methods in Molecular Medicine, vol. 44: Asthma: Mechanisms and Protocols*
Edited by: K. F. Chung and I. Adcock © Humana Press Inc., Totowa, NJ

tures in which, for example, Ag concentration is varied in order to obtain an optimal value. Additionally, the length of culture required to give optimal measurement of proliferation will be determined (*see* **Note 1**) by establishing several cultures, using a fixed Ag concentration, which are harvested and evaluated on a series of successive days. The optimal cell numbers in each culture well will require similar analysis, in order to produce an assay that is as sensitive as possible.

In addition to identifying and defining these relatively crude parameters, the investigator will do well to consider some of the finer points of T-cell biology, when designing an assay. The repertoire of T-cell receptors is extensive, and the circulating T-cell pool contains a vast number of differing T-cell specificities. What this means in real terms is that the frequency of T-cells, with receptors specific for a single Ag, will be small, compared to the whole pool. The frequency of T-cell receptor specificities is related to an individual's exposure to the stimulating Ag, because frequent encounter will stimulate clonal expansion and give rise to a relatively high T-cell frequency *(4)*. Cell frequencies can vary enormously, e.g., from one cell in 1000 (very high frequency) to one cell in one-half million (low frequency). If the investigator is looking for a response to a protein that has never been encountered by the immune system, detecting a T-cell proliferative response will be difficult, if not impossible, since the assay system is unlikely to be able to detect activation of only one cell in one-half million. For this reason, T-cell proliferation assays are usually carried out with Ags that have been previously encountered, so-called "recall Ags." A good example of a recall Ag is purified protein derivative of *Mycobacterium tuberculosis* in populations immunized with the bacille Calmette-Guérin vaccine.

Expanding this point further, within a given protein Ag, there may be more than one T-cell epitope. The exact number will depend on both the size of the protein and the major histocompatibility complex (MHC) molecules expressed by the individual being assayed. The latter are polymorphic cell surface molecules, which comprise an individual's tissue type for the purposes of transplantation. These molecules bind small peptides derived from whole-protein Abs and it is the combination of MHC molecule and bound peptide that is recognized by the T-cell receptor, leading to activation ***(5,6)***. Thus, a single protein may have 20 possible peptide epitopes, but, because of the differing pattern of MHC molecules expressed by different people, one person may only recognize one epitope, but another individual may be able to recognize five. This gives rise to the concept of high and low responders. A person capable of recognizing five epitopes of a protein is likely to have a higher overall frequency of T-cells capable of responding to the whole protein than a person only capable of recognizing one epitope.

In some experimental systems, the investigator will wish to assay the ability of T-cell populations to respond to individual peptide epitopes. In this case, it must be noted that the absolute frequency of T-cells is likely to be very low, and the assay must, therefore, be tailored to detect small responses from infrequent cells. Simple practical issues must be addressed, although, in the author's experience, this is the area most frequently ignored by researchers, leading to poor quality and frequently misleading results. The point can be illustrated with a simple example:

A protein (or peptide) is expected to stimulate a relatively low frequency of T-cells because it carries few T-cell epitopes, and is not encountered frequently. The hypothetical frequency of T-cells capable of responding to this protein is one in 200,000 (2×10^5) cells. Circulating T-cells are usually assayed as part of a peripheral blood mononuclear cell (PBMC) population, of which they form the majority. In an average assay, each culture well of a 96-well plate will contain $1–2 \times 10^5$ cells. There is, therefore, a good chance that some of the culture wells will not contain a single cell capable of responding to the stimulus. In this situation, no statistically significant responses will be detected between cells cultured with no stimulus vs those with, unless a sufficiently large number of culture wells are established. For low-frequency responses, this may need to be 10–20 wells or more. Thus, when examining a primary (i.e., directly ex vivo) T-cell response (in PBMC), it is important to consider the number of cells being assayed, compared to the frequency of responding cells. Twenty wells, each containing 2×10^5 cells, gives a total of 4 million cells. Even with this many cells, it may not be easy "to see the wood for the trees".

The same sorts of problems are less likely to be encountered in situations in which the natural frequency of responding cells is high, or in situations in which the responding cells have been enriched. This usually involves expanding Ag-specific cells during a prior culture period. The resultant cultures are referred to as secondary cultures, as opposed to the primary ex vivo culture. Clearly, because secondary cultures have a higher frequency of responding cells, fewer culture wells will be required to detect statistically significant responses. Additionally, the cells will, to some extent, be synchronized in their activation cycle, and thus variation in the responses between wells cultured under the same conditions will be smaller, reducing the standard deviation (SD) between wells, and leading to greater statistical validity at lower well number. In this situation, it is frequently sufficient to analyze triplicate wells (i.e., three wells in a 96-well plate cultured under the same conditions), since the mean response ± 3 SD will be significantly different from the background control cultures of cells without Ag. Bearing these issues in mind, the following methodology deals with establishing the optimized assay conditions, using the assay and measuring responses.

2. Materials

2.1. Isolation of PBMCs

1. Preservative-free heparin (Leo Laboratories, Bucks, UK).
2. Histopaque (Sigma, Poole, Dorset, UK).
3. Heparinized culture medium: RPMI-1640 L-glutamine-free (*see* **Note 2**), HEPES-buffered, supplemented with 2 m*M* L-glutamine, 100 U/mL penicillin, 100 µg/mL streptomycin (all Sigma), and 10 U/mL preservative-free heparin (Leo).
4. Complete culture medium (*see* **Note 3**): RPMI-1640 L-glutamine-free, bicarbonate-buffered, supplemented with 2 m*M* L-glutamine, 100 U/mL penicillin, 100 µg/mL streptomycin, and 5% normal human AB serum (all Sigma).
5. Serological sterile, plastic pipets: 10 mL and 25 mL (Greiner Laboratories, Stonehouse, Glos., UK).
6. 50-mL Cellstar polycarbonate tubes (Greiner).
7. Sterile, individually wrapped 3 mL pastettes (Greiner).
8. Trypan blue (0.4%) solution in saline (Sigma).

2.2. Proliferation Assays

1. Complete culture medium; RPMI-1640 L-glutamine free, bicarbonate-buffered, supplemented with 2 m*M* L-glutamine, 100 U/mL penicillin, 100 µg/mL streptomycin, and 5% normal human AB serum (all Sigma).
2. Serological sterile, plastic pipets 10 mL and 25 mL (Greiner).
3. Repeater pipet (Eppendorf; through BDH, UK).
4. Repeater pipet tips (Ritips, Greiner).
5. 96-well flat-bottomed (*see* **Note 4**) culture plates (Nalge Nunc International; through Life Technologies, Paisley, Scotland).
6. Ag stock solution at a concentration of 1–10 mg/mL.
7. Tritiated [methyl-^{3}H]-thymidine, sterilized aqueous solution: 925 GBq/mmol (stock solution; Amersham International, Amersham, Bucks, UK). Diluted 1:20 in complete culture medium (working solution).
8. 37°C cell culture incubator gassed with 5% CO_2 in air (e.g., from manufacturers such as Gallenkamp and Lec).
9. Culture harvesting equipment (e.g., Unifilter-96 harvester, Canberra Packard, Pangbourne, Berks., UK).
10. Liquid scintillation counter (for example, TopCount Microplate Scintillation Counter, Canberra Packard).

3. Methods

3.1. Isolation of PBMCs

Many methods have been developed for the convenient separation of circulating T-cells from whole blood, including nylon (glass) wool purification, rosetting with sheep red blood cells (SRBCs), and a variety of methods taking advantage of different buoyant densities among blood cells. More recently, T-cell purification columns have become available (for example, from R&D Systems), which are easy to use and give reproducibly good results. They are, however, expensive, and need not be used for general purposes The use of nylon wool columns is cumbersome, shows variability in terms of purity and yield, and is now mostly passé. Rosetting with SRBCs, although one of the most specific methods for purification of T-cells (rather than lymphocytes *per se*), is also rarely used today. This at least partially results from the fact that the T-cell surface molecule, which acts as a receptor for SRBCs is CD2, a molecule intimately involved in T-cell activation *(7)*. It has been suggested that purification in this fashion may disturb the T-cell population, giving rise to inappropriate activation profiles. Currently, the method of choice for the isolation of PBMC populations is density gradient centrifugation, with products such as Histopaque (Sigma) and Ficoll-paque (Pharmacia). These solutions are mostly carbohydrate-based, and have a density of 1.077 g/L, which allows monocytes, lymphocytes, and basophils to remain at the blood–media interface, while other blood cells pass through to form a pellet. A variable number of platelets may be retained at the interface, along with the mononuclear cells, and it is for this reason that heparinized medium is recommended for initial washing steps, in order to avoid mononuclear cell clumping.

1. Whole peripheral blood is collected into either a heparinized syringe or into a tube containing heparin (final concentration of heparin should be 20 U/mL).
2. Using a wide-bore (i.e., 25 mL) pipet, blood is slowly layered onto an equal quantity (*see* **Note 5**) of Histopaque (at room temperature), taking care not to disturb the interface between the two liquids. Tilting the tube and passing blood slowly down the side of the tube is advisable.
3. Tubes are centrifuged at 700*g* (with the brake in the "off" position) for 20 min at room temperature.
4. Cells at the interface between the separation medium and plasma are collected using a 3 mL pastette. They interface cells form a thin white layer, which can be difficult to see. The pastette bulb should be emptied of air before passing into the solution, in order not to disturb the integrity of the interface. Cells are collected into a tube, together with a mixture of plasma and separation medium. Care should be taken to ensure that all cells are collected, and that not too much of the separation medium is taken up. The latter, by virtue of its density, may make subsequent washing of the cells by centrifugation difficult.
5. Heparinized culture medium is added in at least equal volume to the cell suspension. Close the tube and invert several times to ensure adequate mixing. Centrifuge the suspension at 500*g* for 10 min with the brake on.
6. Discard the supernatant, and resuspend the cell pellet by briskly and firmly tapping the bottom of the tube. Refill the tube with heparinized medium, and add

plasma (*see* **Note 6**) to approx 10% final concentration. Centrifuge the suspension at 300*g* for 10 min with the brake on.

7. Resuspend the cell pellet as before. Bring the volume in the tube up to 10 mL with complete culture medium. Mix gently, and remove 10 µL, using a sterile pipet tip. Mix the 10 µL with 90 µL trypan blue solution, and load a Neubauer (or similar) haemocytometer. Count cells and calculate both cell concentration in the solution and also the total number of cells recovered.
8. If not used immediately, cell suspensions should be stored on ice prior to use in the proliferation assay.

3.2. Proliferation Assays

3.2.1. Determination of Optimum Ag Dose

Proliferation assays should be meticulously planned prior to execution. Component solutions should be prepared at concentrations that take into account subsequent dilution by the addition of other reagents. For example, in the dose-determination experiment described below, the assay includes two component solutions that are added to wells in equal volume (100 µL). As a result, the final concentration of each solution is halved. For this reason, particularly with more complex experiments, it is important to consider the number of solutions being included in the assay and their ultimate concentration therein. For an experiment with two solutions (such as cell suspension and Ag solution), each must be added to the well at twice the required final concentration. Similarly, if three or four components are required, quadruple strength solutions will be required. In the author's experience, a three-component assay is best treated as four, with the fourth solution being culture medium. Such an approach will allow stock solutions to be prepared and stored at convenient concentrations. It is rare that an experiment will have more than four component parts, but, in such a case, solutions of higher concentration can be prepared in a similar fashion.

In addition to preparation of solutions, the layout of the experiment should be decided, recorded in the investigator's notebook, and finally, drawn onto the lid of the 96-well plate, to be used for the assay. The number of wells employed for each culture condition should be decided bearing the earlier considerations in mind. For the example described below, the Ag being titrated to determine optimal dose will be the house dust mite Ag Der p 1 (from *Dermatophagoides pteronyssinus*). This is a recall Ag, because the whole population are exposed on a daily basis. From this one can assume that the frequency of responding T-cells will be relatively high, and thus demonstrable, using a relatively small number of culture wells per Ag dilution. For the purposes of the example, six replicate wells will be used at each Ag concentration. For convenience, a plate plan for the experiment is given in **Table 1**.

Table 1
Plate Plan for Determination of Ag Dose

	Wells 1–6	Wells 7–12
A	Cells with medium alone	Cells with Ag at 0.01 µg/mL
B	Cells with Ag at 0.03 µg/mL	Cells with Ag at 0.1 µg/mL
C	Cells with Ag at 0.3 µg/mL	Cells with Ag at 1.0 µg/mL
D	Cells with Ag at 3.0 µg/mL	Cells with Ag at 10 µg/mL
E	Cells with Ag at 30 µg/mL	Cells with Ag at 100 µg/mL
F		
G		
H		

1. Adjust cell suspension to 2×10^6 mL, and dispense 100 µL into the selected wells on the plate. The procedure can be carried out rapidly and with relative accuracy, using a repeater pipet.
2. Calculate the total quantity of each Ag dilution required, allowing enough solution for subsequent dilutions in the series, and also for wastage and loss in pipeting (approx 5% extra is reasonable for this purpose). Prepare the dilution series as described in **Note 7**.
3. Dispense the Ag solutions with a repeater pipet. The same pipet tip may be used for all solutions, but, if this is to be the case, the solution of lowest concentration should be dispensed first, and so on. Care must be taken to avoid cross-contamination of wells caused by splashing.
4. Incubate the plate for 6 d in the first instance, or, for a time-course study, prepare several identical plates, and incubate for differing periods, such as 4, 5, 6, 7, 8, and 9 d.
5. Between 8 and 16 h before the end of the prescribed culture period, add approx 37 kBq (1 µCi) of tritiated thymidine per well (*see* **Note 8**).
6. Harvest the contents of each well onto a suitable surface, following the manufacturer's instructions.
7. Count the incorporated radioactive label, using a scintillation counter according to the manufacturer's instructions.
8. Determine the mean and SD (or standard error) for each Ag concentration, and plot these values on the y-axis against Ag concentration on the x-axis. An example of a typical dose response curve is shown in **Fig. 1**.

Determination of the optimal cell concentration for use in the assay should also be carried out. High cell concentrations in an assay may favor cytokine production at the expense of the proliferative response. Plates should be prepared so that Ag dose remains constant between plates; cell concentration varies from plate to plate. A suitable range of cell concentrations would be 0.5, 1, 2, 3, 4, and 5×10^6/mL.

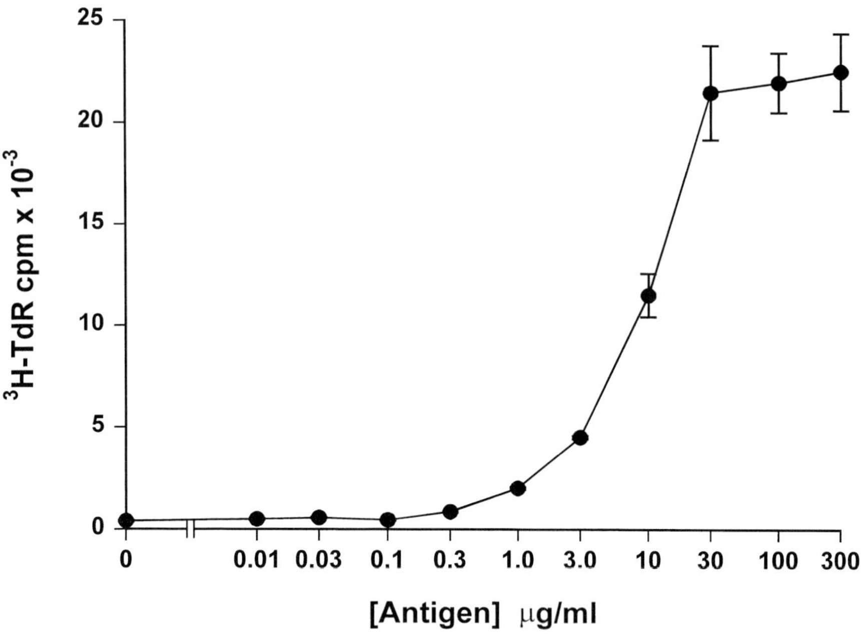

Fig. 1. Dose-response curve of hypothetical Ag. PBMCs are cultured for 7 d in the presence of medium alone or a range of Ag doses to determine optimal Ag concentration for subsequent assays.

3.3. Assay Example: Evaluation of Inhibitory Effects of Corticosteroid (Dexamethasone) and Cyclosporin A, on Allergen-Specific T-Cell Proliferation

For this experiment, two compounds are being evaluated. Their ability to inhibit T-cell proliferation is compared to a baseline value of proliferation in their absence. Furthermore, the proliferative response itself will require a baseline for comparison: This will be cells in the absence of allergen. For the purpose of the example (*see* **Table 2**), it is assumed that optimal concentrations of all components of the assay have been previously determined. Three doses of cyclosporin A (CsA) and dexamethasone (Dex) will be used to provide dose response data **(Fig. 2)**.

1. PBMCs are isolated as previously described. After washing, cells are resuspended at a concentration of 4×10^6/mL in complete culture medium. Because there are up to three components to the assay (cells, Ag, and drug), fourfold stock solutions are required, to allow for a one-quarter dilution (50 μL in a final well volume of 200 μL).
2. 50 μL cell suspension is placed in the appropriate wells of a 96-well plate (*see* **Table 2**).

Table 2
Plate Plan for 50 μL Cell Suspension

	Wells 1–6	Wells 7–12
A	Cells with medium alone	Cells with Ag
B	Cells with Ag and Dex (10^{-9} *M*)	Cells with Ag and Dex (10^{-7} *M*)
C	Cells with Ag and Dex (10^{-5} *M*)	Cells with Ag and CsA (10^{-9} *M*)
D	Cells with Ag and CsA (10^{-7} *M*)	Cells with Ag and CsA (10^{-5} *M*)
E		
F		
G		
H		

3. 50 μL Ag stock solution (at 4× final concentration, to allow for one-quarter dilution effect) is dispensed into appropriate wells. Culture medium is added to those wells not receiving Ag (A1–6).
4. 50 μL of 10^{-9} *M* Dex is added to wells B1–6, 10^{-7} *M* Dex to wells B7–12, and 10^{-5} *M* Dex to wells C1–6.
5. 50 μL of 10^{-9} *M* CsA is added to wells C7–12, 10^{-7} *M* CsA to wells D1–6, and 10^{-5} *M* CsA to wells D7–12.
6. Wells not receiving drug receive 50 μL culture medium.
7. Finally, all wells receive 50 μL culture medium, to give a final volume of 200 μL.
8. Cultures are incubated for 6 d prior to addition of tritiated thymidine and subsequent harvesting, as previously described.

4. Notes

1. T-cells may have different proliferation kinetics when challenged with differing proteins. For example, for the author, cat allergen extract gives peak proliferative responses after 9 d; dust mite allergen extract gives optimal proliferation after 7 d.
2. L-glutamine is labile in solution. Sigma has conducted a study addressing the stability of glutamine solutions at various temperatures. Even at 4°C, after approx 3 wk, only 60% remains, and this figure falls to only 10% after storage for the same period at 35°C. See the Sigma catalog for more details.
3. Some investigators use mercaptoethanol at 5×10^{-5} *M* to enhance proliferative responses in vitro (*see* **ref. *8***).
4. A variety of shapes are available for the 96-well format. The most common are flat-bottomed, U-bottomed, and V-bottomed. For proliferation assays, flat and U are the most useful, V-bottomed being used predominantly in cytotoxicity assays. The issue of which plate to use centers on cell density. T-cell activation requires the interaction of T-cell with Ag-presenting cell, and thus cells must be cultured in close proximity to one another. If a small number of cells are being used in each well, a U-bottomed plate will concentrate the cells in a relatively small area,

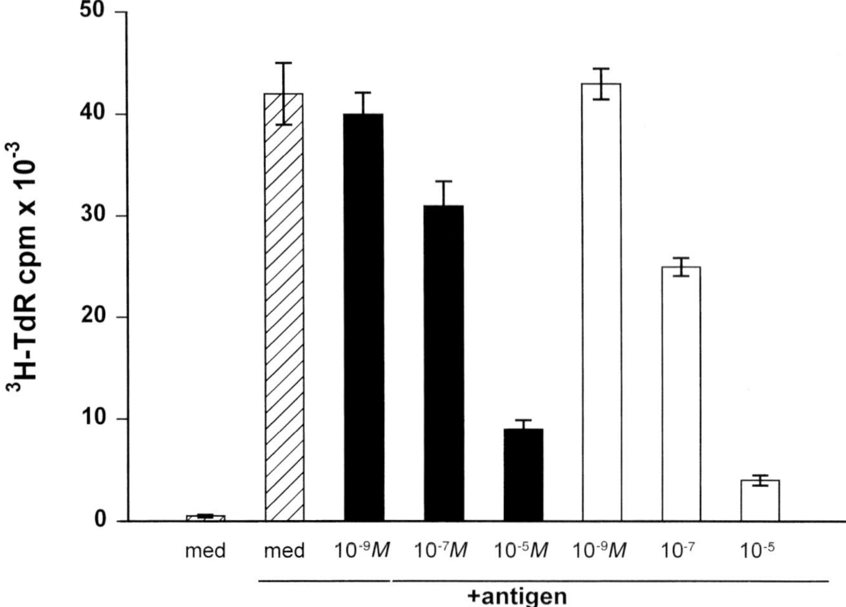

Fig. 2. Inhibition of Ag-specific proliferation by Dex and CsA. Cells were cultured in the absence of Ag or in the presence of Ag (house dust mite extract 20 μg/mL) for 7 d in a humidified incubator gassed with 5% CO_2 in air at 37°C. Dex (black bars) or CsA (open bars) were added over three concentrations indicated as molarity (10^{-9} *M*–10^{-5} *M*).

allowing interaction. Too many cells, however, may lead to overcrowding and subsequent restriction of gas and nutrient exchange for the cells at the bottom of the well. In higher cell-density-situations, therefore, it is advisable to use the flat-bottomed variety. A comparison of both within the same system can yield useful information, when establishing an assay.

5. Manufacturers of density gradient separation media, such as Histopaque and Ficoll-Paque, generally suggest that, prior to layering, blood should be diluted 1:1 with culture medium, and subsequently layered over equal volumes of separation medium. Although this does give the best yields, it is also expensive, and, in many cases (particularly, when cell yield is not vitally important), is not economically viable. In this laboratory, PBMCs are separated from whole blood without dilution. Separation is usually carried out in 50-mL tubes in which 20–25 mL blood is layered onto 15 mL separation medium. This is effectively 140% less media than is recommended per unit whole blood, and provides a considerable saving.
6. When washing cells in heparinized medium, save some of the autologous plasma from the cell separation, which may be added back to the cell suspension at

approx 10%, to act as a protein source for the cells during washing. This means that relatively expensive AB serum or fetal calf serum is not required.

7. The dilution series illustrated in this example goes from 0.01 μg/mL up to 100 μg/mL. Follow these steps:
   a. Calculate the amount of AG solution required for the assay, in this case, six wells of 100 μL, and thus a total of 600 μL per concentration. Allow extra volume for inaccuracy in pipeting and other spillage, i.e., 700 μL should be sufficient.
   b. Make solutions for the top two concentrations: 100 and 30 μg/mL. From these, subsequent 10-fold dilutions will be made to generate the lower concentrations. Be sure to make enough of each to allow sufficient for the wells at that concentration (i.e., 700 μL), and enough for the next dilution in the series.
   c. Make 800 μL of the first two stock solutions. Add 100 μL of each and 900 μL culture medium. Mix well, and remove 100 μL for the next dilution. Add this to 900 μL culture medium, and repeat the process until the series is complete.
   d. The final series should have the first two concentrations at 700 μL, the last two at 1 mL and those in between at 900 μL.

   The volumes can be adjusted to avoid wastage, but the principle will remain the same for any series.
8. Alternative methods for determination of cell proliferation are available. Incorporation of the thymidine analog, 5-bromodeoxyuridine, has been employed ***(9)***, and may be particularly useful when restrictions prevent the use of radioactive isotopes, or when sophisticated liquid scintillation spectroscopy equipment is not available. More recently, vital techniques have been employed to quantify live cells following a period of stimulation in culture (for example, CytoLite, Packard Bioscience, Groningen, Netherlands). It should be stressed, however, that this approach is not suitable for use on heterogeneous populations, such as PBMCs. The technique is effective with more homogenous cell sources, such as T-cell clones or lines.

References

1. Tonegawa, S., Steinberg, C., Dube, S., and Bernardini, A. (1974) Evidence for somatic generation of antibody diversity. *Proc. Natl. Acad. Sci. USA* **71,** 4027–4031.
2. Boniface, J. J., Rabinowitz, J. D., Wulfing, C., Hampl, J., Reich, Z., Altman, J. D., et al. (1998) Initiation of signal transduction through the T cell receptor requires the peptide multivalent engagement of MHC ligands. *Immunity* **4,** 459–466.
3. Larché, M. and Kay, A. B. (1999) T lymphocytes, in *Current Review of Allergic Disease* (Kaliner, S. A. ed.), Current Medicine, Philadelphia PA. pp. 25–38.
4. Winandy, M., Lewalle, P., Deneys, V., Ferrant, A., and De Bruyere, M. (1998) Improved IL-2 detection for determination of helper T lymphocyte precursor frequency in limiting dilution assay. *J. Immunol. Methods* **215,** 81–94.

5. Zinkernagel, R. M. and Doherty, P. C. (1974) Restriction of in vitro T cell-mediated cytotoxicity in lymphocytic choriomeningitis within a syngeneic or semiallogeneic system. *Nature* **248,** 701, 702.
6. Bjorkman, P. J., Saper, M. A., Samraoui, B., Bennett, W. S., Strominger, J. L., and Wiley, D. C. (1987) Foreign antigen binding site and T cell recognition regions of class I histocompatibility antigens. *Nature* **329,** 512–518.
7. O'Flynn, K., Krensky, A. M., Beverley, P. C., Burakoff, S. J., and Linch, D. C. (1985) Phytohaemagglutinin activation of T cells through the sheep red blood cell receptor. *Nature* **313,** 686–687.
8. Iwata, S., Hori, T., Sato, N., Ueda-Taniguchi, Yamabe, T., Nakamura, H., Matsutani, H. and Yodoi, J. (1994) Thiol-mediated redox regulation of lymphocytes proliferation. *J. Immunol.* **152,** 5633–5642.
9. Pera, F., Mattias, P. and Detzer, K. (1977) Methods for determining the proliferation kinetics of cells by means of 5-bromodeoxyuridine. *Cell Tissue Kinet.* **10,** 255–264.

11

Differential Display Analysis of Airway Epithelial Inflammatory Genes

Lisa M. Schwiebert

1. Introduction

Airway epithelial cells (ECs) form a continuous pseudostratified layer in the lung, creating a tight barrier that protects underlying tissue from the external environment. As such, airway ECs have been described classically as barrier cells that are involved in homeostasis; these cells respond to a variety of environmental stimuli, resulting in the alteration of their cellular functions, such as ion transport and movement of airway secretions. Recent evidence, however, suggests that airway ECs may also act as immune-effector cells, in response to noxious endogenous or exogenous stimuli. Several studies have shown that airway ECs express and secrete various immune molecules, such as lipid mediators, oxygen radicals, adhesion molecules, and a wide variety of cytokines, including chemokines *(1)*. Through the expression and production of these immune molecules, the epithelium is now thought to be important in the initiation and exacerbation of inflammatory diseases of the lung, such as asthma.

To learn new information regarding the mechanisms of airway inflammation, DNA differential display-polymerase chain reaction (DD-PCR) analysis may be used to identify novel genes that are relevant to airway diseases, including asthma, as well as to examine the expression of known genes that encode inflammatory molecules in lung ECs *(2)*. DD-PCR, developed initially by Liang and Pardee *(3,4)*, is a powerful technology that permits the identification and cloning of differentially expressed genes on a global scale. This method allows simultaneous analysis of multiple RNA samples per run, thereby revealing genes unique to a given cell type or cellular process. The differential expression of genes may result from a variety of causes, such as cell differentiation,

From: *Methods in Molecular Medicine, vol. 44: Asthma: Mechanisms and Protocols*
Edited by: K. F. Chung and I. Adcock © Humana Press Inc., Totowa, NJ

mutations, viral insertion, and exposure to inflammatory cytokines, including tumor necrosis factor-α (TNF-α) and interleukin (IL)-1β. Moreover, differential gene expression may occur during disease states; therefore, through the characterization of such gene expression, novel gene targets may be identified, and the activity of therapeutic agents may be determined.

2. Materials

2.1. DNA Differential Analysis

1. Diethyl pyrocarbonate (DEPC)-treated water: Add 1 mL DEPC (Sigma, St. Louis, MO) per liter of distilled water. Stir 18–20 h at room temperature (RT) in a fume hood, autoclave, and store at RT in glass bottles. DEPC-treated water is stable for approx 1 mo.
2. DNA precipitation buffer: For this buffer, mix 60 μ*M* sodium (Na) acetate, 100 μg/mL glycogen, and 100% ethanol. This buffer should be made fresh each time.
3. Luria broth (LB) ampicillin–agar: Mix 40 g LB-agar with 1 L distilled water, and autoclave. Cool autoclaved agar to 55°C, and then add 100 μg/mL ampicillin. Pour LB–ampicillin agar into Petri plates, allow to solidify, and store at 4°C, wrapped in aluminum foil. LB–ampicillin agar plates are stable for 1 mo. On the day of transformation, allow plates to warm to RT. One-half hour before plating transformed bacteria, coat plates with 20 μg/mL X-gal (Sigma) and 0.1 m*M* isopropylthiogalactopyranoside (IPTG) (Sigma).

2.2. False-Positive Analysis

1. 6% sequencing gel: Mix 16.6 mL 30% acrylamide, 10 mL 10X TBE (0.9 *M* Tris-base, 0.9 *M* boric acid, 0.02 *M* Na_2 ethylenediamine tetraacetic acid [EDTA]-$2H_2O$), 48 g urea, and bring to 100 mL with distilled water; solution will need low heat to mix completely. Once mixed, filter solution, add 800 μL 10% ammonium persulfate and 30 μL *N,N,N,N*-tetramethylethylenediamine, then pour gel immediately.
2. Hybridization buffer: Prepare a solution that is comprised of 50% formamide, 2X PIPES (0.2 *M* NaCl, 0.01 *M* KCl, 0.04 *M* 1,4-piperazinediethanesulfonic acid, pH 7.5), 0.5% sodium dodecyl sulfate (SDS), and 100 μg/mL sheared, heat-denatured salmon sperm DNA (Sigma). This solution should be made fresh before use.
3. 10X NaCl/sodium citrate solution (SSC): Mix 1.5 *M* NaCl and 0.15 *M* Na_3 citrate-$2H_2O$, pH 7.0. Filter and store at RT; solution is stable for months.

3. Methods

3.1. DNA Differential Display Analysis

The DD-PCR method involves the reverse transcription of mRNAs with oligo-deoxythymidine (oligo-dT) primers anchored to the 5' end of the poly(A) tail, followed by amplification in the presence of random primers, thereby gen-

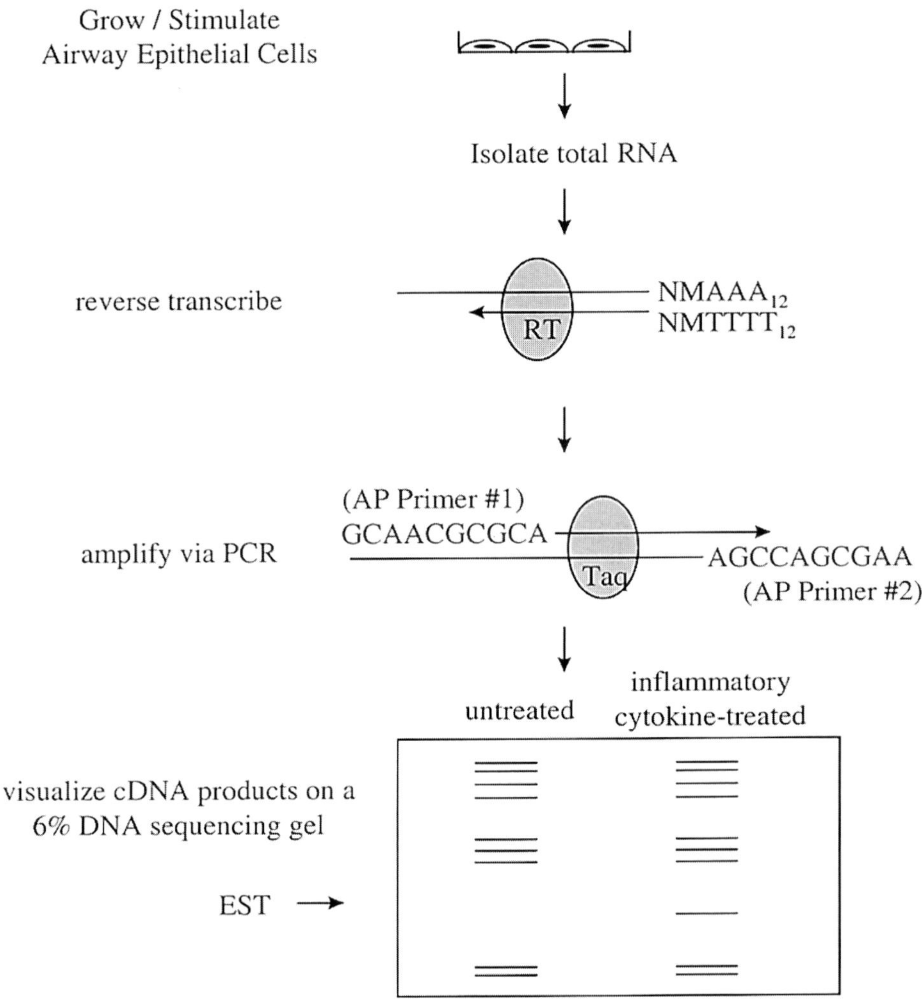

Fig. 1. Schematic illustration of DD-PCR. Total RNA is isolated from airway ECs and then reverse-transcribed. Resulting cDNA products are amplified in the presence of two independent AP primers, and then visualized on a 6% DNA sequencing gel.

erating double-stranded complementary DNA (cDNA) products of varying lengths (**Fig. 1**). By changing primer combinations, up to 15,000 individual mRNA species from mammalian cells may be visualized *(4)*. cDNA products are then visualized on a DNA sequencing gel (**Figs. 1** and **2**), differentially expressed bands (expressed sequence tags [ESTs]) are isolated, and the differential expression of the ESTs is confirmed through Northern blot analysis. DD-PCR has several advantages over existing methods, including subtractive

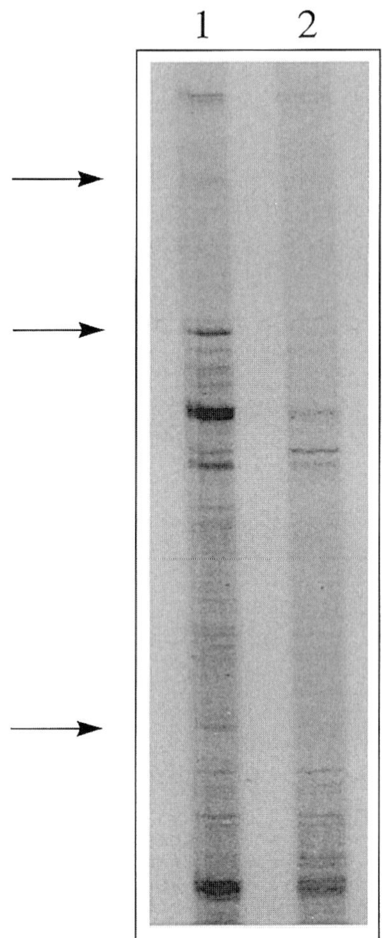

Fig. 2. Visualization of differentially expressed cDNA. Total RNA isolated from IB3-1 airway ECs stimulated with (lane 1) and without (lane 2) TNF-α (100 ng/mL, 20 hours at 37°C) was analyzed via DD-PCR, as described in **Fig. 1.** Differentially expressed ESTs are noted with arrows.

hybridization *(5)*. DD-PCR is also very sensitive, requiring small amounts of total RNA for the visualization of expressed mRNA species in a mammalian cell, and it is highly reproducible, with approx 95% of the bands reproduced from one run to another.

3.1.1. RNA Isolation

1. Total RNA is isolated from airway ECs (untreated, inflammatory cytokine-treated, and so on), using Trizol (Gibco-BRL, Grand Island, NY). Briefly, 2–5

Table 1
DNase-Treated RNA Samples

	Vol/reverse transcription (μL)	Final concentration
DEPC to dH_2O	9.4	
5X reverse-transcriptase buffer	4.0	1X
dNTP	1.6	20 μ*M*
Total RNA (DNA-free)	2.0	0.1 μg/μL
$T_{12}MN$	2.0	1 μ*M*
MMLV-RT	1.0	100 U
Final volume	20 μL	

× 10^6 cells are harvested and pelleted in an Eppendorf tube. Cells are then resuspended in 1 mL Trizol until lysed, 200 μL chloroform is added, and the sample is shaken for 15 s.

2. The sample is allowed to sit at RT for 2 min, then centrifuged at 13,000*g* for 15 min at 4°C, in order to separate the aqueous and nonaqueous phases.
3. Following centrifugation, the aqueous (top) phase is removed and combined with an equal volume of ice-cold isopropanol. The sample is then placed at –80°C for 18–20 h, in order to facilitate RNA precipitation. Precipitated RNA is washed with 200 μL 70% ice-cold ethanol, air-dried for 5 min, and then resuspended in DEPC-treated water.

3.1.2. DD-PCR Amplification

1. Total RNA is treated with DNase I (Gibco-BRL) at 1 U/μg RNA for 15 min at RT. The reaction is then stopped with the addition of 20 m*M* EDTA, and subsequent heating to 65°C for 10 min, in order to inactivate the enzyme.
2. DNase-treated RNA samples are reverse-transcribed in the presence of Moloney murine leukemia virus-reverse transcriptase (MMLV-RT) (GenHunter, Brookline, MA), dNTPs (GenHunter), and oligo-dT $T_{12}MN$ primers (GenHunter), where *M* represents a mixture of the bases G, A, or C, and N represents the bases G, A, T, or C (*see* **Table 1**).

   Reactions are incubated at 37°C for 1 h, then at 95°C for 5 min, in order to inactive the MMLV-RT enzyme.
3. The resulting cDNA products are amplified via PCR in the presence of two different 10-mer primers (AP primers, GenHunter) that bind randomly to the cDNA (*see* **Note 1**). Amplification reactions contained AmpliTaq (Perkin-Elmer), dNTPs, [α-^{35}S]-deoxyadenasine triphosphate (dATP) (1200 Ci/mmol; New England Nuclear, Boston, MA), and two AP primers (GenHunter), using various combinations of the AP primers 1–10 (*see* **Table 2**).

Table 2
Amplification Reactions from AP Primers 1–10

	Vol/reverse transcription (μL)	Final concentration
dH_2O	9.2	
10X PCR buffer	2.0	1X
dNTP	1.6	2 μ*M*
AP primer #1	2.0	0.2 μ*M*
AP primer #2	2.0	0.2 μ*M*
cDNA	2.0	10% of reverse transcription mix
[α-^{35}S]-dATP	1.0	12.5 μCi
AmpliTaq	0.2	1 U
Final volume	20 μL	

Amplification reactions are cycled at 94°C for 30 s, 40°C for 2 min, and 72°C for 30 s for 40 cycles; reactions then undergo a final extension at 72°C for 5 min. All reactions are performed in duplicate.

4. PCR products are then visualized on a 6% DNA sequencing gel run at 1500 V for approx 4 h; following the run, the gel is transferred to Whatman paper and prepared for autoradiography.
5. Upon exposure, bands of interest (ESTs) are selected and isolated. For isolation, ESTs are cut from the transferred gel, soaked in 100 μL distilled water for 15 min at RT, and then heated to 100°C for 15 min. The transferred gel paper is removed and the cDNA (ESTs) is precipitated in DNA precipitation buffer; samples are set on dry ice for 30 min, and DNA is then pelleted and washed with 85% ethanol.
6. Each EST is reamplified with the respective primer pair (*see* **Table 3**).

3.2. False-Positive EST Analysis

The greatest potential pitfall in DD-PCR is the detection of false-positive ESTs, i.e., those cDNA bands that do not represent authentic mRNAs (***2,4***; *see* **Notes 1** and **2**). In order to circumvent this problem, the following approaches have been taken in the method outlined below: All samples for DD-PCR are run in duplicate, in order to ensure that the banding pattern was reproducible; Total RNA samples are treated with RNase-free DNase, in order to remove contaminating DNA species that might compete for reagents during amplification; and false-positive ESTs that migrate at the same position during electrophoresis as true-positive ESTs, and therefore may elute simultaneously, are identified via partial dideoxy sequencing analysis of EST-(pGEM) clones. Because only one EST fragment may be inserted into one molecule of pGEM vector during a ligation, multiple positive clones from an EST-pGEM cloning

Table 3
Reamplification of EST with the Respective Primer Pair

	Vol/reverse transcription (μL)	Final concentration
dH_2O	20.4	
10X PCR buffer	4.0	1X
dNTP	3.2	2 μ*M*
AP primer 1	4.0	0.2 μ*M*
AP primer 2	4.0	0.2 μ*M*
EST	4.0	0.4% of eluted cDNA
AmpliTaq	0.4	1 U
Final volume	40 μL	

event may represent several different EST species. To determine the true-positive EST, 10 EST-pGEM clones are partially sequenced and the sequences compared; the majority of identical sequences are considered to be the true-positive EST.

3.2.1. T-A Cloning

1. Reamplified ESTs are electrophoresed in a 1% agarose gel and purified with the QIAquick Gel Extraction Kit (Qiagen, Chatsworth, CA).
2. Isolated EST cDNA fragments are then cloned into the pGEM-T vector using the pGEM T-A Cloning Kit (Promega, Madison, WI), and selected via blue-white screening. For cloning, EST cDNA fragments are ligated into the pGEM-T vector with T4 DNA ligase (1U/reaction) at an insert:vector ratio of 10:1. JM109 cells (Promega) are transformed with the plasmid and plated on LB–ampicillin agar containing X-gal and IPTG.
3. Positive (white) colonies are expanded in ampicillin-containing (100 μg/mL) Luria broth; plasmid EST DNA is isolated with the Perfect Prep Kit (5 Prime–3 Prime, Boulder, CO).

3.2.2. Single-Base Sequencing

1. To assess the presence of false-positives, 10 positive (white) colonies representing each EST are prepared for dideoxy sequencing of one nucleotide base, using the DNA sequencing kit with Sequenase (United States Biochemical–Amersham, Arlington Heights, IL), and are analyzed on a 6% DNA sequencing gel.
2. Sequences are then compared, and the majority of identical sequences are considered to be the true-positive EST.

3.2.3. Northern Blot Analysis

1. mRNA (poly[A]) is isolated from cells, using the Micro-Fast Track Kit (Invitrogen, San Diego, CA).

2. Two mg mRNA are electrophoresed in a 1% agarose gel containing paraformaldehyde, and transferred to a nylon filter membrane (GeneScreen, New England Nuclear–Dupont, Beverly, MA).
3. The mRNA is then hybridized with a [α-^{32}P]-dATP-labeled EST fragment as a cDNA probe (5×10^5 cpm/mL hybridization buffer; Random Label Kit, Gibco-BRL) at 37°C for 18-20 h.
4. Following hybridization, membranes are washed twice with 2X SSC for 15 min at RT, once with 2X SSC containing 1% SDS at 65°C, and once with 0.1X SSC. Membranes are then prepared for autoradiography.

3.3. Automated DNA Sequencing and Basic Local Alignment Search Tool Analysis

Following false-positive analysis, ESTs are sequenced on both strands, and the resulting sequences are compared with public sequence databases, including GenBank and EMBL, using the basic local alignment search tool (BLAST) algorithm. Through such alignment analysis, it can be determined whether any of the identified ESTs share homology at the nucleotide levels with previously identified genes.

1. The cloned EST fragments are sequenced on both strands, using an automated ABI 373A sequencer according to the manufacturer's procedures and chemistry.
2. Alignments are done with computer software designed by the Genetics Computer Group (University of Wisconsin at Madison).

4. Notes

1. Although DD-PCR is a powerful technique, there are potential problems with this method. First, as stated in **Subheading 3.2.**, false-positive ESTs may be detected. Second, certain combinations of primers may generate ESTs that are located in the 3' end of an expressed gene, and may therefore represent untranslated sequences, making homology analysis difficult. To decrease this possibility, cDNA products are amplified with pairs of random 10-mer primers, instead of with a single random primer and the respective oligo-dT primer for amplification, as described in the original Liang and Pardee protocol ***(3)***. Third, rare mRNAs may not be visualized. Despite the high sensitivity of DD-PCR, it may not detect mRNAs that exist at less than 50 copies/cell ***(4)***.
2. To further reduce the possibility of encountering false-positive ESTs with DD-PCR, additional approaches may be taken. The generation of false-positive ESTs probably results from the random and spurious nature of the priming reactions during the PCR amplification portion of the protocol; therefore, factors that enhance the stringency of these reactions should reduce the incidence of false-positive ESTs. To increase the stringency of the priming reactions, longer random primers (on the order of 16–20-mers), which would necessitate higher annealing temperatures, could be utilized. Alternatively, the annealing temperature of the priming reactions could be increased following the first several cycles, in order to estab-

lish the arbitrary annealing sites along the first-strand fragment, and then lock in these sites during the remaining cycles. Last, the differential expression of specific gene families may be examined using DD-PCR. Such an analysis may be achieved through the design of primers that recognize shared sequences of the desired gene family.

References

1. Schwiebert, L. M., Stellato, C., and Schleimer, R. P. (1996) Epithelium as a target of glucocorticoid action in the treatment of asthma. *Am. J. Respir. Crit. Care Med.* **154,** S16–S19.
2. Schwiebert, L. M., Mooney, J. L., Van, H. S., Gupta, A., and Schleimer, R. P. (1997) Identification of novel inducible genes in airway epithelium. *Am. J. Respir. Cell Mol. Biol.* **17,** 106–113.
3. Liang, P. and Pardee, A. B. (1992) Differential display of eukaroytic messenger RNA by means of the polymerase chain reaction. *Science* **257,** 967–971.
4. Liang, P., Averboukh, L., and Pardee, A. B. (1993) Distribution and cloning of eukaryotic mRNAs by means of differential display: refinements and optimization. *Nucleic Acids Res.* **21,** 3269–3275.
5. Liang, P. and Pardee, A. B. (1998) Differential display. A general protocol. *Mol. Biotechnol.* **10,** 261–267.

12

Analysis of Transcription Factor Activation

NFκB as Regulator of Inflammatory Genes in Epithelial Cells

Robert Newton and Ian M. Adcock

1. Introduction

In addition to being essential for differentiation and maturation, regulated gene expression governs many cellular responses to their local environment. For example, cytokines, viral infection, and numerous other inflammatory stimuli elicit the expression of specific response genes. Such signals are generally transduced to the nucleus, and result in the activation of particular DNA-binding proteins or transcription factors ***(1,2)***. Transcriptional activation requires the basal transcription machinery, consisting of RNA polymerase II and associated general transcription factors, and an array of specific transcription factors or activators that are responsible for conferring both gene and stimulus specificity ***(3)***. The general transcription factors are involved in recognition of core promoter elements, such as the TATA box, and stabilization of RNA polymerase II at the transcription start site ***(4–6)***. Regulated transcription involves binding of sequence-specific transcription factors to their cognate sequences (enhancers and silencers) in the control regions (promoter) of target genes (*see* **Table 1**). These elements are most commonly found in the immediate 5'-region upstream of transcription start. However, more distal regions and elements within the coding region may also be necessary. As a model for inducible activation, this chapter concentrates on the analysis of NF-κB and its role in gene transcription.

First described as a factor that bound to the immunoglobulin κ light-chain enhancer, NF-κB is now recognized as an almost ubiquitous activator of immune and acute-phase genes, and therefore plays an important role in a range of immunological responses ***(7,12)***. This DNA-binding activity consists of

From: *Methods in Molecular Medicine, vol. 44: Asthma: Mechanisms and Protocols*
Edited by: K. F. Chung and I. Adcock © Humana Press Inc., Totowa, NJ

Table 1
Transcription Factor Binding Sites

Factor	Consensus 5'–3' (sense strand)	Site	Ref.
NF-κB (p50, p65 + other rel proteins)	GGG(A/G)NN(T/C)(T/C)CC	κB	*(7)*
AP-1 (fos, jun + other bZIP proteins)	TGA(G/C)TCA	AP-1/TRE	*(8)*
CREB (+ other bZIP proteins)	T(G/T)ACGTCA	CRE	*(9,10)*
C/EBPβ (+ other C/EBP proteins)	T(T/G)NNGNAA(T/G)	C/EBP	*(11)*

bZip, basic-leucine zipper; N, any base.

multiple Rel family transcription factors, which in mammalian cells includes c-Rel (Rel), p50/p105 (NF-κB1), p65 (RelA), p52/p100 (NF-κB2), and RelB *(7)*. Although p50/p65 heterodimers are usually the most abundant NF-κB complexes, other Rel proteins may also bind DNA as hetero- or homodimers. Dimers of NF-κB are held in the cytoplasm as inactive complexes by inhibitory, IκB, molecules, such as IκBα, IκBβ, IκBε, and IκBγ *(7,13)*. Inducing agents result in activation of IκB kinases (IKKs), which phosphorylate and subsequently lead to ubiquitin-dependent degradation of IκB *(14,15)*. This releases NF-κB, which translocates to the nucleus, binds κB elements, and activates transcription. In addition, the p50 and p52 subunits exist as precursor forms, p105 and p100, respectively, which bind transactivation subunits, such as p65 or RelB, and, on activation, proteolytic cleavage releases active p50 or p52 containing heterodimers *(13)*.

In the context of NF-κB (or other transcription factor) activation and a role in gene expression, potential investigators will frequently have expression or functional data showing a particular response as a result of treatment with a given stimulus. It is then usual to demonstrate that the response in question is in fact dependent on regulated gene transcription, i.e., a transcriptional response, as opposed to posttranscriptional, translational, or posttranslational. For example, Northern hybridization or semiquantitative reverse transcription-polymerase chain reaction (RT-PCR) should be performed to show increased steady-state mRNA expression of the gene of interest. Ideally, mRNA half-life studies and nuclear run-on transcription reactions should be performed to determine the contribution of mRNA half-life and actual transcription rate to the observed mRNA induction. Assuming these data point to a transcriptionally regulated process, the investigator may then seek to address the issue of which transcription factors are activated, and whether these are involved in the increased transcription of the gene in question.

The authors here examine some of the strategic considerations and detail the core methodologies required to examine the activation and role of transcription factors in gene regulation.

2. Materials

2.1. Electrophoretic Mobility Shift Assay

All chemicals are from Sigma (Poole, UK) except where stated.

1. Buffer A: 10 m*M* HEPES, pH 7.9, 1.5 m*M* $MgCl_2$, 10 m*M* KCl, 0.5 dithiothreitol (DTT), 0.1% nonidet P40 (NP-40) (BDH, Poole, UK).
2. Buffer C: 20 m*M* HEPES pH 7.9, 25% glycerol, 0.42 *M* NaCl, 1.5 m*M* $MgCl_2$, 0.2 m*M* ethylenediamine tetra-acetic acid (EDTA) pH 8.0, 0.5 m*M* phenylmethylsulfonyl fluoride (PMSF), 0.5 m*M* DTT.
3. Buffer D: 20 m*M* HEPES, pH 7.9, 20% glycerol, 50 m*M* KCl, 0.2 m*M* EDTA, pH 8.0, 0.5 m*M* PMSF, 0.5 m*M* DTT.
4. Bradford Reagent (Bio-Rad, Hemel Hempstead, Herts, UK).
5. $\gamma[^{32}P]$ adenosine triphosphate (ATP), 10 mCi/mL, >5000 Ci/mmol (Amersham Pharmacia Biotech, Little Chalfont, Bucks, UK).
6. NF-κB consensus (underlined) double-stranded oligonucleotide (oligonucleotide) 5'-AGT TGA <u>GGG GAC TTT CCC</u> AGG-3' (sense strand) (Promega, Southampton, UK). AP-1, Sp-1, and Oct 1 consensus probes (Promega).
7. T4 polynucleotide kinase (PNK) and 10X kinase buffer (Promega).
8. Tris-EDTA (TE) buffer: 10 m*M* Tris-HCl, pH 7.5, 1 m*M* EDTA, pH 8.0.
9. Sterile G-25 sephadex in TE (Amersham Pharmacia Biotech).
10. 5X Electrophoretic mobility shift assay (EMSA) buffer: 20% glycerol, 5 m*M* $MgCl_2$, 2.5 m*M* EDTA, 250 NaCl, 50 m*M* Tris-HCl, pH 7.5, 0.4 mg/mL denatured salmon sperm DNA (Sigma), 2.5 m*M* DTT.
11. 10X Gel loading buffer: 50% glycerol, 0.05% bromophenol blue.
12. 10X Tris–boric acid–EDTA (TBE)/L: 108 g Tris-HCl, 55 g boric acid, 20 mL EDTA, pH 8.0, H_2O to 1 L.
13. 40% acrylamide/2.105% *bis*-acrylamide solution (Scotlab, Cotbridge, Strathclyde, UK), *N',N',N',N'*-tetramethylethylenediamine (TEMED), ammonium persulfate (APS).

2.2. Transfection Analysis

1. Tfx50 (Promega).
2. G-418 (Geneticin) (Gibco-BRL, Paisley, UK).
3. Luciferase Assay Kit (Promega).

3. Methods

3.1. Electrophoretic Mobility Shift Assay

As noted above, transcriptional activators, e.g., NF-κB, activator protein (AP)-1, CRE-binding protein (CREB), and CCAAT/enhancer-binding protein

(C/EBP), bind DNA in a sequence-specific manner (**Table 1**). This property allows investigators to assay for the presence of the particular DNA-binding activities by means of the EMSA. In brief, nuclear extracts are prepared from the test sample, and then incubated with a double-stranded, radiolabeled DNA probe containing the relevant consensus recognition sequence. Binding of factors to the probe is analyzed by separation of the free probe from the bound probe by nondenaturing polyacrylamide gel electrophoresis (PAGE). Free probe migrates rapidly through the gel; bound probe is retarded because of the size of the protein. This mobility shift allows the presence of a particular DNA-binding activity to be detected, e.g., between different cell types or following treatment with drugs or stimuli (**Fig. 1A**; *see* **Note 1**).

The use of EMSA and supershift analysis (*see* **Subheading 3.2.**) may allow investigators to determine the presence of particular transcription factors in cells of interest, and test the effect of various stimuli and drugs. Thus, the relationship between transcription factor binding (and composition) and the kinetics of putative response genes can be analyzed. In addition, inhibitor studies can be performed to further test the relationship between transcription factor binding and gene induction (*see* **Note 2**). Furthermore, the construction of appropriate probes can be used to address whether putative sites from a real gene are able to bind particular factors (for example, *see* **refs. *16*** and ***17***; **Fig. 2**).

3.1.1. Preparation of Nuclear Extracts

The protocol for the preparation of nuclear extracts is one modified from Dignam et al. ***(18)***, as described by Osborn et al. ***(19)***. In essence, this procedure uses soft lysis to rupture the plasma membrane. Nuclei are spun out, and high salt is used to extract soluble nuclear proteins.

1. Epithelial cells, grown to confluency in six-well plates (Costar, High Wycombe, Bucks, UK) are typically incubated overnight in serum-free media, prior to treatment with cytokines and drugs, as required. Cells are then harvested by scraping on ice in tissue culture medium (*see* **Note 3**).
2. Pellet cells at 14,000*g*, at 4°C, for 2 min in a benchtop centrifuge, and remove medium.
3. Lyse cells by resuspension in 200 µL of buffer A. Vortex briefly, and incubate on ice for 5–15 min (*see* **Note 4**).
4. Pellet nuclei at 14,000*g*, at 4°C, for 5 min, and discard supernatant (cytoplasmic lysate).
5. Retain nuclear pellet, and resuspend pellet in 15 µL buffer C (*see* **Note 5**). Leave on ice 20–60 min, with occasional agitation.
6. Pellet nuclear debris at 14,000*g*, at 4°C, for 15 min and carefully remove all the supernatant to a fresh tube containing buffer D.

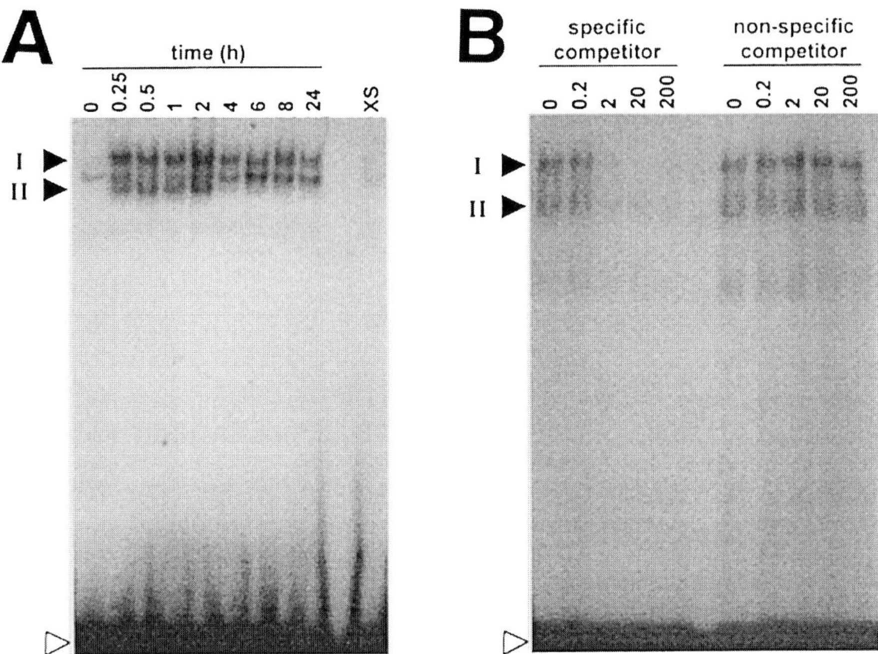

Fig. 1. Activation of NF-κB by interleukin-1β (IL-1β) in A549 cells. **(A)** Cells were treated with IL-1β (1 ng/mL) for the times indicated. Nuclear proteins were harvested and used for EMSA analysis. The two main NF-κB-specific complexes are indicated with solid arrows. Free probe is indicated with an open arrow. XS = competition reaction in which nuclear extracts from IL-1β treated cells (1 h) were incubated as before, except that 100-fold excess unlabeled competitor NF-κB consensus was added. **(B)** Specificity of binding was demonstrated in nuclear extracts from IL-1β-treated cells (1 h). Nuclear extracts were incubated with the indicated fold excesses of either the unlabeled NF-κB consensus probe or with the nonspecific competitor (5'-CGC TTG ATG AGT CAG CCG GAA-3') prior to the addition of the labeled NF-κB probe.

7. Measure protein concentration (*see* **Note 6**). The authors use the Bradford assay (Bio-Rad) and measure the optical density at 600 nm. Generation of standard curves, using bovine serum albumin, allows protein concentrations to be determined.

3.1.2. Generation of Radiolabeled Probe

Radiolabeled DNA probes can be generated by a variety of end-fill and strand-replacement processes involving various DNA polymerase activities ***(20)***. However, probably the most convenient method for radiolabeling oligonucleotides is the 5'-end-labeling of DNA ends, using T4 PNK. Often an investigator will not wish to use commercially available probes, for instance, when analyzing binding

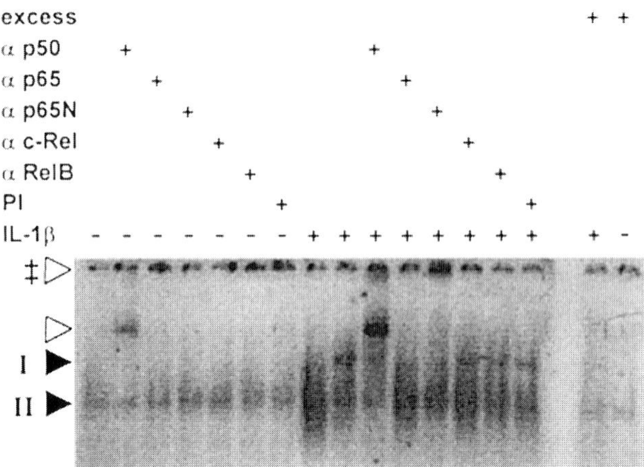

Fig. 2. Supershift analysis. NF-κB p50 and p65 binds the –223/–214 NF-κB site in human COX-2 promoter sequence. Nuclear extracts from either unstimulated or IL-1β-treated cells (1 h) were incubated as indicated with antisera raised against: p50, p65 carboxy terminus (p65C), p65 amino terminius (p65N), c-Rel, RelB or preimmune serum (PI), or 100-fold excess (excess) of unlabeled competitor oligonucleaotide. Binding reactions were performed using a double-stranded probe containing the COX-2 promoter sequence 5'-GAG TGG GGA CTA CCC CCT CT-3' (–228/–209) (NF-κB site underlined). Specific complexes are indicated with solid arrows. Open arrows show supershifted complexes, and ‡ indicates the positions of the wells.

of proteins to putative sites in an uncharacterized promoter, or to allow the incorporation of mutations in order to characterize the binding specificity (**Fig. 2**). In such cases, the appropriate oligo-NT should be synthesized and annealed prior to end-labeling, as described below (*see* **Note 7**).

1. Add: 2 μL consensus double-stranded oligonucleotide (1.75 pmol/μL), 2 μL 10X kinase buffer, 13 μL dH_2O, 2 μL [γ^{32}P]ATP (3000 Ci/mmol at 10 mCi/mL), 1 μL T4 PNK (5–10 U/μL), to a total volume of 20 μL.
2. Incubate 37°C, 30 min.
3. Prepare G-25 spin column by removing the plunger of a 1-mL syringe. Plug the tip end with a pinch of glass fiber, or preferably polymer wool. Pack column with G-25/TE slurry. Allow to settle, topping up as necessary. Spin at 780*g* for 5 min in a swing-out bucket rotor (e.g., Sorvall H_2O 00B, DuPont Ltd., Stevenage, Hertsfordshire, UK).
4. Add 180 μL TE to the labeling reaction, and apply the mix to the G-25 column. Respin at 780*g*, 5 min.
5. Collect effluent from the column (unincorporated NT remains on the column), and monitor to ensure probe has been labeled. Probe can be stored at 4°C for at least one half-life, and two for most applications.

3.1.3. Binding Reactions

The core of EMSA is the binding reaction. For the intensity of the shifted signal observed on a gel to reflect the amount of DNA-binding activity in a sample, it is essential that excess radiolabeled probe is present. If the amount of probe becomes limiting, then, with increased DNA binding, there will be a parallel decrease in free probe at the foot of the gel. In such cases, less nuclear extract or more probe is required. Binding of proteins to the probe may be either specific or nonspecific. Nonspecific binding can be identified by incubation of extracts with excess cold (competitor) probe (**Fig. 1A, B**). Specific complexes will be readily competed out, but nonspecific complexes will remain. Thus, in **Figs. 1A**, **B** and **2**, a band migrating with similar mobility to the lower NF-κB complex is not totally competed out, suggesting some degree of nonspecific binding. Such an approach also allows the sequence-specificity of binding complexes to be determined by the addition of excess competitor probes harboring various point mutations in the putative-binding site.

1. Binding reactions are set up on ice in an Eppendorf tube (*see* **Note 8**). Normally, probe is added 5 min after the nuclear protein, then incubated for a further 90 min. For competition experiments, unlabeled probe, usually a 100-fold excess over the labeled probe, is added 15 min prior to addition of labeled probe: 15–X μL dH_2O, 4 μL 5X EMSA buffer, 4X μL nuclear proteins (1–10 μg), 1 μL radiolabeled probe, to a total volume of 20 μL.
2. Add 2 μL 10X gel-loading buffer.

3.1.4. Nondenaturing PAGE

Nondenaturing PAGE allows separation of free probe from the slower-mobility protein–DNA complexes. Often, the nature of the DNA–protein interaction is weak, and, consequently, low-ionic-strength electrophoresis buffers are used. In addition, rapid running of gels is not recommended, because this may also result in loss of protein–DNA complexes.

1. Assemble gel plates in gel-casting stand (*see* **Note 9**).
2. Typically, a 6% acrylamide gel mix is made: 7.5 mL 40% acrylamide, 41 mL dH_2O, 1.25 mL 10X TBE, 0.6 mL 10% (w/v) APS, 0.6 mL TEMED, to a total volume (sufficient for two gels) of 50 mL. After addition of APS and TEMED, quickly pour the gels, and insert combs, ensuring that no bubbles become trapped. Gels will usually set within 15 min, but it is normal to allow at least 1 h prior to use.
3. When required, remove the combs carefully, and flush out the wells with 0.25X TBE, to remove unpolymerized acrylamide. Add fresh 0.25X TBE to wells.
4. Load samples to the bottom of the each well, using an extended tip.
5. Run gels at in 0.25X TBE at 200 V, until the bromophenol blue reaches the bottom of the gel.

6. At end of the run, separate the gel plates, adhere wet gel to 3MM Whatman paper and cover with Saran Wrap.
7. Place on slab-gel drier at 80°C for 1 h with vacuum.
8. Autoradiograph dried gels with intensifying screens, as required.

3.2. Supershift Analysis

Detection of a mobility shift does not in itself provide conclusive proof of the identity of the bound complex. This can be accomplished by supershift analysis. In essence, an EMSA is performed, except that antibodies (Abs) specific to various transcription factors are coincubated with the nuclear extracts and the radiolabeled probe. Binding of Ab to a protein complexed with the probe will produce a complex of greater size. This will be retarded to a greater extent on PAGE, and gives rise to the term "supershift" (**Fig. 2**). A second possibility is that the Ab may interact in such a manner so as to prevent DNA binding, resulting in depletion of DNA-binding complexes. These alternatives can be seen in **Fig. 2**. The p50 Ab results in a substantial supershift from both NF-κB-specific complexes; the two p65 Abs have depleted of the upper NF-κB-specific binding complex. In either case, supershift or loss of binding, the identity of proteins in the DNA-binding complex may be inferred (see **Note 10**).

1. Prepare nuclear proteins as described in **Subheading 3.1.1.**
2. Set up binding reactions as in **Subheading 3.1.3.**, including competition reactions with excess unlabeled probe. Do not add radiolabeled probe.
3. Add 1–2 μL supershift Ab to the reaction (*see* **Note 11**).
4. Incubate on 2 h on ice.
5. Add 1 μL radiolabeled probe, and continue with binding and running of gels as in **Subheadings 3.1.3** and **3.1.4.**

3.3. Transfection of Epithelial Cells

One problem with EMSA is that transcription-factor DNA-binding activity does not necessarily correlate with transcriptional activation. Unlike NF-κB, which is held inactive in the cytoplasm and translocates to the nucleus following activation, many transcription factors, e.g., AP-1, CREB, and C/EBP, are constitutively present in the nucleus ***(8,9,11,21)***. In the case of AP-1 and related factors, signal transduction processes involving multiple mitogen-activated protein kinase (MAPK) cascades result in active kinases, which then phosphorylate specific transcription factors within the nucleus ***(21)***. For example c-Jun, a component of AP-1, is phosphorylated by members of the Jun N-terminal kinase (JNK) family, and results in enhanced transcriptional activity (***22***; *see* **Note 12**). Thus, considerable DNA-binding activity may be detected independently of stimulus, and only minor changes (if any) observed following cell stimulation ***(9,10,21)***. To address the issue of transcriptional activation of such factors, appropriate transcriptional reporters are required.

Artificial gene reporter systems are now routinely used to assess promoter activation in response to various stimuli and drugs. These are conventional cloning plasmids in which a reporter gene, usually chloramphenical acetyl transferase, or, more recently, firefly luciferase, is placed downstream of a multiple cloning region. Investigators may then clone various putative promoter regions upstream of the reporter gene, to allow assessment of transcriptional activity. Common strategies for a gene of interest would involve the generation of reporter constructs containing the transcription start site (+1), and usually 20–80 bases downstream, along with progressively larger regions of 5' or upstream regions of the putative promoter. Transfection of such deletion constructs into cells of interest may allow determination of the promoter regions required for transcriptional activation (for a good example, *see* **ref.** ***17***; **Fig. 3B**). Specific transcription factor binding sites, e.g., as determined by EMSA, may be mutated by site-directed mutagenesis to verify a role in transcriptional activation (*see* **Fig. 3C**; **Note 13**). In addition, particular elements may be cloned upstream of a minimal promoter (i.e., containing a TATA box plus transcription start) driving an appropriate reporter, to address whether the particular element is capable of driving a transcriptional response. For example, the authors routinely use an NF-κB-dependent reporter, which contains six copies of the consensus κB site upstream of a minimal thymidine kinase promoter driving a luciferase gene (***23,24***; *see* **Fig. 4**; **Note 14**). This has allowed us to examine the activation of NF-κB transcriptional activity in response to various stimuli, and to address the issue of inhibition by anti-inflammatory drugs, such as glucocorticoids or other kinase and enzyme inhibitors ***(23,24)***.

3.3.1. Transient Transfection Analysis

Transfection refers to the transient introduction of essentially naked DNA into a cell. A number of processes, including electroporation and calcium phosphate (CaP) coprecipitation and lipofection, have been developed for this purpose. Of these, CaP coprecipitation and lipofection are most easily applicable to EC monolayers. The CaP method, which involves coprecipitation of the plasmid DNA with CaP, has the advantage of being cheap, but often suffers from low reproducibility, requires more plasmid DNA, and generally gives rise to lower overall transfection efficiencies. This has led to the rapid growth in the number of lipid formulations, which, when complexed with plasmid DNA, are readily adsorbed by the cell, allowing transfer of the DNA to the nucleus. Such transfection procedures are generally quick, reproducible, and produce higher transfection efficiencies. The authors have successfully used

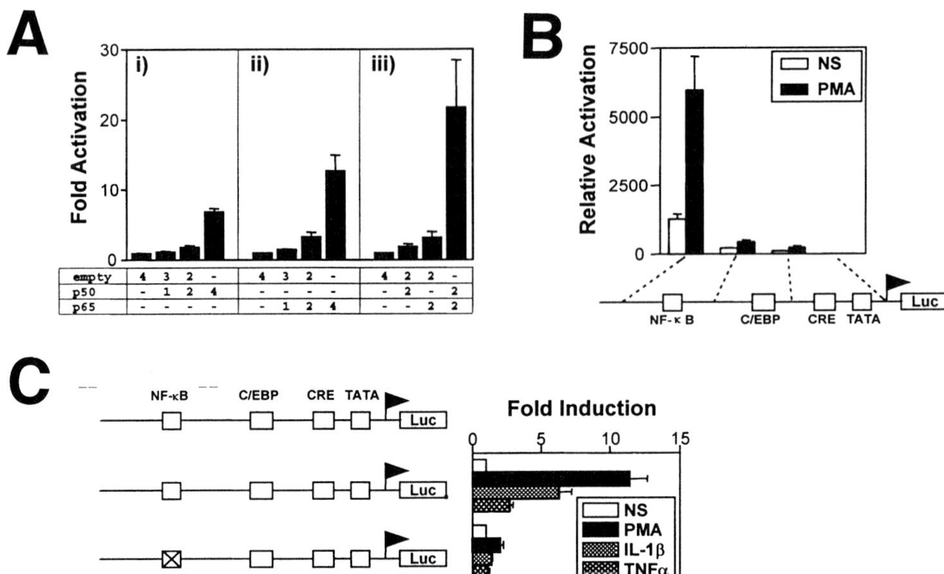

Fig. 3. NF-κB activation of the COX-2 promoter. **(A)** Transfections were carried out using a total of 5 μg DNA, with varying amounts (μg) of the expression vectors RcCMV-p50 (p50) (i), or RcCMV-p65 (p65) (ii), or both together (iii), and empty expression vector (empty) (Invitrogen, Groningen, the Netherlands) as indicated. Data are expressed as fold induction relative to control. **(B)** A549 cells were stably transfected with various parts of the human COX-2 promoter cloned into pGL3basic (Promega), which had been previously modified to contain a neomycin resistance gene, or empty vector. Regions of COX-2 promoter were (relative to transcription start, +1): –358/+49, –189/+49 and –85/+49. Cells in 24-well plates were either not stimulated or treated with the phorbol ester, phorbol 12-myristate 13-acetate (PMA) (10^{-7} *M*) for 6 h prior to harvesting and luciferase assay. **(C)** The –358/+49 construct was subjected to site directed mutagenesis and the NF-κB site (–223/–214) (5'-GGG GAC TAC C-3') was mutated to 5'-GGC CAC TAC C-3' (mutated bases underlined) (indicated by a cross).

lipofectin (Gibco-BRL) and Tfx50 (Promega) for transfection of A549, BEAS-2B, and LA-4 ECs.

1. Grow cells to ~60% confluency in T-75 flasks.
2. Incubate 8 μg of supercoiled reporter plasmid DNA with 40 μL (5.25 mg/mL) Tfx50 for 15 min at room temperature (RT) in 8 mL tissue serum and antibiotic-free culture medium (*see* **Note 15**).
3. Wash cells with serum and antibiotic-free medium.
4. Add DNA–Tfx50–medium mixture to cells.
5. Incubate 2 h at 37°C.

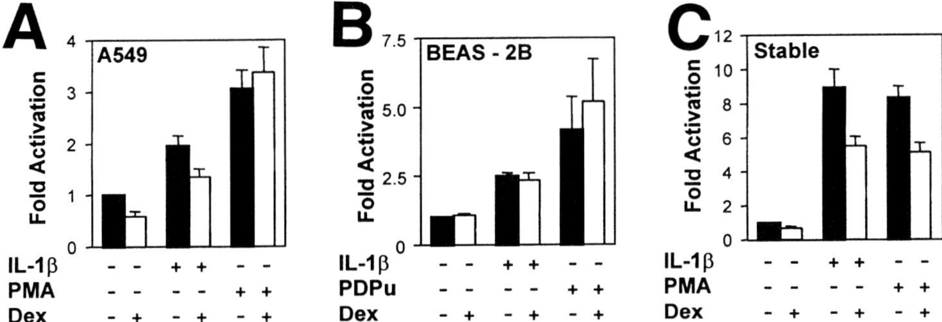

Fig. 4. Activation of NF-κB-dependent transcription and effect of dexamethasone. A549 cells (**A**) or BEAS-2B cells (**B**) were transiently transfected with the NF-κB-dependent reporter, 6κBtk, as described. Cells were treated with dexamethasone (10^{-6} *M*) for 1 h, and stimulated for 6–8 h with IL-1β (1 ng/mL) or the phorbol esters, PMA or phorbol 12,13-dibutyrate (PDBu) (10^{-7} *M*), as indicated. Luciferase data are normalized to total protein and expressed as fold induction. (**C**) A549 cells were stably transfected with the reporter 6κBtk.neo, and cells in 24-well plates retreated, as in (A) and (B) above.

6. Remove media, and replace with fresh serum-containing media, and incubate overnight.
7. Plate cells into six-well plates, and incubate 24–48 h, until confluent.
8. Change to serum-free medium for 12–24 h prior to treating with stimuli and drugs.
9. Harvest cells for luciferase assay.

Using the above protocol, the authors have only achieved relatively modest levels of reporter inducibility (**Fig. 4A,B**; ***16,24***). Although reasons for this are not presently clear, it seems likely that the DNA conformation of transfected plasmids may not mimic the structure of chromosomal DNA. Because this could have multiple effects on stimulus-dependent transcription, such data need to be interpreted with caution.

3.3.2. Stable Transfection

The problems encountered with lack of or low inducibility of reporter constructs in transient transfection analysis led the authors to examine the inducibility of reporter constructs that were stably integrated into the host chromosomal DNA. The procedure is identical with that for transient transfection, except that plasmids to be transfected must carry a selectable marker (usually a neomycin resistance gene), and, after transfection, cells are incubated with the appropriate antibiotic, which results in death of all cells, except those in which the plasmid has become integrated into the host chromosomal DNA. Alternatively, the reporter plasmid may be transfected in the presence of a plasmid containing a selectable marker. In this case, the reporter should be in excess of the selectable plasmid, so that cells that show integration of the marker are likely to have cointegrated the reporter. This second method contains a number of variables, and the preferred method is to have the reporter plasmid carrying the desired selectable marker.

1. Perform **steps 1–6** for transient transfection in **Subheading 3.3.1.**
2. After incubation overnight, trypsinize cells, and plate on to T-162 flask.
3. Add G-418 to a concentration of 0.5 mg/mL (*see* **Note 16**).
4. Change to fresh media (+ G-418) every 2–3 d.
5. Once cell death has occurred and foci of resistant cells are easily visible (2–3 wk), cells can be trypsinized and plated onto new T-162 flasks. Once confluent, cell stocks may be frozen and/or cells plated onto 24-well plates.
6. Once cells in 24-well plates have reached confluency, the media is changed to serum-free medium, and cells are incubated overnight.
7. Change media and treat with stimuli and drugs. Cells are usually harvested for luciferase assay 6–10 h following stimulation.

Using the above procedure, the authors have obtained highly reproducible inducibility of a number of reporter constructs in A549 cells (**Figs. 3B,C** and **4C**).

3.3.3. Overexpression of Signaling Molecules

One further tool in elucidation of promoter function or signal transduction pathways is the ability to overexpress various signaling molecules. Thus, an investigator wishing to examine the function of particular elements in a promoter may cotransfect the reporter construct under investigation, along with eukaryotic expression vectors for transcription factors or their upstream activating kinases, to test for activation of the reporter (**Fig. 3A**). Such experiments may provide convincing data about the ability of particular factors to activate a promoter, but such information should be interpreted with caution. First, overexpression of kinases or transcription factors to unphysiological levels may result in promiscuous activation of signaling pathways and/or transcription. Second, overexpression experiments are typically carried out over 24–48 h, which gives rise to the possibility that the overexpressed gene may be activating the reporter indirectly. However, this approach is often followed up by an analysis using dominant-negative mutants to block the response in question (e.g., *see* **ref. *25***). This approach is often considered to be more robust, because many of the problems associated with overexpression of active signaling components are avoided. In all overexpression experiments, it is important that the total amount of DNA to be transfected remains constant. Therefore, transfections that do not contain the overexpression plasmid should have an equivalent amount of empty expression vector (*see* **Fig. 3A**).

1. Grow cells to ~60% confluency in 6-well plates (*see* **Note 17**).
2. Wash cells with serum and antibiotic-free media.
3. Add DNA to be transfected to serum- and antibiotic-free media.
4. Add Tfx50 reagent at 5 µL/µg/mL media. Typically, 1 mL media is used per well with 0.5 µg reporter plasmid, and from 0.1 to 5 µg of expression plasmid.
5. Add DNA–Tfx50–medium mix to cells, and incubate 2 h at 37°C.
6. Remove media, and add fresh serum-containing medium.
7. Incubate cells for 24–48 h before harvesting for luciferase assay.

3.3.4. Luciferase Assay and Normalization

The presence of luciferase enzyme in cell extracts is readily assayed by the addition of substrate. This assay is highly sensitive, fast, and linear over at least eight orders of magnitude of enzyme concentration (*see* **Note 18**). Because of the variable nature of transient transfection, it is common for investigators to cotransfect a reporter plasmid that gives rise to constitutively high levels of β-galactosidase expression, which can be measured in cell extracts harvested as below and used to normalize the luciferase reading. However, variations in β-galactosidase expression, as a result of stimulation, drugs, or overexpression of signaling molecules, are often observed. Consequently, normalization to protein concentration to control for variations in cell number may also be acceptable. However, this does not control for transfection efficiency, and such variations will therefore show up as experimental error.

1. Harvest cells by scraping on ice in tissue culture medium.
2. Pellet cells at 14,000*g* for 2 min at 4°C.
3. Resuspend in 100–200 µL 1X reporter lysis buffer (Promega).
4. Vortex, and subject cells to one freeze–thaw cycle.
5. Vortex vigorously.
6. Spin down debris at 14,000*g* for 2 min at RT.
7. To 20 µL cell extract to a luminometer vial, add 40 µL luciferase assay reagent (Promega).
8. Determine luminescence using a luminometer.
9. Determine protein concentration of sample using the Bradford assay (Bio-Rad), as above.
10. Normalize luciferase reading to protein.

4. Notes

1. EMSA is essentially a qualitative technique, and is best suited to the detection of large changes (for example, activation of NF-κB by tumor necrosis factor-α), or simply the presence/absence of particular binding activities. This notwithstanding, EMSA can be successfully used in a semiquantitative manner, e.g., in comparison of patient groups ***(26)***. In this instance, prior planning is essential, because

samples prepared and analyzed separately cannot be readily compared. The authors have found that paired samples (i.e., group 1 vs group 2), which are processed and analyzed simultaneously, may yield meaningful data. However, clearly, the best option is to prepare and analyze all samples in a study simultaneously, to allow direct comparison of data.

2. Inhibition of gene expression, but not transcription factor binding, does not exclude a role for the particular transcription factor, because the inhibitor may be acting downstream of transcription factor DNA binding ***(23)*** or on other transcription factors required for gene transcription. Furthermore, possible effects on mRNA processing and stability may also need to be considered.
3. This protocol works well for A549 pulmonary type II cells, i.e., one well (~10 cm^2) of confluent cells will typically yield sufficient nuclear protein for 2–6 binding reactions. For other cell types and lines, the optimal area of cells can be determined empirically, according to the yield of nuclear proteins.
4. The appropriate incubation time varies considerably, depending on the cell type or cell line. This should be determined empirically, by adding buffer A and examining cells by light microscopy using a stain such as Kimura (add: 11 mL toluidine blue [0.05%,], 0.8 mL light green [0.03%], 0.5 mL saponin [saturated], and 5 mL phosphate-buffered saline), which stains the nuclei. The appropriate time is that required to lyse the plasma membrane, but leave the nuclear membrane intact in most cells. In addition, the authors commonly use Gough I buffer (10 m*M* Tris-HCl, pH 7.5, 0.15 *M* NaCl, 1.5 m*M* $MgCl_2$, 0.65% NP-40) in place of buffer A. This not only contains a higher NP-40 level, allowing lysis of more difficult cells, but also, when supplemented with 20–40 U RNasin (Promega), enables preparation of cytoplasmic RNA ***(27)***. RNA prepared by this method is suitable for RT-PCR and Northern analysis.
5. The authors find this step to be critical to the successful isolation of nuclear proteins. The nuclear pellet is usually small and compact, and can be disaggregated with the end of the yellow tip prior to, or simultaneously with, resuspension. Vigorous agitation is essential to release nuclear proteins successfully. Vortexing is not sufficient. The authors drag the tubes up and down an empty Eppendorf rack, to generate a violent, flicking action. This is repeated at intervals during the incubation.
6. The reliability of EMSA depends on the sample preparation and accurate determination of protein concentration. These processes are notoriously variable. The authors therefore routinely perform EMSA on a noninducible transcription factor, for example, Oct 1, in parallel with the factor to be tested, which allows easy identification of loading or processing artifacts, and, in many instances, normalization to the constitutive factor will improve the rigor of experimental data.
7. Generation of double-stranded oligonucleotide probes can be performed by mixing forward and reverse oligonucleotides at a concentration of 100 pmol/μL in TE buffer. This mix is then heated to 100°C for 2 min, and allowed to cool to ~30°C. Annealed probe can be diluted to a working concentration of 2 pmol/μL for radiolabeling.

8. The salmon sperm works well for NF-κB EMSA; however, for CRE, nuclear factor for interleukin 6 (NFIL6), or glucocorticoid response element (GRE) EMSAs, the authors often use an identical buffer, except that the 0.4 mg/mL salmon sperm DNA is replaced with 0.25 mg/mL poly dI/dC (Pharmacia). Binding may also be performed at RT, 30°C, or even 37°C. The optimum will depend on the transcription factor to be analyzed, and, in each case, should be determined empirically. When higher incubation temperatures are used, the incubation time may also be reduced.
9. The authors routinely use a Hoefer SE 600 vertical electrophoresis system for 14 × 16-cm slab gels. Typically, gels are run with 20 well combs and spacers of 1.0 mm thickness.
10. The absence of a supershift or change in DNA binding with a particular AB does not necessarily exclude a factor from the complex. To reach this conclusion, appropriate positive controls would be required.
11. A number of commercial suppliers produce high-concentration (1–2 mg/mL) Abs (for example, Santa Cruz) that are suitable for use in supershift analysis.
12. Activation of particular kinases, for instance, of the MAPK cascades or the IKKs, can be assayed by in-tube or in-gel kinase assay ***(28,29)*** (techniques not addressed here). In addition, a number of commercially available Abs now exist that allow the detection of the phosphorylated, and therefore active, forms of the various kinases and their substrates. Thus, phosphorylated IκBα, c-Jun, JNK, or CREB may be directly analyzed by Western blot analysis (technique not described here) (for example, *see* **ref.** ***28***).
13. Numerous methods now exist for site directed mutagenesis. The authors have found the QuickChange site-direct mutagenesis kit (Stratagene, La Jolla, CA) to work very efficiently.
14. When possible, investigators should seek to obtain reporters that are known to show inducible expression. The cloning and sequencing steps necessary to generate each new reporter can be time-consuming and will not necessarily result in a functional reporter. To this end a number of reporter plasmids, including NF-κB and AP-1, are now commercially available (Clontech, Basingstoke, Hampshire, UK).
15. Transfection conditions should be optimized using a reporter vector, such as pGL3control (Promega), which gives rise to high-level constitutive luciferase expression. A dose-response analysis, using increasing amounts of DNA at a constant DNA:lipid ratio, should be performed to determine the optimal concentration of DNA and the tolerance of the cells to the procedure. In addition, the ratio of DNA to lipid will also affect the transfection efficiency, and should be tested.
16. G-418 at 0.5 mg/mL is effective against A549 cells. Optimal concentrations required for complete cell death should be determined for other cell lines.
17. Reaction could be scaled down for 12- or 24-well plate formats, resulting in savings in reagents.
18. Clearly, it is essential that luciferase readings are performed in the linear part of the assay. This can readily be confirmed by serial dilution of a sample, and subsequent analysis.

References

1. Hunter, T. and Karin, M. (1992) The regulation of transcription by phosphorylation. *Cell* **70,** 375–387.
2. Hill, C. S. and Treisman, R. (1995) Transcriptional regulation by extracellular signals: mechanisms and specificity. *Cell* **80,** 199–211.
3. Roeder, R. G. (1991) The complexities of eukaryotic transcription initiation: regulation of preinitiation complex assembly. *Trends. Biochem. Sci.* **16,** 402–408.
4. Buratowski, S. (1994) The basics of basal transcription by RNA polymerase II. *Cell* **77,** 1–3.
5. Tjian, R. and Maniatis, T. (1994) Transcriptional activation: a complex puzzle with few easy pieces. *Cell* **77,** 5–8.
6. Goodrich, J. A., Cutler, G., and Tjian, R. (1996) Contacts in context: promoter specificity and macromolecular interactions in transcription. *Cell* **84,** 825–830.
7. Siebenlist, U., Franzoso, G., and Brown, K. (1994) Structure, regulation and function of NF-κB. *Annu. Rev. Cell Biol.* **10,** 405–455.
8. Angel, P. and Karin, M. (1991) The role of Jun, Fos and the AP-1 complex in cell-proliferation and transformation. *Biochim. Biophys. Acta* **1072,** 129–157.
9. Roesler, W. J., Vandenbark, G. R., and Hanson, R. W. (1988) Cyclic AMP and the induction of eukaryotic gene transcription. *J. Biol. Chem.* **263,** 9063–9066.
10. Lalli, E. and Sassone Corsi, P. (1994) Signal transduction and gene regulation: the nuclear response to cAMP. *J. Biol. Chem.* **269,** 17,359–17,362.
11. Akira, S., Isshiki, H., Sugita, T., Tanabe, O., Kinoshita, S., Nishio, Y., et al. (1990) A nuclear factor for IL-6 expression (NF-IL6) is a member of a C/EBP family. *EMBO J.* **9,** 1897–1906.
12. Barnes, P. J. and Karin, M. (1997) Nuclear factor-κB: a pivotal transcription factor in chronic inflammatory diseases. *N. Engl. J. Med.* **336,** 1066–1071.
13. Thanos, D. and Maniatis, T. (1995) NF-κB: a lesson in family values. *Cell* **80,** 529–532.
14. Maniatis, T. (1997) Catalysis by a multiprotein IκB kinase complex. *Science* **278,** 818, 819.
15. Yaron, A., Hatzubai, A., Davis, M., Lavon, I., Amit, S., Manning, A. M., et al. (1998) Identification of the receptor component of the IκBα-ubiquitin ligase. *Nature* **396,** 590–594.
16. Newton, R., Kuitert, L. M., Bergmann, M., Adcock, I. M., and Barnes, P. J. (1997) Evidence for involvement of NF-κB in the transcriptional control of COX-2 gene expression by IL-1β. *Biochem. Biophys. Res. Commun.* **237,** 28–32.
17. van de Stolpe, A., Caldenhoven, E., Stade, B. G., Koenderman, L., Raaijmakers, J. A., Johnson, J. P., and van der Saag, P. T. (1994) 12-O-tetradecanoylphorbol-13-acetate- and tumor necrosis factor alpha-mediated induction of intercellular adhesion molecule-1 is inhibited by dexamethasone. Functional analysis of the human intercellular adhesion molecular-1 promoter. *J. Biol. Chem.* **269,** 6185–6192.
18. Dignam, J. D., Lebovitz, R. M., and Roeder, R. G. (1983) Accurate transcription initiation by RNA polymerase II in a soluble extract from isolated mammalian nuclei. *Nucleic Acids Res.* **11,** 1475–1489.

19. Osborn, L., Kunkel, S., and Nabel, G. J. (1989) Tumor necrosis factor α and interleukin 1 stimulate the human immunodeficiency virus enhancer by activation of the nuclear factor κB. *Proc. Natl. Acad. Sci. USA* **86,** 2336–2340.
20 Sambrook, J., Fritsch, E. F., and Maniatis, T. (1989) *Molecular Cloning: A Laboratory Manual,* 2nd ed. Cold Spring Harbor Laboratory, Cold Spring Harbor, NY.
21. Karin, M. (1996) Regulation of AP-1 activity by mitogen-activated protein kinases. *Philos. Trans. R. Soc. Lond. B. Biol. Sci.* **351,** 127–134.
22. Derijard, B., Hibi, M., Wu, I. H., Barrett, T., Su, B., Deng, T., Karin, M., and Davis, R. J. (1994) JNK1: a protein kinase stimulated by UV light and Ha-Ras that binds and phosphorylates the c-Jun activation domain. *Cell* **76,** 1025–1037.
23. Bergmann, M., Hart, L., Lindsay, M., Barnes, P. J., and Newton, R. (1998) IκBα degradation and nuclear factor-κB DNA binding are insufficient for interleukin-1β and tumor necrosis factor-α induced κB-dependent transcription: requirement for an additional activation pathway. *J. Biol. Chem.* **273,** 6607–6610.
24. Newton, R., Hart, L. A., Stevens, D. A., Bergmann, M., Donnelly, L. E., Adcock, I. M., and Barnes, P. J. (1998) Effect of dexamethasone on interleukin-1β (IL-1β) induced nuclear factor-κB (NF-κB) and κB-dependent transcription in epithelial cells. *Eur. J. Biochem.* **254,** 81–89.
25. Malinin, N. L., Boldin, M. P., Kovalenko, A. V., and Wallach, D. (1997) MAP3K-related kinase involved in NF-κB induction by TNF, CD95 and IL-1. *Nature* **385,** 540–544.
26. Hart, L. A., Krishnan, V. L., Adcock, I. M., Barnes, P. J., and Chung, K. F. (1998) Activation and localization of transcription factor, nuclear factor-κB, in asthma. *Am. J. Respir. Crit. Care Med.* **158,** 1585–1592.
27. Gough, N. M. (1988) Rapid and quantitative preparation of cytoplasmic RNA from small numbers of cells. *Anal. Biochem.* **173,** 93–95.
28. Newton, R., Stevens, D. A., Hart, L. A., Lindsay, M., Adcock, I. M., and Barnes, P. J. (1997) Superinduction of COX-2 mRNA by cycloheximide and interleukin-1β involves increased transcription and correlates with increased NF-κB and JNK activation. *FEBS Lett.* **418,** 135–138.
29. Mercurio, F., Zhu, H., Murray, B. W., Shevchenko, A., Bennett, B. L., Li, J., et al. (1997) IKK-1 and IKK-2: cytokine-activated IκB kinases essential for NF-κB activation. *Science* **278,** 860–866.

13

Transient Transgenic Approaches for Investigating the Role of Granulocyte-Macrophage Colony-Stimulating Factor in Pulmonary Inflammatory and Immune Diseases

Zhou Xing, Martin R. Stämpfli, and Jack Gauldie

1. Introduction

Granulocyte-macrophage colony-stimulating factor (GM-CSF), a 23-kDa polypeptide, was originally identified as a hematopoietic growth factor, but has recently been found to be a multifunctional cytokine with many proinflammatory activities *(1,2)*. GM-CSF can be produced by, and act upon, a broad range of cell types, including both immature and mature granulocyte and monocyte lineage cells, dendritic cells, and tissue structural cells. Abundant in vitro observations have suggested that GM-CSF is able to induce both differentiation and activation of these cells *(1)*.

GM-CSF has been found heightened in a number of pulmonary inflammatory and immune diseases, both allergic and nonallergic, including asthma, sarcoidosis, eosinophil pneumonia, lung carcinomas, and idiopathic pulmonary fibrosis *(2)*. However, the precise role of GM-CSF in the pathogenesis of these conditions remains incompletely understood. One invaluable tool that has been frequently used to study cytokine functions in vivo is genetic transgenic animals. However, random incorporation of transgene into the host genome, and early embryogenic exposure to transgene product in transgenics, are among potential concerns. During inflammatory responses, cytokines are often expressed in a transient and tissue-directed manner over an adult host background; therefore, a transient transgene approach would be more desirable for cytokine functional studies in vivo. To study the role of GM-CSF in the pathogenic processes underlying pulmonary fibrosis and asthmatic inflammation, the

From: *Methods in Molecular Medicine, vol. 44: Asthma: Mechanisms and Protocols*
Edited by: K. F. Chung and I. Adcock © Humana Press Inc., Totowa, NJ

authors have engineered a recombinant replication-deficient human type 5 adenovirus (ADV) vector to express murine GM-CSF transgene (AdGM-CSF), and have developed intrapulmonary gene transfer techniques to achieve prolonged, but relatively transient, adjustable levels of GM-CSF transgene expression in adult rodents.

Construction of AdGM-CSF involves insertion of the murine GM-CSF cDNA into the E1 region of the human type 5 ADV genome. Disruption in E1 results in viral replication deficiency, because the E1 region is essential for viral replication *(3)*. A fragment of the murine GM-CSF cDNA is first ligated into the E1 multicloning site of a shuttle plasmid, which accommodates a human cytomegalovirus (CMV) promoter and a SV40 poly(A^+) signal sequences. The resulting construct, containing the left 16% of the ADV genome, is cotransfected into 293 cells, which provide the E1 function *in trans*, along with a second viral rescuing plasmid containing all of the ADV genomic sequences but the left end. The recombinant virus, with murine GM-CSF incorporated in E1 driven by the CMV promoter, is rescued by homologous recombination (**Fig. 1**). The rescued recombinant virus is characterized, amplified, purified, and titrated.

Routinely, purified AdGM-CSF, or a control viral vector that does not contain a transgene, is instilled intratracheally into the lung of rats or intranasally into the lung of mice. Transgene is targeted primarily into bronchial, but not tracheal, epithelial cells and, to a lesser degree, to alveolar epithelial cells and intra-alveolar macrophages *(2)*. Transgene expression results in raised levels of transgene protein, mostly compartmentalized within the lung for approx 12–16 d. Depending on the level of transgene protein in the lung, there will be a small amount of spill-over to the circulation, which is normally 200–400× lower than in the lung.

By using these approaches, the authors have been able to reveal an important role of GM-CSF in the development of airway eosinophilia and fibrosis, and the differentiation and activation of pulmonary dendritic cells, not only in normal naïve animals, but also in models of asthmatic airways inflammation *(4–7)*.

The methods described below may also be applied to constructing recombinant replication-deficient ADV vectors expressing cytokines or growth factors other than GM-CSF, and creating pulmonary transient transgenic mouse or rat models for functional and/or therapeutic studies.

2. Materials

2.1. Construction of AdGM-CSF

1. Plasmid pCDSRα containing the full-length murine GM-CSF cDNA, the shuttle plasmid pACCMV containing 0–17 mu human type 5 ADV genome with a 760-bp human CMV promoter and a 430-bp SV40 splicing junction–poly(A) signal,

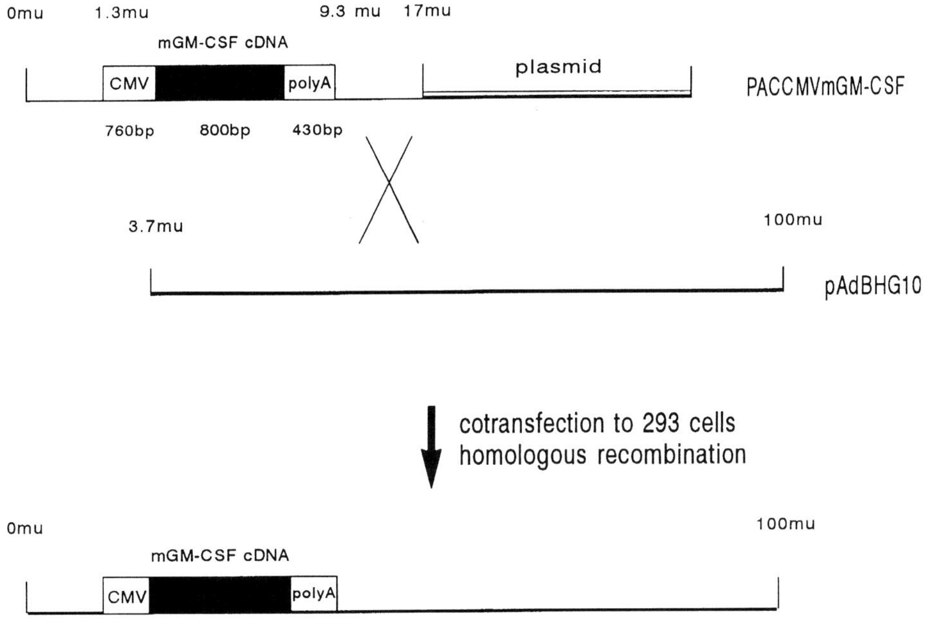

Fig. 1. Construction of recombinant adenoviral vector Ad5E1PACCMVmGM-CSF (AdGM-CSF). The recombinant plasmid PACCMVmGM-CSF was constructed by inserting murine GM-CSF cDNA into the multicloning site of a shuttle vector pACCMV, which harbored a cytomegalovirus (CMV) promoter and a SV40 splicing junction/poly(A) signal. The recombinant ADV AdGM-CSF was generated by homologous recombination after cotransfecting 293 cells with PACCMVmGM-CSF and a virus-rescuing vector pAdBHG10.

and the viral rescuing plasmid pAdBHG10 containing the most rightward sequences (3.7–100 mu) of human type 5 ADV genome with a partial deletion in the E3 region ***(4,8)***.

2. Endonuclease restriction enzymes *Bam*HI, *Dra*I, and *Sal*I; T4 kinase, T4 ligase, and deoxynucleoside-triphosphate (dNTPs) (New England Biolabs).
3. 293 cells, 1X minimum essential medium (MEM)-F-11 culture media containing 10% fetal bovine serum (FBS), 1% penicillin, and streptamycin; 2X MEM-F-11 culture media containing 10% FBS, 0.1% yeast extract, 2% P/S, 2% L-glutamine, and 0.05 μg fungizone/100 mL (kept in 44°C water bath before use).
4. Overlay agarose: 1.0 g agarose + 100 mL distilled water, dissolved in a microwave and kept in a 44°C water bath before use.
5. 1X HEBS buffer, pH 7.1 (4 g NaCl, 2.5 g HEPES, 0.185 g KCl, 0.05 g, Na_2HPO_4, 0.5 g D-glucose in 480 mL distilled water), 2.5 *M* $CaCl_2$.

6. Phosphate-buffered saline $(PBS)^{2+}$ buffer: PBS 100 mL, 1 mL 1% $CaCl_2$, and 1 mL 1% $MgCl_2$.

2.2. Amplification of AdGM-CSF

1. For small-scale amplification, confluent 293 cells in 6-cm dishes; MEM-F11 media containing 5% FBS and 0.05 μg fungizone/100 mL.
2. Cell scraper.
3. For large-scale amplification, expanded 293N3S cells in spinner bottles; Joklik culture media containing 5% FBS, 1% penicillin and streptamycin, and 1% L-glutamine.

2.3. Purification of AdGM-CSF

1. Virus pellet resuspended in 0.1 *M* Tris-HCl, pH 8.0.
2. 5% Na deoxyclolate (DOC), sterilized by filtration through filters.
3. CsCl gradients.
4. 50Ti rotor, SW50.1 rotor buckets, Beckman polyallomer quickseal tubes, Beckman centrifuge tubes (Beckman Instruments Inc., Palo Alto, CA).
5. Top-off solution: 1.8 mL saturated CsCl, 3.2 mL 0.1 *M* Tris-HCl, pH 8.0, and 1 m*M* ethylenediamine tetraacetic acid (EDTA).
6. PD-10 Sephadex columns (Pharmacia Biotech, Baie d'Urfé, Quebec, Canada).
7. Sterile 10% glycerol in PBS.
8. Conductance meter (Yellow Springs Instrument, Becton Dickinson Labware, Franklin Lakes, NJ), sterile round-bottomed polystyrene tubes (Falcon 2058 and 2057, 6- and 14-mL size, respectively).

2.4. Titration of AdGM-CSF

1. 70–80% confluent 293 cells in 6-cm dishes.
2. 2X MEM-F11 culture media and overlay agarose, prepared as described in **Subheading 2.1.**

2.5. Intratracheal Administration of AdGM-CSF

1. Normal rats weighing 280–340 g.
2. AdGM-CSF or a control ADV vector, Addl70-3, properly diluted to a total volume of 300 μL with sterile PBS, pH 7.4.
3. 1-mL syringes attached to 26-gage needles; curved forceps; surgical scalps; anesthetic isoflurane; 50-mL plastic tubes; 70% ethanol; wound clips.

2.6. Intranasal Administration of AdGM-CSF

1. Normal specific pathogen-free mice at the age of 8–14 wk.
2. AdGM-CSF or Addl70–3, properly diluted to a total volume of 30 μL with sterile PBS, pH 7.4.
3. P-20 Pipetteman, autoclaved fine pipet tips, anesthetic isoflurane.

2.7. Analysis of Transgene Expression in the Lung by Polymerase Chain Reaction

1. 2 μg total lung tissue RNA sample for each time-point, kept at –70°C freezer.
2. Sense and antisense murine GM-CSF primers (5'-GTCTCTAACGAGTTCTCC TTCAAG-3' and 5'-TTCAGAGGGCTATACTGCCTTCCA-3').
3. 40 U rRNasin, 0.5 μg random primer, 10 m*M* of each dNTP, 20 U reverse transcriptase, and 25 μL reaction buffer. These reagents are used for reverse transcription.
4. Polymerase chain reaction (PCR) buffer (Promega, Madison, WI), pH 9.0: 10 m*M* Tris-HCl, 50 m*M* KCl, 1.5 m*M* $MgCl_2$, and 0.1% Triton X-100, 1.25 m*M* of each dNTP, 5 μL of each reversed transcribed product, 150 pmol antisense and sense GM-CSF primers, 2.5 U Taq DNA polymerase, and 50 μL mineral oil. These reagents are used for PCR amplification.
5. Apparatus used for gel electrophoresis: agarose gel, gel box, and power supply.

2.8. Analysis of Transgene Protein in the Lung by Enzyme-Linked Immunosorbent Assay

1. Bronchoalveolar lavage (BAL) fluids stored at –20°C freezer.
2. Commercially obtained enzyme-linked immunosorbent assay (ELISA) kits detecting murine GM-CSF.

2.9. Analysis of Cellular Responses in BAL

1. BAL fluids collected in Eppendorf tubes from the lung at various times, and stored on ice.
2. Hemacytometer, cell counter, and microscope.
3. Glass slides, Cytospiner, Hemat-Tek 2000 Slide Stainer (Miles, Swedenboro, NJ).

2.10. Histologic Examination of Lung Tissue

1. 10% formalin.
2. Tissue-processing equipment: tissue processor, H&E stain, Congo red stain, elastic van Gieson stain.
3. Mouse antirat α smooth muscle (α-SMA) actin monoclonal antibody (Sigma, St. Louis, MO); Vectastain Elite ABC mouse immunoglobulin G staining kit (Vector Laboratories, Burlingame, CA).

2.11. Mouse Models of Asthmatic Airway Inflammation

1. Specific pathogen-free Balb/c mice at the age of 6–8 wk.
2. Ovalbumin (OVA) (Sigma), aluminum hydroxide (Aldrich, Milwaukee, WI).
3. Plexiglas chamber; Bennette/Twin nebulizer; medical air tank with an air-flow regulator.

3. Methods

3.1. Construction of AdGM-CSF

Construction of AdGM-CSF is fairly a straightforward procedure. Both the shuttle plasmid pACCMV and viral rescuing plasmid pAdBHG10 may be obtained from the authors upon request. The nature of promoter sequences is of importance in determining the level of transgene expression. The 760-bp human CMV promoter, which the authors had in AdGM-CSF, or a murine CMV promoter, were the best choice ***(9)***. Because AdGM-CSF has a defective E1 region, and is therefore replication-deficient, the rescuing of this recombinant virus has to be implemented in a complementary cell line, 293 cells, which has been transformed to express the E1a gene whose function allows viral replication ***(10)***.

1. Digest pCDSRα plasmid with *Bam*HI and *Dra*I at 37°C for 1 h to release an 800-bp fragment of murine GM-CSF cDNA.
2. Digest pACCMV plasmid with *Sal*I at 37°C for 1 h to linearize the plasmid, and the ends are repaired with T4 kinase and dNTPs; this plasmid is then subjected to a second digestion with *Bam*HI at 37°C for 1 h, to generate the 3' complementary ends.
3. Subclone the GM-CSF cDNA into the *Bam*HI–*Sal*I site in pACCMV plasmid by ligation with T4 ligase at 16°C overnight.
4. Transform the ligation product (pACCMVGM-CSF) into *Escherichia coli* cells, and grow cells in a small-scale culture overnight in the presence of ampicillin. Purify plasmid DNA and check the presence and orientation of GM-CSF cDNA by restriction digestion and gel electrophoresis.
5. Purify the recombinant plasmid, pACCMVGM-CSF, on a large scale, and store purified DNA in Tris–EDTA (TE)8 buffer at –20°C until use.
6. Prepare 293 cell monolayer (60–80% confluence) in 60-mm culture dishes the night before cotransfection.
7. To prepare DNA precipitates, add 1 mL 1X HEBS, pH 7.0, to a 14-mL clear, round-bottomed tube, add 20 μg each of pACCMVGM-CSF and pAdBHG10, and then add 50 μL 2.5 *M* $CaCl_2$ drop-wise, with a fine pipet tip, while mixing slowly by gentle agitation, and incubate at room temperature (RT) for 15 min.
8. Add 0.5 mL DNA precipitates to each 293 cell dish with 5 mL culture media, and incubate in a CO_2 37°C incubator for 16 h (*see* **Note 1**).
9. Remove the media, add 10 mL overlay media (prepared by mixing overlay agarose with 2X MEM-F11 media, 1:1, just prior to use), and let solidify in the hood for about 10 min before returning to CO_2 incubator (*see* **Note 1**).
10. Incubate for 1–2 wk, check for viral plaques daily after 5 d incubation, and pick up plaques with a pipet tip into PBS^{2+} buffer in individual cryotubes, and store at –70°C until amplification.

3.2. Amplification of AdGM-CSF

Initial characterization of viral plaques is highly recommended. To this end, harvested plaques are subjected to a small-scale amplification. A verified plaque will then be chosen and subjected to a large-scale amplification procedure using spinner culture bottles.

3.2.1. Small-Scale Amplification and Characterization of AdGM-CSF

1. Add 100–250 µL viral plaque preparation in PBS^{2+} to a 60-mm dish of confluent 293 cells in 3–5 mL culture media.
2. Incubate in a CO_2 incubator for 3–5 d until the cell monolayer is approx 100% lysed.
3. Scrape adherent cells into the media, and collect cells and media into a tube, centrifuge at 4°C for 10 min to pellet, collect supernatant, and save for large-scale amplification of virus.
4. Add 0.5 mL pronase–sodium dodeoyl sulfate (SDS) solution (0.05 mL 5 mg/mL pronase in 0.01 *M* Tris-HCl, pH 7.5, 0.01 mL 0.5 *M* EDTA, pH 8.0, 0.025 mL 10% SDS, 0.415 mL 1 *M* Tris-HCl, pH 7.5) to the pellet, pipet and incubate at 37°C for 3–4 h.
5. Extract viral DNA by the standard phenol extraction method, and dissolve DNA in 50 µL TE8 buffer.
6. Digest 5 or 10 µL viral DNA with 100 U *Hin*dIII at 37°C for 2–14 h, analyze the resultant DNA fragments by electrophoresis and Southern hybridization with a murine GM-CSF cDNA (**Fig. 2A,B**; *see* **Note 2**).

3.2.2. Large-Scale Amplification of AdGM-CSF

1. Use supernatants saved from small-scale amplification to infect 293 monolayers in 2–3 150-cm^2 flasks containing 30–40 mL culture media, and culture for 3–4 d until the monolayer is 70–80% lysed, collect supernatants, clear by centrifugation for 10 min, and store at –70°C.
2. Transfer two flasks of confluent 293N3S cells to two 1-L spinner bottles with 850 mL Joklik culture media, and allow to grow in a 37°C warm room under constant stirring.
3. Follow cell density beginning at 4–5 d, until it reaches $>2 \times 10^5$ cells/mL, then transfer the cell content from each spinner bottle to a 3-L spinner bottle with a total volume of media built up to 3 L, and allow to grow for additional 4–5 d, until the density reaches 2×10^5 cells/mL.
4. Transfer the cell content from each bottle to three 1-L centrifuge bottles, and centrifuge at 600*g* for 15 min at RT in a centrifuge with brakes off.
5. Save 50% of supernatants for later; resuspend cell pellet in 300 mL virus inoculum media (Joklik media containing 1% FBS, 1% penicillin and streptamycin, and 1% L-glutamine), and transfer to an 1-L spinner bottle, add approx 80 mL virus-containing supernatant saved from **step 1**, and incubate in a 37°C warm room for 1.5 h.

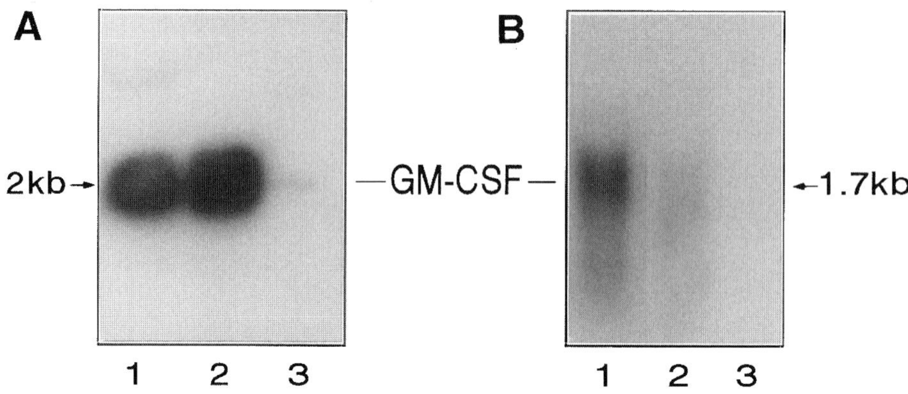

Fig. 2. **(A)** Characterization of AdGM-CSF by *Hin*dIII digestion. The viral genomic DNA was extracted from purified AdGM-CSF, and digested with *Hin*dIII. The resultant fragments were gel-separated, and further hybridized to a murine GM-CSF cDNA probe. Lanes 1 and 2, 5 and 10 µg viral genomic DNA from AdGM-CSF, respectively; lane 3, 5 µg viral genomic DNA from a wild type ADV as a control. **(B)** Characterization of AdGM-CSF by examination of transgene-derived mRNA. 293 cells were infected with 10 PFU/cell of AdGM-CSF, or Addl70-3 as a control, and total RNA was extracted and hybridized to a murine GM-CSF cDNA probe. Lanes 1 and 2, cells infected with AdGM-CSF for 24 and 48 h, respectively; lane 3, Ccells infected with Addl70-3 for 24 h.

6. Transfer back to a 3-L spinner bottle containing a total volume of media built up to 3 L, and incubate at 37°C, with constant stirring, for about 3–4 d.
7. Check inclusion body, until 90% of cells contain the inclusion bodies: Incubate a cell pellet in 0.5 mL 1% Na-citrate for 10 min at RT, add 0.5 mL Carnoy's fixative, and incubate for additional 10 min at RT, add 1 mL 1% Na-citrate, centrifuge at 80*g* for 10 min at RT, resuspend pellet in five drops of 1% Na-citrate, add one drop of cell suspension onto a glass slide, air-dry for 1 h, add 1 drop of Orcein, cover slip, and examine under a microscope.
8. Harvest cells by centrifuge in 1-L bottles in an MSE centrifuge.
9. Save five 40-mL tubes of virus-containing supernatants, and store at –70°C for future large-scale preparation; discard the remaining supernatants (*see* **Note 3**).
10. Resuspend pellets with 15 mL 0.1 *M* Tris-HCl, pH 8.0 (save 2 mL as crude virus for future infection), and store at -70% until viral purification.

3.3. Purification of AdGM-CSF

Add 1.3 mL 5% Na DOC (final concentration 0.5%) to 13 mL viral suspension, incubate at RT for 30 min, with a couple of agitations, then add 143 µL 2 *M* $MgCl_2$ (final concentration 0.02 *M*) and 10 mg/mL DNase I, to a final concentration of 50 μg/mL, and incubate at 37°C for 45 min, with gentle mixing each 10 min. After these steps, the preparation is subjected to two consecutive banding procedures.

3.3.1. First Banding

1. Add 1/10 vol of 5% Na DOC (0.5% final concentration) to the virus suspension, and incubate at RT for 30 min, with occasional agitations.
2. Add 1/100 vol of 2 *M* $MgCl_2$ to the preparation (final concentration 0.02 *M*), and 1/200 vol of 10 mg/mL DNase I, to a final concentration of 50 μg/mL, and incubate at 37°C for 45 min, with gentle mixing each 10 min.
3. Centrifuge at 1500*g* for 15 min at 4°C in a Beckman TJ-6 centrifuge, and transfer the supernatant to another tube; discard the pellet.
4. Prepare CsCl step gradients, and, to each Ultra Clear centrifuge tube (Beckman Instruments, Inc., Palo Alto, CA) (three tubes are required for a 3-L spinner bottle content), add the following step gradients: 0.5, 3, and 3 mL of $CsCl_2$ with a density 1.5, 1.35, and 1.25, respectively.
5. Load 5 mL sample supernatant, saved above, onto the gradients in each tube, and balance all tubes with 0.1 *M* Tris-HCl, pH 8.0, and centrifuge in a SW41 Ti rotor at 150,000*g* at 10°C for 1 h, with the brakes off.
6. Collect the virus band to a 14-mL tube by using a 3-mL syringe attached to a 20-gage needle (see **Note 4**).

3.3.2. Second Banding

1. Add the top-off solution to the collected virus band, to a final volume of 4.8 mL; mix, and transfer the content to a Beckman centrifuge tube (13 × 51 mm).
2. Balance the tubes with top-off solution, and engage tubes into the buckets.
3. Centrifuge in a SW50.1 rotor at 120,000*g*, 4°C, for 16–18 h, with the brakes off.
4. Clamp the tube on a retort stand, with a beaker containing bleach placed below the tube to collect the waste; collect the viral band by piercing a hole with a 20-needle gage.
5. Subject the viral band to PD-10 column chromatography to remove CsCl: Adjust the volume of virus obtained from **step 4** to 2.5 mL with PD-10 buffer, equilibrate each PD-10 column with 25 mL PD-10 buffer, load 2.5 mL viral sample on the PD-10 column, collect each 0.5-mL fraction into separate 6-mL tubes, add 3.5 mL PD-10 buffer to the column, and continue to collect each 0.5-mL fraction; repeat this once more; measure conductance by using 50 μL of each fraction, and pool fractions, 7–11 of which normally contain CsCl-free virus.
6. Collect AdGM-CSF in 0.5-mL aliquots into cryovials, and store at –70°C until titration.

3.4. Titration of AdGM-CSF

1. Make serial dilutions of virus with PBS^{2+} buffer, ranging from 10^8 to 10^{10}.
2. Remove the media from cultured 70–80% confluent 293 cells.

3. Add 200 µL of each diluted virus dropwise evenly to the cell monolayer, and leave dishes at RT for 45 min in the hood.
4. Prepare overlay solutions, and warm up at 44°C, mix 2X MEM-F11 with overlay agarose, 1:1, just before use.
5. Add 10 mL overlay solution to each dish, allow to solidify in the hood, and return to the CO_2 incubator and incubate for 5–10 d. Count plaques, and calculate the concentration (*see* **Note 5**).

3.5. Intratracheal Administration of AdGM-CSF in Rats

Intratracheal (IT) administration of AdGM-CSF is a straightforward procedure. Since the rat has a relatively long passage of the upper airway, ADV vectors delivered in such a way will remain within the respiratory system without spilling over to the gastrointestinal (GI) tract. In mice, the IT route can be an option for the delivery of AdGM-CSF as well, alternative to the intranasal (IN) route, except that the IT procedure will be much more delicate in mice. Virus delivered through IT or IN route targets the transgene primarily to the bronchial epithelium and, to a lesser extent, to the alveolar epithelium and alveolar macrophages ***(5,11)***.

1. Anesthetize rats, and place them on a slanted board. Anesthesia is maintained with a nose cone.
2. A frontal midline incision is made with a blade, sterilized with 70% ethanol; the skin and muscle layers are blunt-separated with sterile forceps, to expose the trachea.
3. A dose of 10^9 PFU AdGM-CSF, or a control vector diluted with PBS, to a final volume of 300 µL is instilled into the trachea by using a 26-gage needle and 1-mL syringe. The soft tissues are allowed to rejoin, and 2–3 wound-healing clips are dispensed to close the skin (*see* **Note 6**).

3.6. Intranasal Administration of AdGM-CSF in Mice

IN delivery is a noninvasive, simple way to administer ADV vector to the lung of mice. In comparison, the IT procedure in mice requires more skill. From time to time, however, a small amount of vector will inevitably be taken into the GI tract. Nonetheless, in most of the studies that the authors have carried out, this is not a problem that will confound the experimental results ***(5,7,12)***.

1. Mice are anesthetized, and restrained in a hand, with the head up.
2. A desirable dose of AdGM-CSF or a control vector, diluted in a total of 30 µL PBS, is applied, in two aliquots, to the nostril, slowly, so that the mouse can breathe the content into the airway. The second aliquot is delivered to the mouse that has rested for a short while in an anesthetic chamber (*see* **Note 7**).
3. Mice are released back to the cage, and should recover soon thereafter.

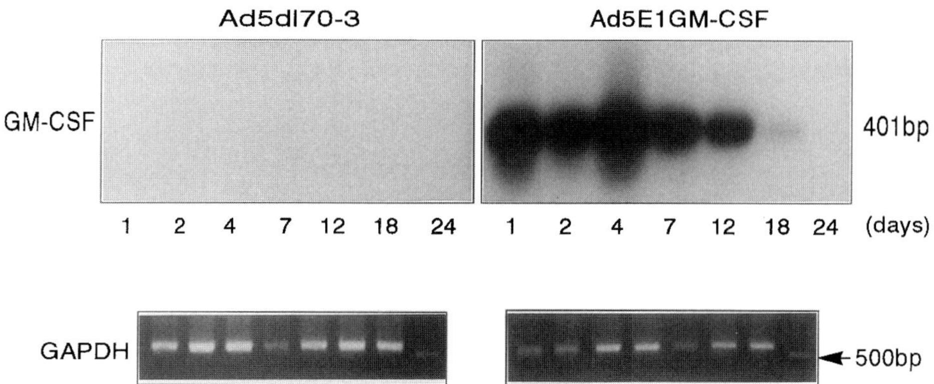

Fig. 3. GM-CSF transgene expression in rat lung by RT-PCR and Southern hybridization. A dose of 10^9 PFU AdGM-CSF, or Addl70-3 as a control, was intratracheally injected into rat lung, and total lung RNA was extracted at d 1, 2, 4, 7, 12, 18, and 24 post-gene transfer and amplified by RT-PCR, using specific primers for murine GM-CSF. The PCR products (401 bp) were hybridized to a murine GM-CSF cDNA probe. The same total RNA samples were also amplified by RT-PCR for rat GAPDH as an internal control, and the PCR products (555 bp) were visualized by ethidium bromide staining.

3.7. Analysis of Transgene Expression in the Lung by PCR

The level and kinetics of transgene mRNA expression may be analyzed by a number of means, including Northern analysis ***(11)***, *in situ* hybridization ***(11)***, and PCR ***(4,13)***; each method has its own pros and cons, but PCR analysis is a faster and more straightforward way.

1. To 2 μg total lung RNA, add 40 U of rRNasin, 0.5 μg random primer, 10 m*M* of each dNTP, and 20 U reverse transcriptase, and incubate in a total of 25 μL reaction mixture buffer for 1 h at 42°C.
2. To 5 μL reverse transcription product, add 1.25 m*M* of each dNTP, 150 pmol of both antisense and sense murine GM-CSF primers, 2.5 U *Taq* DNA polymerase and PCR reaction mixture buffer, to a total volume of 100 μL, and top with 50 μL mineral oil.
3. 40 cycles of PCR amplification are performed using a DNA thermal cycler.
4. PCR products are subjected to gel electrophoresis; the expected size of PCR products specific for murine GM-CSF mRNA should be 401 bp.
5. Optionally, the gel may be transferred onto a nylon membrane and subjected to Southern hybridization by using a murine GM-CSF cDNA probe, in order to demonstrate the specificity of PCR products (**Fig. 3**).

3.8. Analysis of Transgene Protein in the Lung by ELISA

The level of GM-CSF in BAL fluids (*see* **Subheading 3.9.** for BAL procedure) can be easily measured by using specific ELISA kits, by following steps described by the manufacturer. For the purpose of localizing transgene protein in the lung, however, immunohistochemistry (IHC) should be carried out.

3.9. Analysis of Cellular Responses in BAL

This involves carrying out the BAL procedures and cytologic analysis. Easy access to cellular constituents in the intra-alveolar compartment of the lung allows easy quantification of the cellular responses in various animal models.

3.9.1. Bronchoalveolar Lavage

The following BAL procedure is carried out in mice. The only difference to BAL in rats is that the entire lung does not have to be moved out of the thoracic cavity, and BAL is carried out *in situ* ***(4,11,14)***.

1. At various time-points after virus delivery, mice are sacrificed and bled via the lower abdominal artery and vein.
2. From the abdominal cavity, the diaphragm is perforated by using a pair of scissors, thc thoracic cavity is opened, and the lungs are carefully removed, with a portion of trachea attached.
3. The trachea is cannulated with a polyethylene tube (Becton Dickinson, PE50) attached to a 25-gage needle and 1-mL syringe.
4. The lungs are lavaged twice with 0.25 mL and 0.20 mL PBS, respectively.
5. Approximately 0.3–0.4 mL instilled fluid will be recovered into an Eppendorf tube (*see* **Note 8**).
6. Leave BAL fluids on ice.

3.9.2. Cytologic Analysis

1. Spin to pellet each BAL sample in a microcentrifuge at 800*g* for 5 min at RT or 4°C.
2. Save and store supernatant at –20°C for cytokine ELISA assay.
3. Resuspend the pellet in 500–800 µL PBS, depending on the size of pellet.
4. Count cell number on a hemocytometer.
5. Make a cytospin on a glass slide with about 100 µL cell suspension and stain cells by using a Hemat-Tek 2000 Slide Stainer (*see* **Note 9**).
6. Count about 300–500 cells on each cytospin for differential cell types, and calculate percentages of differentials and absolute cell numbers, based on total cell counts.

3.10. Histologic Examination of Lung Tissue

Although BAL cell analysis provides quantitative information on differential cell types in the lung, it provides information only on the types of cells present within the airways and alveolar spaces, and may not adequately represent the level and type of tissue responses. Thus, complementary to BAL analysis, conventional histologic examination of lung tissue is of importance, and should be carried out on a routine basis. In addition, to provide more specific information on cell types, extracellular matrix components or cell surface markers, specific histochemical or IHC staining will be required.

3.10.1. Conventional Histologic Examination and Histochemical Staining

1. After BAL, both sides of lungs are perfused slowly with 0.2 mL 10% formalin, and the trachea is then tied up with suture and the lung is placed into an Eppendorf tube with 10% formalin, in case only the conventional histology is desired, or into a 15-mL plastic tube containing at least 10 mL 10% formalin, in case both conventional histology and IHC are to be performed (*see* **Note 10**).
2. Fix the lung in formalin for about 20–24 h (see **Note 10**).
3. Subject the fixed lung to tissue processing, including paraffin-embedding, sectioning, and conventional H&E staining.
4. If eosinophil identification is desired, Congo red histochemical staining can be carried out with hematoxylin counterstaining. Eosinophils are stained pink to red ***(4,7)***.
5. If identification of collagen and elastin is desirable, elastic van Gieson staining should be carried out. Collagen and elastin are stained pink and black, respectively ***(4,14)***.

3.10.2. IHC Staining for Identification of Myofibroblasts

αSMA serves as a hallmark for the myofibroblast phenotype ***(15)***. In normal lung, only vascular or bronchial smooth muscle cells are stained positive for αSMA. Following transgene expression of fibrogenic cytokines, however, there is a marked increase in the number of myofibroblastic cells in fibrosing foci throughout the lung parenchyma ***(4,14)***.

1. Rat lung tissue sections are deparaffinized in toluene for 5 min, twice, and dipped up and down in 95% ethanol 20×.
2. Soak in ethanol–formal solution for 5 min, and in running water for 10 min.
3. Treat sections with 0.3% hydrogen peroxide in Tris-buffered saline for 30 min.
4. Wash twice, 5 min each, with Tris-buffered saline.
5. Incubate sections with blocking serum 1 for 30 min.
6. Incubate with anti-αSMA monoclonal antibody or the control mouse mouse immunoglobulin G1 antibody at 1:800 dilution overnight.
7. After wash, incubate with sera 2 and 3 in Vectastain kit for 60 and 30 min, respectively.
8. Incubate with substrate–chromogen solution for 8 min.
9. The final immunoreactive product is identified as a red-brown-colored deposit.

3.11. Mouse Models of Asthmatic Airway Inflammation

In addition to studying the functional activities of GM-CSF in normal rodent lung, mouse models of allergic airways inflammation may be used to directly address the role of GM-CSF in pathogenic processes. The advantage is that normally very little endogenous GM-CSF is induced in these models *(17)*, which allows a unique opportunity to study the role of GM-CSF in the pathogenesis of this cytokine in asthma. To this end, the authors have established and used two models. One is regarded as a model of asthmatic airway inflammation, in which a typical allergic airways eosinophilia is induced upon peritoneal sensitization and airway challenge with OVA *(17)*. The other is regarded as a model of airway antigenic tolerance, in which repeated aerosol exposures of OVA only induce an airway response comprising lymphocytes and neutrophils, but not eosinophils *(7)*. The latter model allows study of whether GM-CSF plays a role in allergic airway antigen sensitization, allowing an asthmatic airway eosinophilic inflammatory response to take place *(7)*.

3.11.1. Mouse Model of Asthmatic Airway Inflammation

1. Mice are sensitized intraperitoneally with 0.5 mL 8 µg OVA adsorbed overnight at 4°C to 4 mg aluminum hydroxide in PBS at d –17 and –12.
2. Twelve days after the second sensitization (d 0), the mice are placed in a Plexiglas chamber (10 × 15 × 25 cm) and exposed to aerosolized OVA (5 mg/mL in 0.9% saline) challenge twice, 4 h apart, with each lasting for 1 h (aerosolized OVA is produced by a Bennet nebulizer, at a flow rate of 10 L/min).
3. AdGM-CSF or a control vector is delivered intranasally to these mice 1 d before OVA challenge. The dose of AdGM-CSF should be small enough (0.03×10^9 PFU), in order to achieve small, but significant GM-CSF levels compartmentalized to the lung (**Fig. 4**).
4. Mice are sacrificed at d 1, 5, 14, and 21 postaerosol challenge for analysis.

3.11.2. Mouse Model of Airway Antigenic Tolerance

1. A small dose of AdGM-CSF or a control vector (0.03×10^9 PFU) is intranasally delivered to mice 1 d prior to the first OVA aerosol exposure.
2. Mice are exposed to aerosolized OVA for 20 min/d for 10 consecutive days. Mice are then sacrificed 48 h later, for analysis.

4. Notes

1. 293 cells should not be too old, and, whenever possible, one should try to save some young passage cells for the purpose of cotransfection. After adding DNA precipitates onto the cell monolayer, cells may not look very healthy because of $CaCl_2$ contained in the buffer. Transfection process can take either 6 or 8 h or overnight, which is not crucial. In the initial days of incubation after introducing overlay agarose to the culture, the cell monolayer should gradually become confluent, a sign of healthy growth beneath the overlay agarose. If cells appear to be rounding up and becoming detached, it may suggest that cells are too old, and cotransfection is probably not going to work. At this point, one needs to consider setting up a new transfection experiment. From this step onward, recombinant

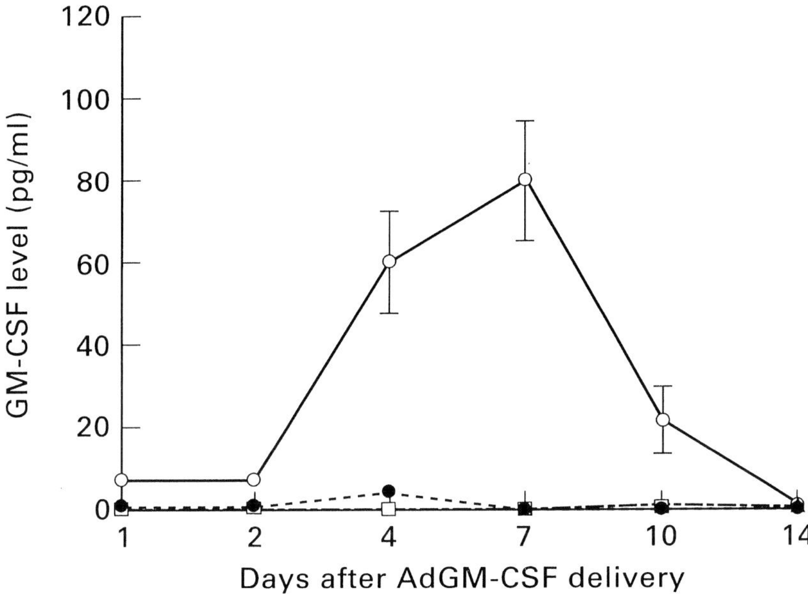

Fig. 4. Compartmentalized GM-CSF transgene protein in mouse lung. The level of GM-CSF in bronchoalveolar lavage (BAL) fluids or sera collected at various times postgene transfer were analyzed by ELISA. A dose of 0.03×10^9 PFU AdGM-CSF or Addl70-3 was delivered intranasally to naïve mice. Open circles: BAL from AdGM-CSF-treated mice; closed circles: sera from AdGM-CSF-treated mice; open squares: BAL from Addl70-3-treated mice (control).

ADV should be treated as a level II biohazardous agent: The appropriate disinfectant is bleach.

2. The resultant viral DNA preparation also contains a small quantity of cellular DNA, which is normally overwhelmed by the large amount of viral-derived DNA, because of rapid amplification of virus within cells ***(10)***. The *Hin*dIII digestion may not always yield outstanding ADV DNA fragments, as visualized in the gel. If this is the case, one needs to further clean up the DNA preparation and carry out an overnight incubation with *Hin*dIII. If the problem still exists, one may decide to reinfect 293 cells and proceed with total-cell RNA extraction, and then carry out Northern hybridization by using a murine GM-CSF cDNA probe to verify the presence and the transcription of the transgene (**Fig. 2B**). This can be followed by a large-scale amplification of virus. Upon obtaining the purified virus, one can go back to carry out *Hin*dIII digestion with purified virus, to obtain the ideal-looking viral DNA fragments.
3. Occasionally, one may find that, after several batches of adenovectors are produced, the expression level of transgene appears to deteriorate in vivo. This may result from a wild-type ADV recombination event occurring during repeated

amplifications using the same batch of virus-containing supernatants. To circumvent this problem, it is advisable that, for each large-scale amplification, one always starts with a small-scale amplification by inoculating 293 cells with a small aliquot of the original plaque(s) saved in PBS^{2+}, or of the first batch of amplified virus.

4. One may see multiple bands, but the virus band should be situated at the lowest position below the interface of two gradients, with densities of 1.35 and 1.25, respectively.
5. Routinely, the authors titrate the virus on two separate occasions, and average two results for the final titer.
6. The dose of AdGM-CSF may be adjusted, depending on the questions to be pursued. During IT instillation, it is of importance to ensure that anesthesia is not too deep, and that the rat is breathing regularly. Generally speaking, IT delivery gives rise to a deeper distribution of virus in the lung than IN delivery.
7. It is common that the mouse inhales the first aliquot smoothly, but has a bit of difficulty in taking in the second aliquot. Do not let the mouse be anesthetized too far, or more viral content will end up in the GI tract. For most studies that the authors have carried out to date, a dose of 0.03×10^9 PFU AdGM-CSF is used. This dose gives rise to a compartmentalized level of GM-CSF in the lung and a negligible level in the peripheral blood.
8. Removing the lung from the thoracic cavity is to ensure an even, effective lung lavage, since the mouse lung has a much shorter upper airway, which often results in an uneven delivery of lavage buffer, if BAL was performed with the lung unseen in the chest. The lung should be hung in the air, with the trachea pointing up during instillation. Instillation of PBS should be slow, and one should witness the inflation of two sides of the lung while instilling. Withdrawal of lavage fluids should be gentle as well, and it will be more effective if gentle massage or tapping is applied to the lung while retrieving. The amount of retrieval is always smaller after the instillation of the first PBS aliquot than after the second.
9. Cells on a cytospin should not be too dense, or else differential counting will be difficult.
10. Fixation by perfusion is essential to the preservation of intra-alveolar cells. The authors find that the loss of information on tissue responses is minimal if a lavaged lung is further processed and used for the purpose of histologic observation. However, for certain studies, it may be desirable to carry out such histologic observations on unlavaged lung tissues. In addition, if IHC is to be carried out on paraffin-embedded sections, it is essential to fix the lung in a large volume of 10% formalin for no longer than 24 h at RT ***(13)***.

References

1. Ruef, C. and Coleman, D. L. (1990) Granulocyte-macrophage colony stimulating factor: pleiotropic cytokine with potential clinical usefulness. *Rev. Infect. Dis.* **12,** 41–62.

2. Xing, Z., Braciak, T., Ohkawara, Y., Sallenave, J.-M., Foley, R., Sime, P. J., et al. (1996) Gene transfer for cytokine functional studies in the lung: the multifunctional role of GM-CSF in pulmonary inflammation. *J. Leukocyte Biol.* **59,** 481–488.
3. Bramson, J. L., Graham, F. L., and Gauldie, J. (1995) The use of adenoviral vectors for gene therapy and gene transfer in vivo. *Curr. Opin. Biotech.* **6,** 590–595.
4. Xing, Z., Ohkawara, Y., Jordana, M., Graham, F. L., and Gauldie, J. (1996) Transfer of granulocyte-macrophage colony-stimulating factor gene to rat lung induces eosinophilia, monocytosis, and fibrotic reactions, *J. Clin. Invest.* **97,** 1102–1110.
5. X.-Lei, F., Ohkawara, Y., Stämpfli, M. R., Gauldie, J., Croitoru, K., Jordana, M., and Xing, Z. (1998) Compartmentalized transgene expression of granulocyte-macrophage colony-stimulating factor (GM-CSF) in mouse lung enhances allergic airways inflammation. *Clin. Exp. Immunol.* **113,** 157–165.
6. Wang, J., Snider, D., Hewlett, B. R., Lukacs, N. W., Gauldie, J., Liang, H., and Xing, Z. (2000) Transgenic expression of GM-CSF induces the differentiation and activation of a novel dendritic cell population in the lung. *Blood,* in press.
7. Stämpfli, M. R., Wiley, R. E., Neigh, G. S., Gajewska, B. U., Lei, X.-F., Snider, D. P., Xing, Z., and Jordana, M. (1998) GM-CSF transgene expression in the airway allows aerosolized ovalbumin to induce allergic sensitization in mice. *J. Clin. Invest.* **102,** 1704–1714.
8. Bett, A. J., Haddara, W., Prevec, L., and Graham, F. L. (1994) An efficient and flexible system for construction of adenovirus vectors with insertions or deletions in early regions 1 and 2. *Proc. Natl. Acad. Sci. USA* **91,** 8802–8806.
9. Sime, P. J., Xing, Z., Foley, R., Graham, F. L., and Gauldie, J. (1997) Transient gene transfer and expression in the lung. *Chest* **111,** 89S–94S.
10. Graham, F. L. and Prevec, L. (1991) Gene transfer and expression protocols, in *Methods in Molecular Biology* (Murray, E. J. and Walker, J. M., eds.), Humana Press Inc., Clifton, NJ, pp. 109–127.
11. Xing, Z., Braciak, T., Jordana, M., Croitoru, K., Graham, F. L., and Gauldie, J. (1994) Adenovirus-mediated cytokine gene transfer at tissue sites: overexpression of IL-6 induces lymphocytic hyperplasia in the lung. *J. Immunol.* **153,** 4059–4069.
12. Wang, J., Palmer, K., Lotvall, J., Milan, S., Lei, X. F., Matthaei, K. I., et al. (1998) Circulating, but not local lung, IL-5, is required for the development of antigen-induced airways eosinophilia. *J. Clin. Invest.* **102,** 1132–1141.
13. Xing, Z., Gauldie, J., Tremblay, G. M., Hewlett, B. R., and Addison, C. (1997) Intradermal transgenic expression of granulocyte-macrophage colony-stimulating factor induces neutrophilia, epidermal hyperplasia, Langerhans' cell/macrophage accumulation and dermal fibrosis. *Lab. Invest.* **77,** 615–622.
14. Sime, P. J., Xing, Z., Graham, F. L., Csaky, K. G., and Gauldie, J. (1997) Adenovector-mediated gene transfer of active transforming growth factor β-1 induces prolonged severe fibrosis in rat lung. *J. Clin. Invest.* **100,** 768–776.
15. Desmouliere, A. (1995) Factors influencing myofibroblast differentiation during wound healing and fibrosis. *Cell Biol. Int.* **19,** 471–476.

16. Xing, Z., Tremblay, M. G., Sime, P. J., and Gauldie, J. (1997) Overexpression of granulocyte-macrophage colony-stimulating factor induces pulmonary granulation tissue formation and fibrosis by induction of transforming growth factor beta-1 and myofibroblast accumulation. *Am. J. Pathol.* **150,** 59–66.
17. Ohkawara, Y., X-Lei, F., Stämpfli, M. R., Marshall, J. S., Xing, Z., and Jordana, M. (1997) Cytokine and eosinophil responses in the lung, peripheral blood, and bone marrow compartments in a murine model of allergen-induced airways inflammation. *Am. J. Respir. Cell Mol. Biol.* **16,** 510–520.

14

Quantitative Analysis of RANTES mRNA in Endobronchial Biopsies Using Polymerase Chain Reaction

Neville Berkman

1. Introduction

Inflammation of the airways is considered to be the key pathogenetic factor in asthma, airway hyperreactivity and clinical symptoms are considered secondary phenomena *(1–3)*. Biopsies of the bronchial wall of asthmatics demonstrate infiltration with inflammatory cells, primarily eosinophils, T-lymphocytes, and monocytes/macrophages *(4–6)*. The mechanisms leading to airway infiltration are complex and have not been fully elucidated; however, several proinflammatory mediators are considered important, including leukotrienes, prostaglandins, cytokines, and others *(7,8)*.

RANTES (regulated on activation, normal T-cell expressed and secreted) belongs to a group of small chemotactic cytokine molecules called chemokines. These 8–10 kDa proteins share a high degree of homology (20–70%), and are subdivided into four groups, based on the position of their cysteine residues *(9–11)*. RANTES belongs to the family of β-chemokines, which contains four cysteine residues, of which the first two are adjacent to each other (C–C chemokines). Other members of the C–C chemokine family include eotaxin, macrophage inflammatory proteins-1α and -β and monocyte chemoattractant proteins 1–5 *(11)*.

The specific activity profile of RANTES suggested to the author that this chemokine may be important in asthmatic inflammation. RANTES induces migration and activation of human eosinophils *(12,13)*, and selectively attracts $CD4^+$ lymphocytes and specifically $CD45RO^+$ memory T-cells *(14)*. The author and others have demonstrated that several cell types present in the airway, including airway epithelial cells, smooth muscle cells, endothelial cells, eosi-

From: *Methods in Molecular Medicine, vol. 44: Asthma: Mechanisms and Protocols*
Edited by: K. F. Chung and I. Adcock © Humana Press Inc., Totowa, NJ

nophils, and lymphocytes, are able to produce RANTES, and that this chemokine is upregulated in response to in vitro stimulation with proinflammatory cytokines, such as tumor necrosis factor-α and interferon-γ. ***(15–18)***.

The author therefore hypothesized that RANTES would be upregulated in asthmatic airways, and may account in part for chemoattraction and activation of airway inflammatory cells. Using quantitative polymerase chain reaction (PCR), the author demonstrated that RANTES mRNA expression in endobronchial biopsies is enhanced in asthmatics, compared to normal controls ***(19)***.

The PCR method used for the above studies is described here. This highly sensitive and reliable method of quantitative PCR enables one to compare mRNA expression from multiple small samples of human tissue ***(19,20)***. This method can be used when smaller-than-microgram quantities of total RNA are available, and allows analysis of several different RNAs from the same tissue. This procedure involves the extraction of RNA from tissue or cells, reverse transcription of RNA, and simultaneous PCR of all relevant samples, together with known standards using primers for the target gene (RANTES) and a control gene (β-actin or glyceraldehyde 3-phosphate dehydrogenase [GAPDH]). Southern blotting of cDNA samples and standards was then performed using radioactive ^{32}P, and samples were measured using a β-counter. Standards are plotted (counts vs starting DNA) to create a standard curve, and samples are plotted on the standard curve to determine amount of starting target DNA. This is corrected for amount of total starting cDNA by expressing this value relative to the amount of β-actin DNA (***19***; *see* **Note 1**).

2. Materials

2.1. RNA Extraction

1. Hand held glass tissue homogenizer.
2. Guanidinium thiocyanate (Sigma, Poole, UK).
3. 0.75 *M* sodium (Na) citrate, pH 7.0.
4. Sarcosyl solution (10%).
5. Mercaptoethanol (Sigma).
6. 2 *M* Na acetate, pH 4.0.
7. Water saturated phenol (not neutralized).
8. Chloroform:isoamyl alcohol (49:1).
9. Isopropanol.
10. Ethanol (75%).
11. Glycogen (Boeringer-Mannheim, Lewes, UK).

Obviously, all precautions for working with RNA need to be observed to prevent degradation: All work is done while wearing gloves, materials and solutions should be kept separately for RNA work only; water should be RNase-free or diethyl pyrocarbonate-treated.

Caution: Guanidinium thiocyanate and mercaptoethanol are highly corrosive and toxic, and should best be used while working in a flowhood and while wearing gloves.

2.2. Reverse Transcription

1. Oligo-deoxythymidine (Oligo-dT) (100 μg/mL). Can be stored at –20°C (Promega, Southhampton, UK).
2. Deoxynucleotide triphosphates (dNTPs) (Promega). Prepare a mix by adding to 20 μL of each nucleotide (come as 100 mmol concentrations) (20 × 4), 120 μL water, to give 200 μL stock mix of 10 mmol.
3. $MgCl_2$ (25 mmol).
4. Avian myeloblastosis virus reverse transcriptase (AMV-RT) (Promega). Store at –20°C.
5. AMV-RT buffer: 50 m*M* KCl, 10 m*M* Tris-HCl, pH 9.0, 0.1% Triton X-100.
6. Recombinant ribonuclease (RNase) inhibitor (Promega). Store at –20°C.

2.3. Creating Standards

2.3.1. Obtaining Starting cDNA

1. For materials for PCR, *see* **Subheading 2.5.**
2. GeneClean (BIO 101, La Jolla, CA), Jetsorb (AMS Biotechnology, UK), or similar kit.

2.3.2. Cloning of PCR Product

2.3.2.1. Ligation of PCR Product to Plasmid

1. pGEM-T vector system (Promega).
2. T4 DNA ligase. Store –20°C.
3. T4 DNA ligase 10X buffer: 300 m*M* Tris-HCl, pH 7.8, 100 m*M* $MgCl_2$, 100 m*M* dithiothreitol, 10 m*M* adenosine triphosphate (ATP). Store –20°C in single-use aliquots.

2.3.2.2. Cloning

1. Luria-Bertoni (LB) plates with ampicillin–IPTG–X-Gal (Ambion, Austin, TX), not more than 30 d old. You will need four plates (two for each ligation reaction, and two for transformation efficiency).
2. LB plates with ampicillin: Add 32 g LB agar (Sigma L-2897) to 1 L H_2O, and autoclave. Allow to cool to 50°C, and add ampicillin to a final concentration of 50 μg/mL. Pour 30–35 mL into 85-mm Petri dishes, and allow to set. Store at 4°C for up to 1 mo.
3. LB plates with ampicillin–IPTG–X-Gal: 100–120 μL 100 m*M* IPTG and 20–30 μL of 50 mg/mL X-Gal may be spread over the surface of an LB-ampicillin plate and allowed to absorb for 30 min at 37°C, prior to use.
4. IPTG stock solution (0.1 *M*): To 1.2 g, add water to 50 mL, and store at 4°C.

5. X-Gal: 100 mg 5-bromo-4-chloro-3-indolyl-β-D-galactoside. Dissolve in 2 mL *N,N'*-dimethyl formamide. Cover with aluminium foil, and store at –20°C.
6. (SOC) medium (100 mL): 2.0 g Bacto-Tryptone, 0.5 g Bacto-Yeast extract (Sigma), 1 mL 1 *M* NaCl, 0.25 mL 1 *M* KCl, 1 mL 2 *M* Mg^{2+} stock (1 *M* $MgCl_2$/ 1 *M* $MgSO_4$), filter-sterilized, 1 mL 2 *M* glucose, filter-sterilized).

   Add first four ingredients to 97 mL distilled water and stir to dissolve. Autoclave and cool to room temperature (RT). Add Mg and glucose to a final concentration of 20 mM. Bring to 100 mL with sterile distilled water. Filter medium through 0.2-µm filter unit. Final pH should be 7.0.
7. LB broth (Sigma L-3022): 20 g in 1 L.
8. Competent cells (*see* **Note 2**).

2.3.3. Miniprep

1. Glycerol.
2. Promega Wizard Miniprep DNA purification system. This contains the following solutions:
   a. Cell suspension solution: 50 m*M* Tris-HCl, pH 5.0, 10 m*M* ethylenediamine tetra-acetic acid (EDTA), 100 mg/mL RNase A.
   b. Cell lysis solution: 0.2 *M* NaOH, 1% sodium dodecyl sulfate (SDS).
   c. Neutralizing solution: 1.32 *M* potassium acetate, pH 4.8.
   d. Tris-EDTA (TE) buffer: 10 m*M* Tris-HCl, pH 7.5, 1 m*M* EDTA.
   e. Column wash solution: 200 m*M* NaCl, 20 m*M* Tris-HCl, pH 7.5, 5 m*M* EDTA; dilute with 95% ethanol, as described by manufacturer.
3. Vacuum manifold (Promega). Alternatively, a 2-mL syringe works equally well.

2.3.4. Confirming That the Cloned Insert Is Correct

1. Restriction enzymes *Apa*I and *Sac*I. Store at –20°C.
2. Restriction enzyme buffer.
3. DNA size marker (100-bp ladder).
4. Facilities for sequencing.

2.3.5. Preparing Known cDNA Standards

Circleprep (Bio 101) or Wizard Midiprep DNA purification system (Promega).

2.5. PCR Reaction

1. Primers for RANTES: Forward: TCATTGCTACTGCCCTCTGC
   Reverse: CCTAGCTCATCTCCAAAGAG (242 bp).
   β-actin: Forward: GTGGGGCGCCCCAGGCACCA
   Reverse: CTCCTTAATGTCACGCACGATTTC (572 bp).

   Primers are kept at working solutions of 2.5 pmol/µL in sterile water.
2. dNTP mix containing deoxyadenosine triphosphate (dATP), deoxythymidine triphosphate (dTTP), deoxyguanosine triphosphate (dGTP), and deoxycytosine triphosphate (dCTP) at a final concentration of 2 m*M* (20 µL each of 100 m*M* dNTPs is added to 920 µL water, to give a working stock solution of 2 m*M*).

3. *Taq* polymerase (store at –20°C).
4. $MgCl_2$ (25 m*M*).
5. 10X *Taq* buffer: 500 m*M* KCl, 100 m*M* Tris-HCl, and 1% Triton X-100.
6. Mineral oil (Sigma).

2.6. Southern Blotting

1. Hybond-N nylon membrane (Amersham, Amersham, UK).
2. Whatman paper.
3. Denaturing solution: 0.5 *M* NaOH, 1.5 *M* NaCl.
4. Neutralizing solution: 0.5 *M* Tris-HCl, 3 *M* NaCl, pH 7.5.
5. 20X standard sodium citrate (SSC): 3 *M* NaCl 175 g/L; 0.3 *M* Na_3citrate·$2H_2O$ 88 g/L; adjust pH to 7.0 with 1 *M* HCl.
6. Prehybridizing/hybridizing buffer: 10% dextran sulfate, 6X SSC, 0.5% SDS, 5 m*M* EDTA, 0.2% Na pyrophosphate, salmon sperm DNA 0.1 mg/mL, and 10X Denhardt's solution.

   For 1 L: dexran sulfate (100 g); 20X SSC (300 mL); 10% SDS (50 mL), 0.5 *M* EDTA, pH 8.0; (10 mL) 10% Na pyrophosphate 20 mL, salmon sperm DNA 20 mL (of 5 mg/mL), 100X Denhardt's solution (100 mL), H_2O 500 mL.
7. Multiprime labeling kit (Amersham).
8. cDNA 50 ng (obtained from Midiprep).
9. [^{32}P]-dCTP (Amersham).
10. Sephadex G-50 spin column.
11. Scintillation fluid.

3. Methods

3.1. RNA Extraction

Endobronchial biopsies are obtained from segmental or subsegmental bronchi at the time of bronchoscopy. This procedure has consistently been shown to be safe in asthmatic patients, even following allergen challenge, and should be performed according to American Thoracic Society guidelines ***(21)***. Two biopsies are immediately placed in a single 2-mL microcentrifuge tube containing guanidinium thiocyanate prepared as described below. The microcentrifuge tube is immediately placed in liquid nitrogen, then transferred to –70°C for storage. Bronchoalveolar lavage (BAL) can be performed during the same procedure, and additional biopsies can be obtained for other studies, such as immunohistochemistry.

RNA extraction based on the method of Chomczynski and Sacchi ***(22)*** is a simple and now widely used technique. Several companies market a single reagent monophasic solution of phenol and guanidinium thiocyanate for RNA extraction (Tripure, Boehringer-Mannheim; Tri-Reagent-Molecular Research Center Inc., Cincinnati, OH), but these are fairly expensive, and, if large numbers of samples are analyzed, it is cheaper to prepare reagents oneself.

All samples should be analyzed/extracted at the same time to ensure uniformity.

1. Prepare guanidinium thiocyanate mix by adding 293 mL ddH_2O, 17.6 mL 0.75 *M* Na citrate (pH 7.0), and 26.4 mL of 10% sarcosyl solution to a 250-g guanidinium thiocyanate bottle. These are dissolved using a stir bar, and the solution is then stable for several months at RT. For working solution, 0.36 mL mercaptoethanol is added per 50 mL of the above mix. This is allegedly stable for 1 mo at RT, but is best prepared fresh as required.
2. 800 µL of this mix is placed in a 2-mL microcentrifuge tube (*see* **Note 3**), and two endobronchial biopsies are immersed in the solution; the closed microcentrifuge tube is snap-frozen in liquid nitrogen. This should be done immediately in the bronchoscopy room, because biopsies should be as fresh as possible. Biopsies are stored at –70°C, until RNA extraction.
3. The guanidinium thiocyanate mix containing the tissue biopsies is defrosted and transferred to a glass hand-homogenizer, and the biopsies are homogenized. The guanidinium thiocyanate solution is then returned to a microcentrifuge tube, and the next sample is homogenized. It is best to bake the glass homogenizer prior to use (180°C for 3–4 h), and between samples, the homogenizer is rinsed twice with RNase-free distilled water, then with 100% ethanol.
4. Add 80 µL 2 *M* Na acetate, pH 4.0, and vortex.
5. Add 800 µL phenol and vortex.
6. Add 160 µL chloroform-isoamyl alcohol (premixed in a ratio of 49:1 by volume), and vortex 15 s.
7. Leave on ice 10–15 min.
8. Spin for 15 min at 13,000 rpm (microcentrifuge).
9. Remove top phase leaving ±20% (*see* **Note 4**).
10. Add another 200 µL guanidinium thiocyanate mix, and vortex.
11. Add 20 µL 2 *M* Na acetate, pH 4.0, and vortex.
12. Add 800 µL phenol, and vortex.
13. Add 160 µL chloroform-isoamyl alcohol, vortex 15 s.
14. Repeat **steps 7–9**.
15. Add glycogen as carrier (1–2 µL).
16. Add 800 µL isopropanol.
17. Leave overnight at –20°C to precipitate RNA.
18. Spin 30 min at 13,000 rpm. The RNA should be visible as a white pellet at the bottom of the microcentrifuge tube. Pour off liquid.
19. Wash by adding 1 mL 75% ethanol, vortex, spin 10–15 min, and pour off ethanol. Repeat this wash a second time.
20. Dry the RNA using a freeze-dryer, a Speed-Vac concentrator (Savant Instruments, Inc.), or by allowing to stand in a flowhood for 5–10 min. Beware of overdrying the RNA, which may then not dissolve in water.
21. Add 40 µL H_2O to dissolve RNA, and store at –70°C until use.

3.2. Reverse Transcription

Total volume for reaction: 40 µL.

1. Mix 18 µL RNA in water with 0.4 µg (4 µL 100 µg/mL) oligo-dT.
2. Heat at 65°C for 5–10 min.
3. Cool on ice for 5 min.
4. Prepare a mix containing the following per sample of RNA:
   a. 4 µL nucleotide mix (10 mmol). This will give a final concentration of 1 m*M* of each deoxynucleotide.
   b. 8 µL 25 mmol $MgCl_2$, to give a final concentration of 5 m*M*.
   c. 4 µL buffer 50 m*M* KCl, 10 m*M* Tris-HCl, pH 9.0, 0.1% Triton X-100.
   d. 1 µL AMV-RT (15 U).
   e. 1 µL Recombinant ribonuclease inhibitor.
5. Add mix to RNA + oligo-dT (18 µL per sample).
6. Quick-vortex, and spin down.
7. Incubate 42°C for 60–90 min.
8. Heat 80°C 10 min.
9. Ice 5 min.
10. Dilute cDNA in water (160 µL to give a total volume of 200 µL).

3.3. Creating Standards

3.3.1. Obtaining Starting cDNA

In order to create a standard curve for quantifying PCR products from biopsy samples, standard PCR is performed using cDNA from a sample tissue likely to express the required mRNA. RANTES and β-actin are ubiquitously expressed, so most tissues can be used to obtain a PCR product (peripheral blood mononuclear cells, endobronchial biopsies, BAL cells, or other). The PCR products are run on a gel, and, if of correct length (as predicted from primers, for RANTES, 242 bp; for β-actin, 572 bp), the band is excised from the gel and cleaned using GeneClean, Jetsorb, or a similar kit (*see* detailed PCR method in **Subheading 3.5.**)

3.3.2. Cloning of PCR Product

Cloning of the PCR product into a pGEM5Z vector is performed using the T-vector system (Promega), which makes use of a plasmid with T-overhangs at the insertion site, and takes advantage of the fact that PCR products produced with *Taq* polymerase tend to have extra deoxyadenosine on their ends. This greatly improves efficiency of ligation, and allows insertion into plasmid without the need to go through additional steps of adding sticky ends or designing primers with restriction sites upstream and then performing restriction enzyme digestion prior to cloning. The vector contains a multiple cloning site

Table 1
Ligation Reaction

	Standard reaction (μL)	Positive control (μL)	Background control (μL)
T4 DNA ligase buffer	1	1	1
pGEM-T vector (50 ng)	1	1	1
PCR product	X	—	—
Control insert DNA	—	2	—
T4 DNA ligase (3 Weiss units/μL)	1	1	1
Deionized water to a total volume of	10	10	10

within the coding region of the enzyme β-galactosidase to allow easy color identification of recombinants.

3.3.2.1. Ligation of PCR Product to Plasmid

The ratio of vector DNA (plasmid) to insert DNA (PCR product) for optimum ligation varies for different inserts, and is determined empirically (trial and error). The author uses molar ratios of 1:1 and 1:3 for initial experiments (*see* **Note 5**). The vector is approx 3 kb in size, and is supplied at 50 ng/μL. The amount of insert to include is calculated from the equation:

$$\frac{\text{ng of vector} \times \text{size (kb) of insert}}{\text{size (kb) of vector}} \times \text{insert:vector molar ratio} = \text{ng of insert}$$

1. Briefly centrifuge tubes containing vector, and insert DNA.
2. Set up ligation reactions using 0.5-mL tubes (with low DNA-binding capacity) (**Table 1**).
3. Mix the reactions by pipeting and incubate overnight at 4°C.

3.3.2.2. Cloning

1. Prepare LB plates with ampicillin–IPTG–X-Gal, and allow to equilibrate to RT.
2. Centrifuge tubes from ligation reaction, and transfer 2 μL to two sterile 1.5-mL microcentrifuge tubes on ice (beware of DNA binding to the tube). Set up another tube on ice, with 0.1 ng uncut plasmid, for determination of transformation efficiency.
3. Remove tube of frozen JM109 cells from –70°C, and place in an ice bath until just thawed. Mix gently by flicking tube.
4. **Carefully** transfer 50 μL cells into tubes prepared in **step 2** (100 μL cells for determination of transformation efficiency). Avoid excessive pipeting, because the cells are very fragile.
5. Gently flick the tubes to mix, and place on ice for 20 min.

6. Heat-shock the cells for 45–50 s in a water bath at exactly 42°C (DO NOT SHAKE).
7. Immediately return the tubes to ice for 2 min.
8. Add 950 µL RT SOC medium to the tubes containing ligation reaction mix and 900 µL to tubes containing uncut plasmid (LB may be used, but gives lower yield).
9. Incubate for 90 min at 37°C, with shaking (150 rpm).
10. Plate 100 µL onto duplicate plates. For the transformation control, a 1:10 dilution with SOC medium is recommended for plating. For a higher number of colonies, pellet cells (centrifuge 1000*g* for 10 min), resuspend in 200 µL SOC medium and then plate (100 µL/plate).
11. Incubate the plates overnight (16–24 h) at 37°C. Promega estimates yield of 100 colonies/plate. Longer incubation (at 4°C) may facilitate blue-white screening (*see* **Note 6**).
12. Choose 2–4 white colonies from each plate, and put into separate sterile tubes containing 10 mL LB plus ampicillin (white colonies are recombinants). Allow to grow overnight at 37°C on a shaker.

3.3.3. Miniprep

The following morning, if bacteria have grown in the LB, take several 700-µL aliquots from each colony. Add 300 µL 50% glycerol, and store at –70°C.

Perform miniprep using Promega Wizard Miniprep DNA purification system, or something similar. This technique is quick and consistently gives good results. The purified plasmid can be used directly for DNA sequencing or restriction digestion, which is not always possible without a further organic extraction phase with other similar kits. The system relies on a silica-based resin, which binds DNA. The miniprep starts with 1–3 mL overnight culture, and yields 1–10 µg plasmid DNA.

1. Pellet 1–3 mL (the author has used up to double) by centrifugation at top speed. Resuspend pellet in 200 µL cell resuspension solution, and transfer to a microcentrifuge tube.
2. Add 200 µL cell lysis solution, and mix by gently inverting the tube until the cell suspension becomes clear.
3. Add 200 µL neutralizing solution, and mix by inverting the tube several times.
4. Spin at top speed in microcentrifuge 5 min.
5. Decant the cleared supernatant to a new tube.
6. Add 1 mL Wizard DNA purification resin to the tube, and mix by inverting tube. It is important to thoroughly mix the resin prior to removing an aliquot. If necessary, warm the resin to 25–37°C for 10 min to remove aggregates.
7. Attach the syringe barrel of a 2–3-mL disposable syringe to the Luer-Lok extension of each minicolumn.
8. Pipet the resin–DNA mix into the syringe barrel, and gently push the slurry into the minicolumn with the syringe plunger.

9. Detach the syringe from the minicolumn, and remove the plunger from the syringe. Reattach the syringe barrel to the minicolumn, and pipet 2 mL of column wash solution into the syringe. Push through minicolumn, using syringe plunger.
10. Remove syringe, and transfer minicolumn to 1.5-mL tube. Spin for 2 min at top speed to dry the resin.
11. Transfer the minicolumn to a new tube. Apply 50 µL water or TE buffer to the minicolumn, and wait 1 min. To elute the DNA, spin the minicolumn at top speed for 20 s.
12. Remove, and discard the column. Spin again for 20 s to pellet any remaining resin, and carefully collect supernatant (containing plasmid DNA).

For large plasmids, heating the water or TE (65–80°C) improves the yield. Promega markets a vacuum manifold that can be used to attach minicolumns and thereby allows processing several samples simultaneously.

3.3.4. Confirming that the Cloned Insert Is Correct

Having obtained purified plasmid, the next step is to determine whether it contains the correct insert.

1. Measure/determine the amount of DNA obtained from the miniprep using spectrophotometry.
2. Perform an enzyme digest as follows: Cut 1 µg plasmid DNA using *Apa*I and *Sac*I. Both enzymes can be added simultaneously, and are effective using the same enzyme buffer and incubation temperature (37°C). Plasmid DNA (1 µg) + 2 µL enzyme buffer + 1 µL *Apa*I and 1 µL *Sac*I + H_2O to a volume of 20 µL. Allow to digest 2 h.
3. Run on a minigel, as follows: Lane 1:DNA size marker (100 bp ladder); lane 2: 1 µg uncut β-actin plasmid; lane 3: cut β-actin plasmid; lane 4: uncut RANTES plasmid; lane 5: cut RANTES plasmid. It is preferable to run several of the clones for each insert.

   If a single clear band of correct size is seen, the clone is likely to contain the correct insert. The band should be ±80 bp longer than the predicted PCR product, because of the presence of the multiple cloning site sequences at the edges of the plasmid vector (325 bp for RANTES, 655 bp for β-actin).
4. Plasmids containing inserts of the correct predicted length are then sequenced to confirm that the insert is the correct gene product. The plasmid DNA obtained from the miniprep is usually sufficient for sequencing.

   Unless the laboratory is performing sequencing on a fairly regular basis, it is easier and faster to get this done by a company or laboratory set up for sequencing. For short inserts (<300–400 bp), sequencing from one direction is usually adequate. For longer inserts, sequencing from both directions may be preferable. It is not infrequent to get single base pair alterations (when using *Taq* polymerase), but these are of no consequence for purposes here. Remember that the strand sequenced may be the complementary strand, and not the forward strand. Detailed methodology for sequencing should be obtained elsewhere ***(23)***.

3.3.5. Preparing Known cDNA Standards

Once a clone (or clones) containing the correct insert has been identified, bacteria should be grown overnight in 100 mL volume of LB + ampicillin, and midiprep or circleprep performed (Circleprep: BIO 101). Wizard Midiprep DNA purification system (Promega) is identical to the Miniprep system described in **Subheading 3.3.3.** although scaled-up for larger volumes and greater plasmid yield.

The midiprep starts with 25–100 mL overnight culture and yields 10–200 µg plasmid DNA (this can vary greatly, depending on the plasmid copy number, volume of culture, and bacterial strain used). After midiprep has been performed, the plasmid containing the required insert is obtained.

A large-scale reaction using restriction enzymes *Apa*I and *Sac*I is then set up: 100 µg plasmid + 15 µL 10X buffer + 7.5 µL *Apa*I + 7.5 µL *Sac*I + water, to a total volume of 150 µL. Allow to digest overnight.

After digestion, the target band is cut, cleaned, and quantified.

A correction for the additional sequences on the standard DNA can be performed by correcting as follows: weight (µg) of target DNA = weight obtained above × PCR product length:insert length (PCR length + 83). There are 83 bp between the insert site and the restriction site on the cloning vector. Dilute RANTES and β-actin DNA in half-log concentrations from 10^{-3} to 10^{-10} µg ready for use in the quantitative PCR step. Thus, standards will be 10^{-3}, $10^{-3.5}$, 10^{-4}, $10^{-4.5}$, 10^{-5}, $10^{-5.5}$, 10^{-6}, $10^{-6.5}$, 10^{-7}, $10^{-7.5}$, 10^{-8}, $10^{-8.5}$, 10^{-9}, $10^{-9.5}$ and 10^{-10} µg.

3.4. Determine Number of Cycles for PCR

It is imperative that samples be measured on the linear phase of amplification. To determine this, cDNA is taken from all samples, mixed together, and subjected to PCR at two-cycle increments from 20 to 40 cycles (20, 22, 24, and so on). This step should be performed separately for RANTES and β-actin. Product is then quantified using densitometry and plotted on a log scale. The number of cycles for subsequent experiments can then be determined. For RANTES, 28 cycles was used, and, for β-actin 24 cycles.

3.5. PCR Reaction

All samples, as well as standards, are run simultaneously for the number of cycles determined above, i.e., 24 cycles for β-actin and 28 cycles for RANTES. A single mastermix for all ingredients for PCR (other than cDNA) is used, to allow for maximum uniformity.

The author used biopsies from eight normal volunteers and samples from eight asthmatics, to give a total of 16. All samples and standards should be run in duplicate. There are 15 standards and 16 samples run in duplicate = 62 samples.

PCR was performed using:

1. 3 μL (7.5 pmol) each of forward and reverse primers.
2. 3 μL dNTP mix (2 m*M*), to give a final concentration of 0.2 m*M*.
3. *Taq* polymerase 1.5 U (0.3 μL).
4. 1.8 μL MgC12 25 m*M* (final concentration 1.5 m*M*).
5. 3 μL 10X *Taq* buffer (final concentration 50 m*M* KCl, 10 m*M* Tris-HCl, and 0.1% Triton X-100).
6. 6.9 μL H_2O.
7. 10 μL cDNA.

Final volume of 30 μL. It is preferable to use a PCR machine with a heated lid to avoid the need to overlay samples with a drop of oil. Conditions for PCR:

1. 95°C for an initial 5 min (hot start).
2. Denaturation 95°C for 45 s.
3. Annealing 56°C for 45 s.
4. Extension at 72°C for 90 s.
5. Repeat **steps 2–4** 23 or 27×.
6. Final extension was at 72°C for 10 min.

3.6. Southern Blotting

1. Mark out squares of 1.5 × 1.5 cm in diameter on Hybond-N nylon membrane (Amersham).
2. Following PCR, dot-blot 5 μL product onto Hybond-N nylon membrane (Amersham). This is best done in duplicate, for each PCR tube to give four dot-blots per standard and per sample. Allow to dry for 10 min.
3. Denature: Soak two sheets of Whatman paper in denaturing solution (0.5 *M* NaOH, 1.5 *M* NaCl). Place nylon membrane on the Whatman paper, DNA side up, for 5 min (until wet).
4. Then neutralize: Soak two sheets of Whatman paper in neutralizing solution (0.5 *M* Tris-base, 3 *M* NaCl, pH 7.5). Place nylon membrane on the Whatman paper, DNA side up, for 5 min (until wet).
5. Wash by transferring nylon membrane to Whatman paper soaked in 3X SSC for 10 min.
6. Allow to dry.
7. Fix the DNA to the nylon membrane by UV crosslinking.

   Filters are then hybridized with [^{32}P]-labeled RANTES or β-actin cDNA probe generated with a random primer labeling kit (Amersham).
8. Place 20 mL prehybridization solution in hybridization chamber, and allow to prehybridize at 60–65°C for at least 4 h (or overnight).
9. Prepare probe using 50 ng cDNA and multiprime labeling kit (Amersham): 50 ng cDNA; dNTPs: 4 μL each of dATP, dGTP, and dTTP; 5 μL buffer; 5 μL primer; 5 μL [^{32}P]-dCTP; 1 μL enzyme (Klenow); H_2O to a volume of 50 μL. First add cDNA and H_2O. Pierce microcentrifuge tube lid, and boil 5 min, then place on

ice for 2 min. Spin down, and add other ingredients in the above order (enzyme last). Spin down, and allow to incubate at 37°C for 60–90 min. This reaction can be scaled-up or -down, depending on the number of hybridization chambers used.

10. Pass the labeled probe through a Sephadex G-50 spin column. The volume containing the probe is made up to 200 µL, placed in a 5-mL syringe barrel containing Sephadex G-50. The syringe barrel is placed within a 15-mL Falcon tube (or similar) and spun 200*g* for 5 min.
11. Boil probe for 5 min, place on ice for 2 min, then add entire amount of probe (without counting) to the filters, or to 20 mL preheated prehybridization solution, and leave at 60–65°C overnight.
12. After hybridization, rinse filters in 2–3× in 3X SSC/0.1% SDS, then washed in 0.1X SSC/0.1% SDS at 65°C for 40 min.
13. Filters were then cut into their 1.5 × 1.5-cm squares, placed in plastic vials containing scintillation fluid, and counted on a β-counter.
14. Number of counts for each standard are averaged and plotted against starting DNA, to create a standard curve (log counts vs µg DNA) **(Fig. 1)**. Samples are also averaged and plotted on the standard curve, to give amount of starting DNA. This is performed for both RANTES (target gene) and for β-actin (control gene). Each sample is expressed as amount of starting RANTES DNA per pg β-actin. Values for asthmatics are then compared with those of normals (*see* **Note 7**) **(Fig. 2)**.

4. Notes

1. Competitive PCR, using an internal standard of different length to the target gene or containing an additional restriction site, is at least as sensitive and accurate as the method described. Nevertheless, accurate quantitation, using competitive PCR, requires running several PCR reactions for each sample, which is not always possible when the amount of cDNA per sample is a limiting factor.
2. JM109 cells are typically used for this reaction, and competent cells are provided with the pGEM-T vector system. In the author's experience, these cells quickly become less efficient, and fresh cells are best used for this reaction. If a low yield of colonies is obtained, the efficiency of transformation of the competent cells should be determined, and should be at least 10^8 CFU/µg DNA. Transformation efficiency is calculated as follows: 100 µL competent cells are transformed with 0.1 ng uncut plasmid DNA, and this reaction is added to 900 µL SOC medium (0.1 ng/mL). From that volume, a 1:10 dilution with SOC medium is made, and 100 µL is plated on two plates (0.001 ng DNA/100 µL). Transformation efficiency (Z) is:

$$\text{number of CFU on plate}/0.001\ \text{ng} = Z\ \text{CFU/ng} = Z \times 10^3\ \text{CFU/µg DNA} \qquad (1)$$

   Alternatively, XL-1 cells seem to work well, although a transformation step needs to be performed to make these cells competent. Any cells can be used, provided they allow blue-white screening and ampicillin selection.
3. These volumes are suitable for use in a 2-mL tube. For a 1.5-mL tube, 650 µL guanidinium thiocyanate is used. Other volumes are reduced accordingly.

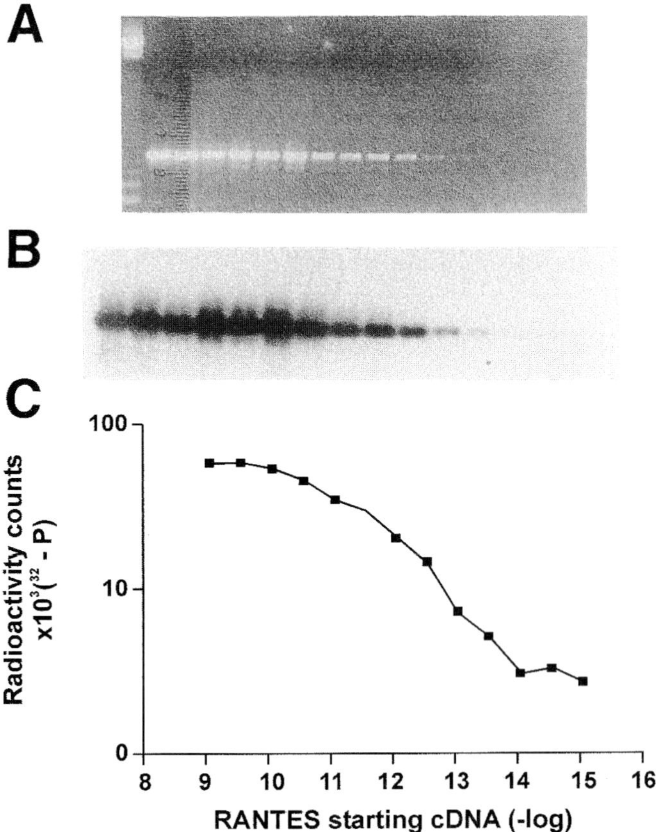

Fig. 1. Construction of a standard curve, relating radioactivity counts to the amount of starting cDNA for RANTES. Standard amounts of RANTES cDNA ranging from 10^{-8} to 10^{-15} g were subjected to PCR for 28 cycles. PCR product was electrophoresed in an ethidium bromide-stained agarose gel **(A)**, transferred to nylon membrane, and hybridized using a 30P-labeled probe **(B)**. PCR product (5 μL) was simultaneously dot-blotted onto nylon membranes, Southern-blotted, and counted on a β-counter **(C)**. All samples were subjected to PCR in duplicate and each duplicate was dot-blotted in duplicate so that plotted values are means of four. The curve is linear between 10^{-14} and $10^{-9.5}$ g. A similar standard curve was constructed for β-actin.

4. It is best to leave a larger amount of upper-phase, and to repeat the phenol extraction phase (**steps 10–15**), to minimize chances of contamination with genomic DNA.
5. More is not necessarily better. The manufacturer ranges from 3:1 to 1:3, although ratios in the range of 8:1 to 1:8 can be used. The amount of insert DNA is estimated by comparing with known standards on an ethidium-bromide-containing gel plate.

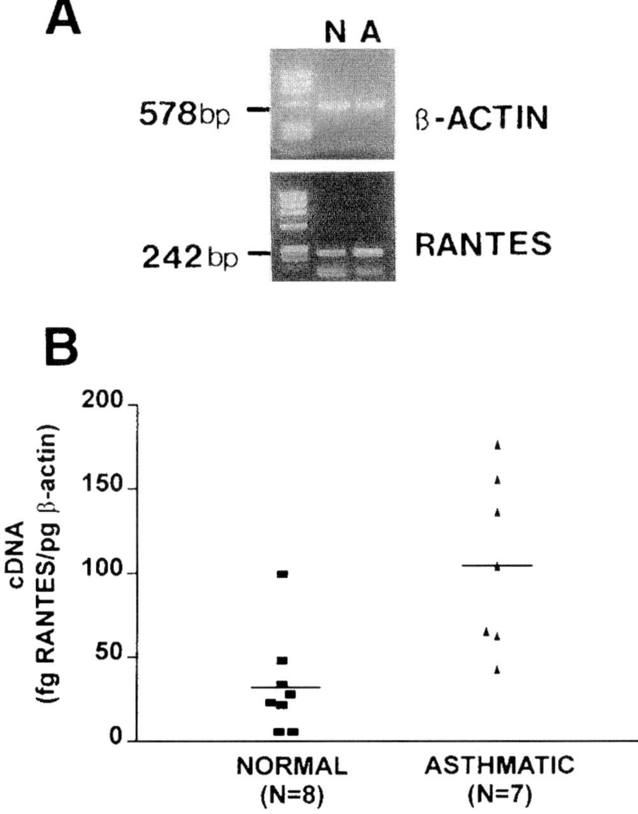

Fig. 2. **(A)** A representative example of an ethidium bromide-stained gel showing PCR product for RANTES obtained from an asthmatic (A) and a normal control (N). PCR performed using primers for β-actin shows similar amounts of cDNA in the two individuals. **(B)** cDNA obtained from endobronchial biopsies of asthmatics ($n = 7$) and normal controls ($n = 8$) was subjected to PCR using primers for RANTES and for β-actin. PCR was performed simultaneously with standard DNAs. Five microliters of product was dot-blotted onto nylon membranes, hybridized using a ^{32}P-labeled probe, and counted on a β-counter. Counts were converted into amounts of starting cDNA using the standard curves and plotted as the ratio of target DNA (fg RANTES) to control DNA (pg β-actin). All samples were subjected to PCR in duplicate and each duplicate was dot-blotted in duplicate, so that plotted values are means of four. Mean values (horizontal bar) were 33.7 ± 11 in normals and 110 ± 18 in asthmatics ($p < 0.003$).

6. Colonies containing the insert are white, because of disruption of β-galactosidase. It is not infrequent, however, for clones containing insert to be blue, as detailed in the users protocol.

   A control fragment of 542 bp is supplied by the manufacturer, and has been designed for minimum blue colonies. This positive control is critical, and should give 100 colonies (if 10^8 CFU/μg DNA are transformed), of which >60% are white.

Several problems may arise during the cloning procedure: If no colonies are seen on the plates, transformation has failed; if only blue colonies are observed, ligation has been unsuccessful; if only a low number of colonies or few white colonies are obtained, ligation conditions are not optimal. Possible explanations include inadequate ligation time, suboptimal insert:vector ratio, the presence of an inhibitor in the PCR product, the absence of an A overhang on the PCR product, or the presence of pyrimidine dimers because of UV exposure. Thus, ligation should be reattempted using adequate ligation time, additional vector:insert mixes, and PCR fragments generated with *Taq* polymerase (and therefore with A overhangs). If the presence of an inhibitor is suspected, PCR product can be mixed with positive control (if necessary, repurify PCR fragment). If all else fails, presence of pyrimidine dimers in the PCR product, because of UV exposure, should be suspected, and the DNA should be remade, taking care to avoid UV as much as possible (use only longwave UV source).

The characteristics of the insert can greatly affect the cloning efficiency and number of clones obtained.

The manufacturer also recommends a background control using vector without insert. This control should yield blue colonies only, similar in number to that seen in reaction. If the PCR plate has far more blue colonies than background control, the recombinants are probably among the blue colonies.

7. Standards and samples can be calculated and plotted as concentrations, rather than in micrograms, but this would not alter results in any way. The issue of using β-actin as a control gene is somewhat controversial, but the author has found that β-actin gives results similar to those obtained with GAPDH.

References

1. Djukanovic, R., Roche, W. R., Wilson, J. W., Beasley, C. R. W., et al. (1990) Mucosal inflammation in asthma. *Am. Rev. Resp. Dis.* **142,** 434–457.
2. Poulter, L. W., Power, C., and Burke, C. (1990) Relationship between bronchial immunopathology and hyperresponsiveness in asthma. *Eur. Respir. J.* **3,** 792–799.
3. Walker, C., Kaegi, M. K., Braun, P., and Blaser, K. (1991) Activated T cells and eosinophilia in bronchoalveolar lavages from subjects with asthma correlated with disease severity. *J. Allergy Clin. Immunol.* **88,** 935–942.
4. Bousquet, J., Chanez, P., Lacoste, J. Y., et al. (1990) Eosinophilic inflammation in asthma. *N. Engl. J. Med.* **323,** 1033–1039.
5. Poston, R., Chanez, P., Lacoste, J. Y., et al. (1992) Immunohistochemical characterization of the cellular infiltration of asthmatic bronchi. *Am. Rev. Respir. Dis.* **145,** 918–921.
6. Azzawi, M., Bradley, B., Jeffrey, P. K., et al. (1990) Identification of activated T lymphocytes and eosinophils in bronchial biopsies in stable atopic asthmatics. *Am. Rev. Respir. Dis.* **142,** 1407–1411.

7. Van Oosterhout, A. J. M. and Nijkamp, F. P. (1993) Role of cytokines in bronchial hyperresponsiveness. *Pulm. Pharmacol.* **6,** 225–236.
8. Kay, A. B. (1991) Asthma and inflammation. *J. Allergy Clin. Immunol.* **87,** 893–910.
9. Schall, T. J. (1991) Biology of the RANTES/ SIS cytokine family. *Cytokine* **3,** 165–183.
10. Baggiolini, M. and Dahinden, C. A. (1994) CC chemokines in allergic inflammation. *Immunol. Today* **15,** 127–133.
11. Luster, D. A. (1998) Chemokines: chemotactic cytokines that mediate inflammation. *N. Engl. J. Med.* **338,** 436–445.
12. Rot, A., Krieger, M., Brunner, T., Bischoff, S. C., Schall, T. J., and Dahinden, C. A. (1992) RANTES and macrophage inflammatory protein Iα induce the migration and activation of normal human eosinophil granulocytes. *J. Exp. Med.* **176,** 1489–1495.
13. Kameyoshi, Y., Dorschner, A., Mallet, A. I., Christophers, E., and Schroder, J. M. (1992) Cytokine RANTES released by thrombin-stimulated platelets is a potent attractant for human eosinophils. *J. Exp. Med.* **176,** 587–592.
14. Schall, T. J., Bacon, K., Toy, K. J., and Goeddel, D. V. (1990) Selective attraction of monocytes and T lymphocytes of the memory phenotype of cytokine RANTES. *Nature* **347,** 669–671.
15. John, M., Hirst, S. J., Jose, P. J., Robichaud, A., Berkman, N., Witt, C., et al. (1997) Human airway smooth muscle cells express and release RANTES in response to T help 1 cytokines: regulation by T helper 2 cytokines and corticosteroids. *J. Immunol.* **158,** 1841–1847.
16. Devergne, O., Marfaing-Koka, A., Schall, T. J., Leger-Ravet, M. B., Sadick, M., Crevon, M. C., Kim, K. J., and Schall, T. T. (1994) Production of the RANTES chemokine in delayed-type hypersensitivity reactions: involvement of macrophages and endothelial cells. *J. Exp. Med.* **179,** 1689–1694.
17. Marfaing-Koka, A., Devergne, O., Gorgone, G., Portier, A., Schall, T. J., Galanaud, P., and Emilie, D. (1995) Regulation of the production of the RANTES chemokine by endothelial cells. Synergistic induction by IFN-γ plus TNF-α and inhibition by IL-4 and IL-13. *J. Immunol.* **154,** 1870–1878.
18. Berkman, N., Robichaud, A., Krishnan, V. L., Roesems, G., Robbins, R. A., Jose, P. J., Barnes, P. J., and Chung, K. F. (1996) Expression of Rantes and macrophage inflammatory protein 1-alpha in airway epithelial cells: effect of corticosteroids and interleukin-4, 10 and 13. *Immunology* **87,** 599–603.
19. Berkman, N., Krishnan, V. L., Gilbey, T., Newton, R., O'Connor, B., Barnes, P. J., and Chung, K. F. (1996) Expression of RANTES mRNA and protein in airways of patients with mild asthma. *Am. Rev. Respir. Crit. Care Med.* **154,** 1804–1811.
20. Melby, P. C., Darnell, B. J., and Tryon, V. V. (1993) Quantitative measurement of human cytokine gene expression by polymerase chain reaction. *J. Immunol. Methods* **159,** 235–244.
21. National Institutes of Health (1992) Workshop summary and guidelines. Investigative use of bronchoscopy, lavage and bronchial biopsies in asthma and other airways disease. *Eur. Respir. J.* **5,** 115–121.

22. Chomczynski, P. and Sacchi, N. (1987) Single-step method of RNA isolation by acid guanidinium thiocyanate-phenol-chloroform extraction. *Anal. Biochem.* **162,** 156–159.
23. Ausubel, F. M., Brent, R., Kingston, R. E., et al., eds. (1994) *Current Protocols in Molecular Biology*, Wiley, New York.

15

Intracellular Cytokine Staining for Analysis by Flow Cytometry

Anthony J. Frew, Jacqueline Madden, and Petros Bakakos

1. Introduction

To determine the function of a particular cell type, it is necessary either to have a large number of similar (ideally identical) cells or to use extremely sensitive methods to detect the activity of a single cell. Lymphocytes present special difficulties, because they have very precise antigen (Ag) recognition requirements, and, under physiological conditions, they will only be activated if they are exposed to their particular Ag. Polyclonal mitogens, such as phytohemagglutinin (PHA) or anti-CD3, will activate most T-cells, but may not elicit a truly physiological response in terms of cytokine production, and so on. Moreover, the biological readout (release of cytokines into culture supernatant) will represent the net balance of the integrated response of all the activated cells, minus any consumption of cytokines by the cultured cells.

Cloning T-cells by limiting dilution allows detailed examination of the progeny of a single T-cell, but cloning requires prolonged passage over several weeks, which may alter the functional properties of the cell, although it should not affect its Ag specificity. T-cell clones are therefore useful for examining Ag-recognition requirements but are less likely to reflect the functional properties of the original cell from which the clone is derived.

There are now well-established methods to identify messenger RNA (mRNA) within single cells in smears or tissue sections, using techniques of *in situ* hybridization *(1)*. However, early attempts to show cytokine proteins within T-cells ran into difficulty, because the amount of cytokine retained within each cell is relatively small. Indeed, immunological studies of human bronchial biopsies yielded a number of unexpected observations, in that the overwhelming majority of cells that stained for interleukin-4 (IL-4) protein

From: *Methods in Molecular Medicine, vol. 44: Asthma: Mechanisms and Protocols*
Edited by: K. F. Chung and I. Adcock © Humana Press Inc., Totowa, NJ

turned out to be mast cells rather than T-cells *(2)*. Mast cells also often contain IL-5 and IL-6; eosinophils may contain IL-5 and transforming growth factor-β. The chief reason for this inability to identify cytokines within the cytoplasm of T-cells is that, instead of storing cytokines and releasing them upon stimulation, the T-cell manufactures cytokines to order, and then releases them more or less immediately *(3)*. Moreover, the translation of mRNA into cytokine protein is subject to posttranscriptional regulation *(4)*, so simply assessing mRNA cytokine profiles is not sufficient to assess the actual type and amount of cytokines that the cell will produce upon stimulation.

To circumvent these problems, a number of techniques have been developed to retain cytokines within the lymphocyte cytoplasm and then stain them for analysis. All these methods have three components: stimulation, retention, and analysis. Each of these components has an important bearing on the eventual experimental result, and careful attention is needed to these technical aspects, especially when comparing data from different models analyzed in different ways (*see* **Notes 1** and **2**).

1.1. Stimulation

In principle, one is usually interested in assessing the potential of the cell at the time it is obtained from the donor, or perhaps at the end of a period of culture. Cells that are resting will require more intense stimulation, and usually more time, before sufficient cytokine accumulates to permit analysis, compared to cells that are already being stimulated in culture. In general, one is interested in determining the identity and quantity of the cytokines that have already been induced, rather than newly induced products, so that it is often appropriate to use stimuli such as phorbol esters, which bring about translation of pre-existing mRNA without inducing new transcription. Other nonspecific mitogens, such as PHA, anti-CD3, and combinations of CD2 and CD28 monoclonal antibodies (mAbs) can also be used, but will probably lead to different patterns of cytokine translation, because of activation of different subcellular pathways *(5)* (*see* **Note 3**).

1.2. Cytokine Retention

Small amounts of certain cytokines (e.g. interferon-γ [IFN-γ]) can be identified in T-cells, without retention, but most cytokines are undetectable in nonparalyzed cells. To retain the cytokine proteins in the cytoplasm, an ionophore is used, which paralyzes transport through the Golgi apparatus. Normally, all secretory proteins are translated in the rough endoplasmic reticulum, then packaged into secretory vesicles in the Golgi. Some additional posttranslational modifications also occur here, e.g., glycosylation and removal of signal peptide; the retained protein may differ antigenically from the secreted form. Most Ag epitopes seem to be expressed in both the secreted and retained protein, but the failure of some anticytokine MAbs to work in this system is probably attributable to their recognition of epitopes expressed on the secreted form, but not on the precursor molecule (*see* **Note 4**).

Monensin, a metabolite of *Streptomyces cinnamonensis,* was the first anti-Golgi agent used for intracytoplasmic cytokine retention ***(6)***. Monensin is very effective, but is also an irreversible cellular poison, so that the cell cannot be recovered after incubation with monensin. Some investigators favor Brefeldin A, which works in a similar way ***(7,8)***.

1.3. Staining Technique

To identify retained cytokine proteins, it is necessary to fix and permeabilize the cell. Fixation (e.g., with paraformaldehyde) serves two purposes: It prevents the cell lysis that would otherwise follow permeabilization, and it also fixes the cytokine proteins within the cell. Permeabilization of the cell membrane (e.g., with saponin) allows MAbs to penetrate the cell and bind to the retained cytokines. For simplicity, directly conjugated antibodies (Abs) have advantages, compared to unconjugated Abs, although it is true that indirect immunofluorescent methods are more sensitive. Typically three-color flow cytometry is then used to allow accurate identification of different cell types or subsets, or simultaneous analysis of two cytokines (**Fig. 1**). Cells may be assessed as positive/negative on the basis of fluorescence intensity, or the pattern or staining can be assessed with the aid of computerized image analysis, in which case, cytokine-specific patterns can be identified (***9***, **Note 2**).

1.4. Applications

The authors' first studies applied the above techniques to bronchoalveolar lavage (BAL) and peripheral blood T-cells from asthmatic subjects, atopic nonasthmatic subjects, and normal healthy controls. *A priori*, the expectation was to find an increased production of T-helper type-2 (Th2) cytokines (IL-4 and IL-5), but, in fact, the principal feature associated with asthma was an increased proportion of BAL T-cells that produced IFN-γ. IL-2 production was similar in all three study groups, and only a small minority of BAL T-cells stained for IL-4 or IL-5 (**Fig. 2**; ***11***). Although there was a trend for an increased proportion of IL-4 producing BAL T-cells in atopic asthma, this was variable between subjects and not statistically significant. In further work, the authors found that this lack of Th2 cytokine production did not appear to result from the use of stimuli that did not favor IL-4 production; similar results were obtained with anti-CD3 and bispecific anti-CD2 MAbs, although the combination of CD2 and CD28 MAbs did increase the proportion of IL-4-producing cells (**Fig. 3**; ***12***).

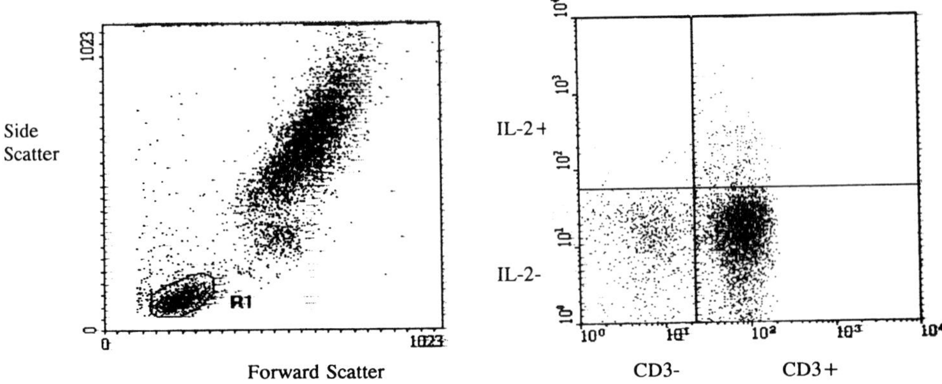

Fig. 1. Two-dimensional plots of forward-scatter (FSC) and side-scatter (SSC) are used to identify the lymphocytes in a blood sample, and an electronic gate is applied (left panel). The gated cells are then analyzed for CD3 expression and IFN-γ staining (right panel).

One of the pieces of evidence supporting an active role of T-cells in asthma was the observation that activated ($CD25^+$) T-cells could be identified in the bronchial mucosa and BAL from patients with asthma ***(13)***. However, a crucial issue in the interpretation of this observation has been the functional significance of the expression of CD25 in vivo, as opposed to in vitro. Intracellular (IC) cytokine staining allows exploration of this, by assessing the cytokine production of $CD25^+$ T-cells from BAL samples. The majority of IFN-γ and IL-2-producing cells are actually $CD25^-$ ***(14)***, and it therefore appears that CD25 expression in vivo may be an indicator of anergy, i.e., cells that have been partially activated and switched off, rather than cells that are currently activated and producing, or about to produce, cytokines ***(15)***. The cells that do produce cytokines upon phorbol myristate acetate (PMA) stimulation are mostly $CD69^+$; this observation that presents questions about CD69 and its possible use as a marker for in vivo T-cell activation ***(16)***.

The authors have also applied these techniques to study the function of T-cells leaving particular T-cell receptor (TCR)-Vβ determinants. This work is at an early stage, but preliminary data indicate that clonal populations of T-cells do exist in BAL, and can be identified by TCR-Vβ staining and genetic analysis ***(17)***. Functional analysis of TCR-Vβ subsets has shown different cytokine profiles among cells belonging to clonal subpopulations, compared to subsets showing polyclonal usage of Vβ genes (**Fig. 4**; ***18***). Here at last evidence was found that certain selected T-cell subpopulations may show increased production of IL-4 and IL-5. This difference is more marked after

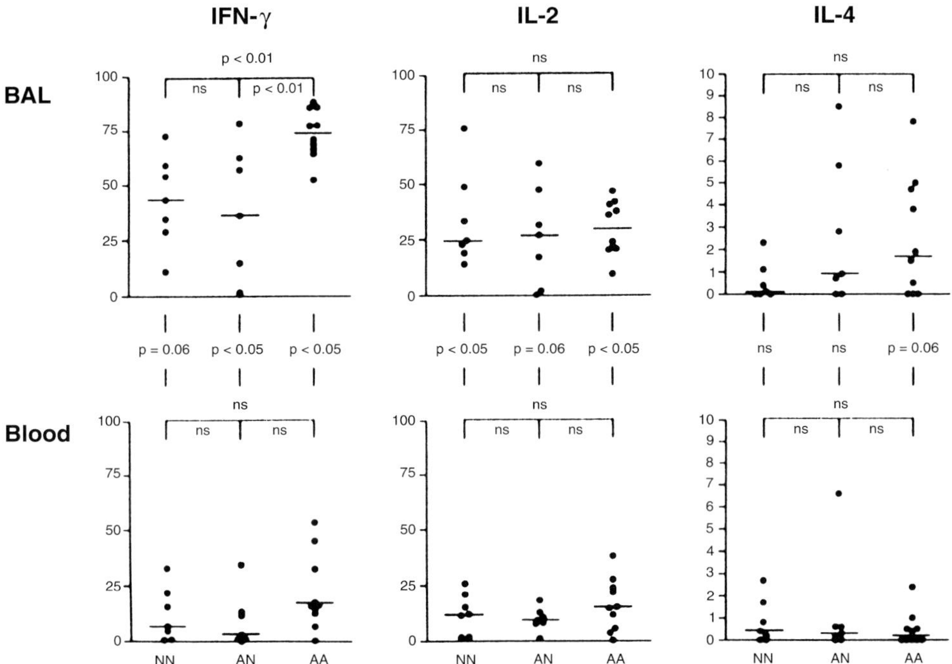

Fig. 2. The proportion of T-cells producing IL-2, IFN-γ, and IL-4 in peripheral blood and BAL from patients with atopic asthma (AA), patients with atopic rhinitis but no asthma (NA), and normal nonatopic healthy controls (NN). Reproduced with permission from **ref. *11***.

allergen challenge, suggesting that it is driven by, or related to, relevant stimuli. Given that clonal expansion is usually driven by Ag, these observations may indicate the presence of a small number of T-cells that recognize relevant Ags/allergens and respond by producing Th2-type cytokines, which in turn favor immunoglobulin E (IgE) production and eosinophilia associated with allergic asthma.

Others have also applied IC cytokine staining techniques to address various aspects of the allergic and asthmatic inflammatory processes. Th clones, derived from mice transgenic for the ovalbumin-specific DO11.10 TCR, were shown to respond differently to Ag exposure, depending on the cytokine content of the culture supernatant *(7)*. Addition of IL-12 or anti-IL-4 MAb caused cells to move toward IFN-γ production; Th2-type cells (IL-4 producing) were generated in standard cultures, presumably as the result of endogenous IL-4 production.

IC cytokine staining has also been used to show that IL-13 is produced by activated human T-cells, and that its production is modulated by both IL-4 and

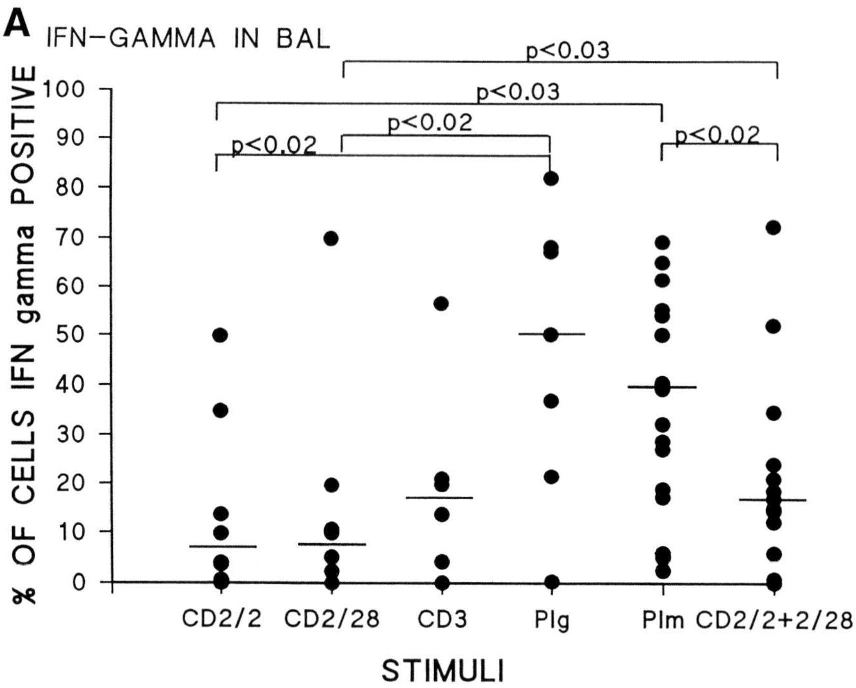
A IFN-GAMMA IN BAL
% OF CELLS IFN gamma POSITIVE
100
90
80
70
60
50
40
30
20
10
0
p<0.03
p<0.03
p<0.02
p<0.02
p<0.02
CD2/2
CD2/28
CD3
PIg
PIm
CD2/2+2/28
STIMULI

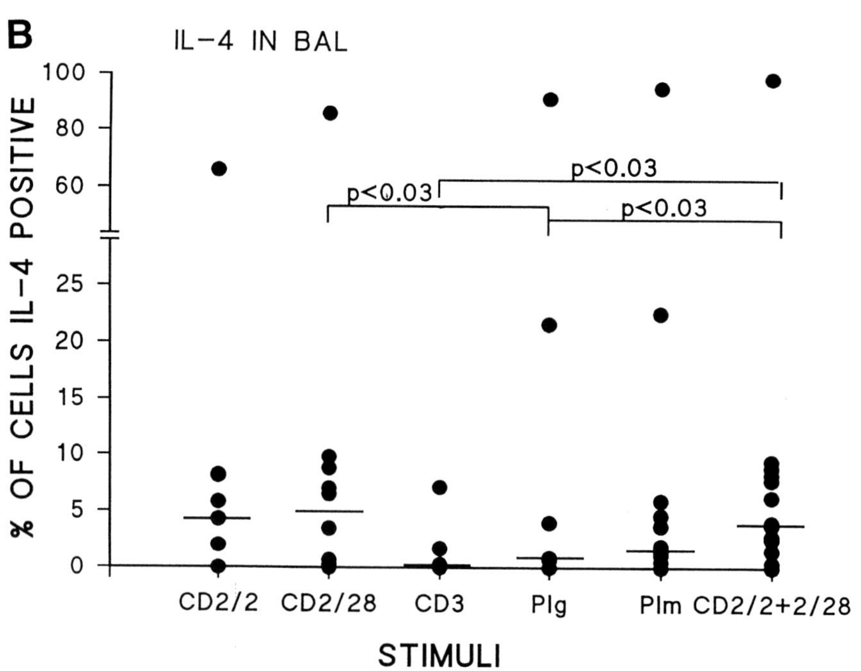
B IL-4 IN BAL
% OF CELLS IL-4 POSITIVE
100
80
60
25
20
15
10
5
0
p<0.03
p<0.03
p<0.03
CD2/2
CD2/28
CD3
PIg
PIm
CD2/2+2/28
STIMULI

IL-12. Among $CD45RO^+$ cells, IL-13 production was associated with IL-4 production, but, in $CD45RA^+$ cells only IL-13 was produced ***(19)***. Because IL-13 can substitute for IL-4 in facilitating B-cell isotype switching to IgE, these data provide further support of T-cell regulation of IgE production.

Others ***(20)*** have used monensin to study cytokine profiles among the human $CD4^+$ $CD27^-$ memory T-cell subpopulation. In this subset, virtually no cells coproduced IL-5 and IFN-γ, but a modest proportion (0.1–8.0%) produced both IL-4 and IFN-γ. Compared with the $CD4^+CD27^+$ subset, the $CD4^+CD27^+$ subset contained more cells that were $IL\text{-}5^+$ $IFN\text{-}\gamma^-$, $IL\text{-}4^+$ $IFN\text{-}\gamma^-$, or $IFN\text{-}\gamma^+IL\text{-}4^-IL\text{-}5^-$, indicating that the $CD4^+CD27^-$ subpopulation is a more differentiated population containing both Th2-like and Th1-like cells. In this study, most $IL\text{-}5^+$ cells also produced IL-4 (66–84%), but the proportion of $IL\text{-}4^+$ cells producing IL-5 was less consistent (3–64%). Others have reported differential time-courses for IL-4 and IL-5, with relatively few cells coproducing these two cytokines on initial stimulation. However, IL-4 and IL-5 were both produced more often by T-cells that had been cultured for at least 14 days with two or more restimulation cycles ***(21)***. Moreover, even in the cultured cells, the frequency of $IL\text{-}4^+IL\text{-}5^+$ cells was no greater than would be expected by chance, given the increased proportions of $IL\text{-}4^+$ cells and $IL\text{-}5^+$ cells. This study provides strong evidence that IL-4 and IL-5 are regulated independently, despite genes being adjacent on chromosome 5q31–33. In general terms, there is a good correlation between an increase in the number of cells staining for IL-4 and the amount of IL-4 released into the supernatant in parallel cultures. The relationship between IFN-γ-producing cells and IFN-γ release is, however, less clear cut ***(21)***. These data allow one to conclude that IL-4 production is either on, or off. Thus, an increase in IL-4 release will reflect entrainment of more cells. In contrast, increased release of IFN-γ seems to reflect increased production and secretion per activated cell, as well as an increase in the frequency of cells producing IFN-γ.

By combining IC cytokine staining with other techniques, it is possible to address immunological mechanisms in great detail. Thus, it has been established for some time that 10-d treatment with corticosteroids leads to an increase in total and specific serum IgE. This in vivo observation has an in vitro correlate, in that peripheral blood mononuclear cells obtained at the end of the steroid course show augmented IgE production, both spontaneous and

Fig. 3. *(opposite page)* Stimulus-dependence of **(A)** IFN-γ and **(B)** IL-4 production by BAL T-cells from nonasthmatic subjects. Stimuli used were bispecific Abs against two determinants of CD2 (CD2/2), a combination of CD2 and CD28 MAbs (CD2/28), a CD3 MAb, PMA, and ionomycin in two concentrations (PIg and PIm) and a combination of CD2/2 and CD2/28 MAbs (CD2/2 + 2/28).

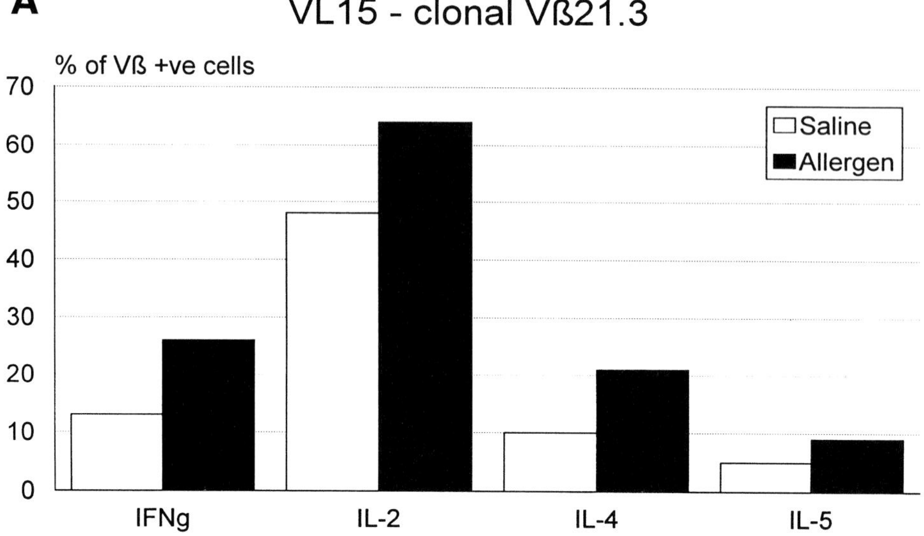

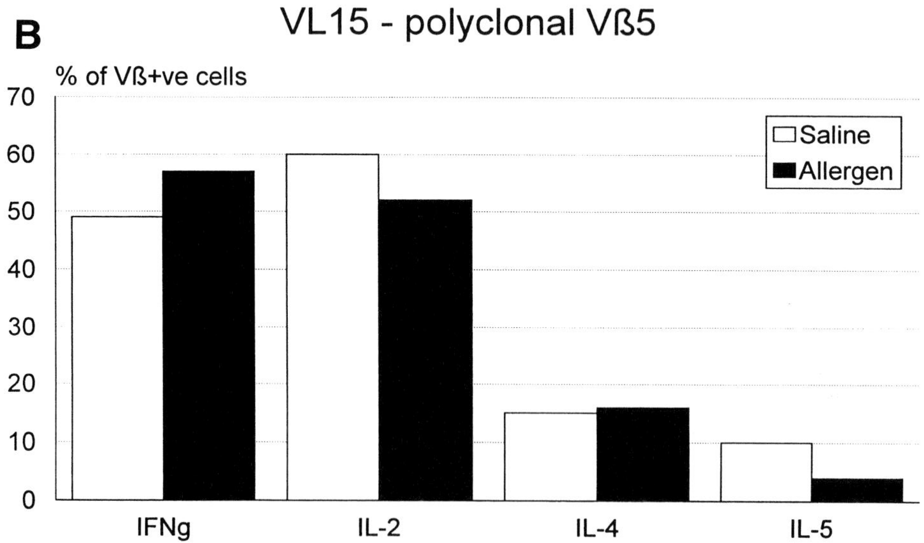

Fig. 4. The proportion of T-cells producing IL-2, IFN-γ, IL-4, or IL-5 within a clonal subpopulation of BAL T-cells expressing Vβ 21.3 (**A**), and within a polyclonal subpopulation of BAL T-cells expressing Vβ6 (**B**). Both sets of data come from the same lavage samples in the same subject 24 h after segmental allergen challenge. Note the much lower proportion of IFN-γ-producing cells in the clonal population (at both allergen and saline sites) and the increased proportion of IL-4-producing cells in the clonal population from the allergen-challenged site, compared with the saline site.

IL-4-induced. IgE synthesis reflects the balance between IL-4 and IFN-γ production, and, although neither cytokine could be detected spontaneously, significant quantities of both cytokines were detected in supernatants after concanavalin A stimulation. IL-4 production did not change, but IFN-γ production decreased to 22% of baseline after steroid treatment. The frequency of IFN-γ-producing cells also decreased, by 39%, indicating both a reduction in the frequency of IFN-γ-producing cells and a reduction in the amount of IFN-γ produced per cell. Further analysis revealed an even larger decrease in the number of IFN-γ-producing natural killer cells *(22)*.

It has long been established that cell-mediated immune responses are depressed in patients with atopic dermatitis. IC cytokine staining has been used to explore the cellular basis of this observation. Although these patients have very high IgE titers and an increased IL-4/:IFN-γ ratio in the supernatant of T-cells stimulated by polyclonal mitogen in vitro, the proportion of IL-4-producing cells is not increased, compared to control subjects. There was, however, a reduced proportion of $CD4^+$ T-cells producing IFN-γ, but no difference in the numbers of $CD8^+$ cells producing IFN-γ. IL-2 production was markedly decreased in all subsets. Taken together, these results indicate a general depression (or repression) of Th1 cells and Tc_1 cells with the maintenance of Th2 cells *(23)*. Although this study did not address IL-5 production, cloning studies indicate that $IL\text{-}5^+IFN\text{-}\gamma^+CD8^+$ T-cells may be important in some forms of allergic disease, and these cells may account for the observed disparity between IL-2 and IFN-γ production by $CD8^+$ cells.

2. Materials

2.1. Cell Samples

1. Heparinized whole blood (can be kept at room temperature for short period).
2. Other samples should be washed and resuspended at 1×10^6 cells/mL in RPMI-1640.

2.2. Stimulation

1. 24-well flat-bottomed plates (Falcon, Becton-Dickinson).
2. Culture buffer: RPMI-1640; 2 m*M* L-glutamine, 1 m*M* sodium pyruvate, 100 U/mL penicillin, 100 µL/mL streptomycin, 20 µ*M* mercaptoethanol, and 5% AB serum.
3. Stimulation buffer: as culture buffer, supplemented with PMA (20 ng/mL), ionomycin (2 µ*M*), and monensin (5 µ*M*).
4. Washing buffer: phosphate-buffered saline (PBS).
5. Fixation buffer: PBS with 4% paraformaldehyde.
6. Permeabilization buffer: PBS with saponin 0.1%, HEPES 0.01 *M*.
7. MAbs: directly conjugated Abs are required, although one biotin-labeled Ab may be used to enhance sensitivity.

3. Methods

3.1. Getting Ready

1. The washing buffers and stimulation buffers should be prepared in advance, according to the above recipes.
2. The stock solutions are kept at +4°C until needed.

3.2. Sample Preparation

1. For peripheral blood samples, stimulation and staining may be performed on heparinized whole blood.
2. Use 200 μL aliquots for each cytokine or control. The blood can be kept at room temperature for a while but should not stand for several hours.
3. If it is thought that granulocytes or monocytes may influence the result, then density-gradient centrifugation and/or carbonyl iron depletion may be used, although these techniques may themselves risk altering the activity of the blood T-cells.
4. Purified cell samples from bronchial lavage, synovial fluid, cell culture, and so on, should be centrifuged at 600*g* for 10 min at +4°C, to separate the cells.
5. Cells are then resuspended in RPMI-1640, counted, and adjusted to 1×10^6 cells/mL.

3.3. Stimulation

1. Make up 200-μL blood samples to 1 mL in culture medium (*see* **Subheading 2.2.**).
2. Plate out in 24-well flat-bottomed plates.
3. For other samples place 1×10^6 cells directly in the wells in 1-mL volume to give a 1×10^6 cells/mL suspension.
4. Each well then receives 1 mL stimulation buffer, giving a final concentration of 10 mg/mL PMA, 1 μ*M* ionomycin, and 2.5 μ*M* monensin.
5. The samples should mix adequately in the plate.
6. Culture the samples for 5 h at 37°C in a humidified atmosphere of 5% CO_2 in air.

3.4. Washing and Fixation

1. At the end of 5 h incubation, the cells and culture medium are aspirated into polypropylene tubes.
2. The wells are washed out with PBS, and the washings added to the aspirated cells.
3. The tubes are centrifuged (600*g* for 10 min), washed in PBS, then fixed for 10 min in ice-cold PBS containing 4% paraformaldehyde.
4. After a further wash in PBS, the cells can be stored overnight at +4°C.

3.5. Staining

1. Fixed cell samples are resuspended in 100 μL saponin buffer (PBS containing 0.1% saponin and 0.01 *M* HEPES).
2. The saponin lyses any remaining red cells, and allows subsequent entry of the MAbs.

3. Anticytokine Abs are diluted in saponin buffer (*see* **Note 4**) and added in 10-µL aliquots, together with 10 µL peridin–chlorophyll–protein conjugate-labeled anti-CD3.
4. After 20 min, the cells are washed in saponin buffer, resuspended in PBS, and analyzed immediately on a flow cytometer.
5. Stained samples may be kept briefly at +4°C in the dark, before analysis, but the fluorescence quenches rapidly, and the authors advise careful quality control assessment if there is to be any consistent delay in analysis.

3.6. Cytometric Analysis

1. The exact protocol used for cytometric analysis will depend on composition of the sample and the question being asked (*see* **Notes 2** and **3**).
2. For samples with many T-cells, and a frequently produced cytokine, 10,000 cells may be collected and stored for later analysis.
3. For BAL samples, and for less frequently produced cytokines, it will usually be necessary to set a live electronic gate to secure sufficient T-cells, and hence improve the precision of the eventual results generated.
4. The lymphocyte peak is selected by gating on the forward- and side-scatter plots.
5. The the remaining cells are analyzed for expression of the various fluorochromes carried on the MAbs.
6. For most purposes, the authors use an anti-CD3 MAb to confirm the identity of T-cells, leaving two channels for analysis of cytokine production and/or T-cell subsets (**Fig. 1**).

3.7. Retrieval of Live Cells

Manz et al. ***(10)*** have devised an alternative system that allows retrieval of live cells after functional analysis.

1. Biotinylate the cell surface by suspending cells in 1 mg/mL sulfosuccinindyl-6-(biotinamido) hexanoate.
2. Bind Ab-avidin complexes to the biotin before stimulating the cells.
3. Any relevant cytokine released from the cell should then bind to the biotin–avidin–Ab matrix on the cell surface.
4. The cytokine can then be labeled and stained for flow cytometry and cell-sorting as described above for CD3.
5. Transfer of secreted products from one cell to another is limited by conducting the experiment with the cells embedded in a gel.
6. Positively selected cells can be sorted, retrieved, and washed prior to use in further experiments.

4. Notes

1. The special advantages of this method include the ability to enumerate the frequency of cells producing a particular cytokine, to correlate cytokine production with surface phenotype, and to study the effects of drugs and other therapies on T-cell function.

2. Like any technique, the results obtained require careful interpretation.
3. It is important to remember, first, that in vivo T-cells become activated by specific Ags, rather than by polyclonal mitogen, and, second, in disease states, the function of a cell is not simply the result of its cytokine production, but is affected by its location and its neighbors, as well as by the number and status of cytokine receptors and the subcellular signaling mechanisms of the target cell.
4. Because the cytokine is retained in the Golgi apparatus, its epitope patterns may be different from the normal secreted molecule. Therefore, some MAbs that work well in fluid phase may not perform well in intracytoplasmic assays. Careful titration and evaluation of each Ab is required, and, ideally, there should be a positive control in each experiment (e.g., a T-cell clone that is known to produce the cytokine of interest). This is not always easy to achieve.

References

1. Ying, S., Durham, S. R., Corrigan, C. J., Hamid, Q., and Kay, A. B. (1995) Phenotype of cells expressing mRNA for TH2 type (IL-4 and IL-5) and TH1 type (IL-2 and IFN-γ) cytokines in bronchoalveolar lavage and bronchial biopsies from asthmatic and normal control subjects. *Am. J. Respir. Cell Mol. Biol.* **12,** 477–487.
2. Bradding, P., Roberts, J. A., Britten, K. M., Montefort, S., Djukanovic, R., Mueller, R., et al. (1994) Interleukins-4, -5, -6 and TNF-alpha in normal and asthmatic airways. Evidence for the human mast cell as an important source of these cytokines. *Am. J. Respir. Cell Mol. Biol.* **10,** 471–480.
3. Powers, G. D., Abbas, A. K., and Muller, R. A. (1988) Frequencies of IL-2 and IL-4 secreting, T., cells in naive and antigen-stimulated lymphocyte populations. *J. Immunol.* **140,** 3352–3357.
4. Ledever, J. A., Lion, J. S., Todd, M. D., Glimcher, L. H., and Lichtman, A. H. (1994) Regulation of cytokine gene expression in, T., helper cell subsets. *J. Immunol.* **152,** 77–86.
5. Leung, J. C. K., Lai, C. K. W., Chui, Y. L., Ho, R. T. H., Chan, C. H. S., and Lai, K. N. (1992) Characterisation of cytokine gene expression in CD4+ and CD8+ T cells after activation with phorbol myristate acetate and phytohaemagglutinin. *Clin. Exp. Immunol.* **90,** 147–153.
6. Jung, T., Schauer, U., Heusser, C., Reumann, C., and Rieger, C. (1993) Detection of intracellular cytokines by flow cytometry. *J. Immunol. Methods* **159,** 197.
7. Ferrick, D. A., Schrenzel, M. D., Mulvania, T., Hsieh, B., Ferlin, W. G., and Lepper, H. (1995) Differential production of interferon-γ and interleukin-4 in response to Th1 and Th2-stimulating pathogens by γδ T-cells in vivo. *Nature* **373,** 255.
8. Openshaw, P. J. M., Murphey, E. E., Hoskan, N. A., Maino, V., Davis, K., Murphey, K., and O'Gara, A. (1995) Heterogeneity of intracellular cytokine synthesis at the single cell level in polarised T helper 1 and T helper 2 populations. *J. Exp. Med.* **182,** 1357–1367.

9. Björk, L., Fehniger, T. E., Andersson, U., and Andersson, J. (1995) Computerised assessment of production of multiple human cytokines at the single cell level using image analysis. *J. Leuk. Biol.* **59,** 287–295.
10. Manz, R., Assenmacher, M., Pflüger, E., Miltenyi, S., and Radbruch, A. (1995) Analysis and sorting of live cells according to secreted molecules relocated to a cell-surface affinity matrix. *Proc. Natl. Acad. Sci. USA* **92,** 1921–1925.
11. Krug, N., Madden, J., Redington, A. E., Lackie, P., Schauer, U., Holgate, S. T., Frew A. J., and Howarth, P. H. (1996) T-cell cytokine profile evaluated at the single cell level in BAL and blood in allergic asthma. *Am. J. Respir. Crit. Care Med.* **14,** 319–326.
12. Madden, J., Krishna, M. T., Redington, A. E., Holgate, S. T., Frew, A. J., and Howarth, P. H. (1999) Time-course and stimulus-dependence of BAL T-cell cytokine production evaluated at the single cell level. *Cytokine* **11,** 456.
13. Robinson, D. S., Bentley, A. M., Hartnell, A., Kay, A. B., and Durham, S. R. (1993) Activated memory T helper cells in bronchoalveolar lavage fluid from patients with atopic asthma:relation to asthma symptoms, lung function and bronchial responsiveness. *Thorax* **48,** 26–32.
14. Madden, J., Frew, A. J., Krishna, M. T., Redington, A. E., Holgate, S. T., and Howarth, P. H. Flow cytometric assessment of the relevance of T-cell subset and activation markers to cytokine protein production capacity in asthma. *Am. J. Respir. Crit. Care. Med.*, in preparation.
15. Schall, T. J., O'Hehir, R. E., Goeddel, D. V., and Lamb, J. R. (1992) Uncoupling of cytokine mRNA expression and protein secretion during the induction phase of T-cell anergy. *J. Immunol.* **148,** 381–387.
16. Hol, B. E. A., Hintzen, R. Q., van Lier, R. A. W., Alberts, C., Out, T. A., and Jansen, H. M. (1993) Soluble and cellular markers of T-cell activation in patients with pulmonary sarcoidosis. *Am. Rev. Respir. Dis.* **148,** 643–649.
17. Dasmahapatra, J., Hodges, E., Smith, J. L., Lanham, S., Krishna, M. T., Holgate, S. T., and Frew, A. J. (1998) T-cell receptor V-beta gene usage in bronchoalveolar lavage and peripheral blood T-cells from asthmatic and normal subjects. *Clin. Exp. Immunol* **112,** 363–374.
18. Jung, T., Wijdenes, J., Neumann, C., de Vries, J. E., and Yssel, H. (1996) Interleukin-13 is produced by activated human CD45RA+ and CD45RO+ T-cells: modulation by IL-4 and IL-12. *Eur. J. Immunol.* **26,** 571–577.
19. Dasmahapatra, J., Smith, J. L., and Frew, A. J. (1997) Effect of local allergen challenge on TcR Vβ usage in BAL T-cells from human airways. *Clin. Exp. Allergy* **27,** 1359.
20. Elson, L. H., Nutman, T. B., Metcalf, D. D., and Prussin, C. (1995) Flow cytometric analysis for cytokine production identifies Th1, Th2 and Th0 cells within the human CD4+CD27-lymphocyte subpopulation. *J. Immunol.* **154,** 4294–4301.
21. Jung, T., Schauer, U., Rieger, C., Wagner, K., Einsle, K., Neumann, C., and Heusser, C. (1995) Interleukin-4 and interleukin-5 are rarely co-expressed by human T-cells. *Eur. J. Immunol.* **25,** 2413–2416.

22. Zieg, G., Lack, G., Harbeck, R. J., Gelfand, E. W., and Leung, D. Y. M. (1994) In vivo effects of glucocorticoids on IgE production. *J. Allergy Clin. Immunol.* **94,** 222–230.

23. Jung, T., Lack, G., Schauer, U., Uberuck, W., Renz, H., Gelfand, E. W., and Rieger, C. H. L. (1995) Decreased frequency of interferon-gamma and IL-2-producing cells in patients with atopic diseases measured at the single cell level. *J. Allergy Clin. Immunol.* **96,** 515–527.

16

Localization of IL-4 and IL-5 mRNA by *In Situ* Hybridization in Bronchial Biopsies

Yutaka Nakamura, Pota Christodoulopoulos, and Qutayba Hamid

1. Introduction

Cytokines are important biochemical mediators essential in initiating and maintaining inflammatory reactions associated with allergic disease in man. Although cytokines can be secreted from a variety of different cell types, considerable attention has been focused on T-lymphocyte-derived cytokines, which have been clearly implicated in the modulation of the immune system. Bronchial asthma is associated with persistent infiltration of the airways with activated $CD4^+$ T-lymphocytes, as well as other inflammatory cells exhibiting a T-helper type-2 (Th2)-like cytokine profile *(1–3)*.

It is evident that Th2-type cytokines, particularly interleukin-4 (IL-4) and IL-5, perform important regulatory roles in asthma, because their gene expression has been localized in vivo at the level of the tissue. These cytokines have been shown to be the driving force behind eosinophil activation, immunoglobulin E production, and stimulation of the endothelium to produce mediators important in allergic inflammation. The localization of IL-4 and IL-5 mRNA in endobronchial biopsies from asthmatic subjects, has been well documented using the technique of *in situ* hybridization (ISH) *(4–7*; **Fig. 1**). ISH has been used extensively to localize cytokine mRNA in tissue sections from normal and diseased individuals *(7–9)*. This approach is valuable in cytokine research, because there is in vitro evidence suggesting that cytokines are synthesized *de novo* and released very rapidly. Thus, the chances of detecting their immunoreactivity in lymphocytes or other cells are limited. The localization of cytokine mRNA at the tissue level indicates the expression and activation of the gene and the potential ability of the cell to produce cytokines. Thus, the *in situ*

From: *Methods in Molecular Medicine, vol. 44: Asthma: Mechanisms and Protocols*
Edited by: K. F. Chung and I. Adcock © Humana Press Inc., Totowa, NJ

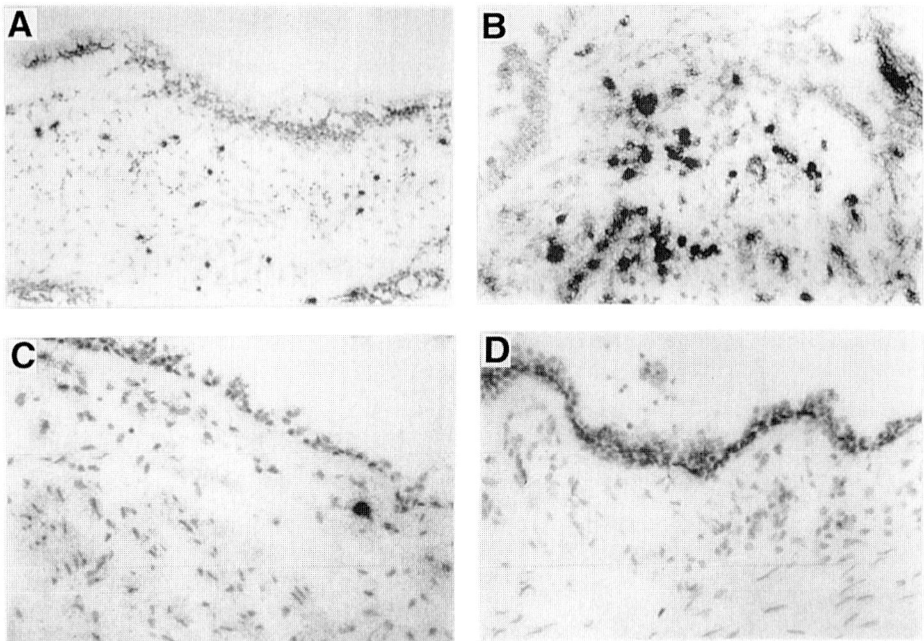

Fig. 1. Representative autoradiographs of ISH of bronchial biopsy specimens using ^{35}S-labeled cRNA probes. Bronchial biopsy specimen from atopic asthmatic hybridized with antisense riboprobes for IL-4 **(A)**, IL-5 **(B)**, and IL-12 **(C)**. Note the strong hybridization signals for IL-4 and IL-5 mRNA compared to IL-12 mRNA, which is normally expressed in Th1 mediated diseases. **(D)** Autoradiograph of bronchial mucosa from normal subject. The section was hybridized with IL-5 cRNA probe. No hybridization signal was detected.

detection of cytokines has provided valuable information on the mechanisms responsible for allergic inflammation. Investigating beyond the presence of activated cells within the tissues, *in situ* localization has enabled both the cellular source and relative contribution of cytokines to be assessed, as well as indicating the possible pathways involved.

ISH in general can be defined as the cellular localization of specific nucleic acid sequences (DNA or RNA), using a labeled complementary strand. The two nucleic acid forms, DNA and RNA, are found in both the nucleus and the cytoplasm, and the technical approach to the demonstration of these molecules in each anatomical location is different. ISH was first introduced in 1969, and was used primarily for the localization of specific DNA sequences ***(10)***. In more recent years, ISH has been applied to localize mRNA, the intermediate molecule in the transfer of genetic information from genomic DNA to functional polypeptide. The regulation of gene expression, through transcriptional activation and inactivation within a cell, is reflected by the cellular content and distribution of the specific message. In disease states, it can be used for temporary studies in relation to physiological, pathological, and developmental processes. This chapter deals with the practical aspects of using RNA probes for the localization of mRNA in clinical material, with particular emphasis on radiolabeled probes.

1.1. Principles of Cytokine mRNA Hybridization

The general principle of ISH is based on the fact that labeled single-stranded RNA or DNA containing complementary sequences (probes) is hybridized intracellularly to mRNA under appropriate conditions, thereby forming a stable hybrid. This will be detected according to the type of labeling of the probe. Different probes are available to detect mRNA, including double- and single-stranded DNA, oligonucleotides, and single-stranded RNA probes. Single-stranded RNA probes have been used extensively in recent years for detection of cytokine mRNA by both isotopic and nonisotopic methods. The use of RNA probes has a number of advantages beyond other types of probes ***(11,12)***, including the ability to synthesize a probe of relatively constant size (*see* **Note 1**), the high stability and affinity of RNA hybrids, and the ability of RNase to remove the unhybridized probe during the posthybridization washing stages. All of these favor the high specificity and sensitivity of RNA probes. To construct a labeled RNA probe, the DNA sequences of interest are subcloned into an RNA expression vector (e.g., pGEM), transfected into *Escherichia coli* bacteria, extracted, and then linearized prior to the in vitro transcription (**Fig. 2**).

1.2. In Vitro Transcription and Probe Labeling

In order to synthesize a single-stranded, radiolabeled RNA probe, the cDNA attached to a promoter site must be transcribed in the presence of labeled nucleotide and the appropriate RNA polymerase (SP6, T7, or T3 polymerase) (***13***; **Fig. 3**). Following transcription, the labeled probe is extracted from the mixture, and the incorporation of the label is assessed. The probe can be used immediately, stored for a limited time in case of radiolabeled probes, or stored for an unlimited time, in the case of nonradiolabeled probes. Two types of labeling can be used for RNA probes: isotopic or nonisotopic. Several types of isotopes can be applied for labeling RNA, including ^{3}H, ^{33}P, ^{32}P, and ^{35}S, and the hybridization signal is detected using autoradiography. Radiolabeled probes have several advantages, including: The efficiency of the probe synthesis can be monitored easily; radioisotopes are readily incorporated into the synthesized RNA; and autoradiography represents the most sensitive detection system available. However, problems that have occurred with the radiolabeled

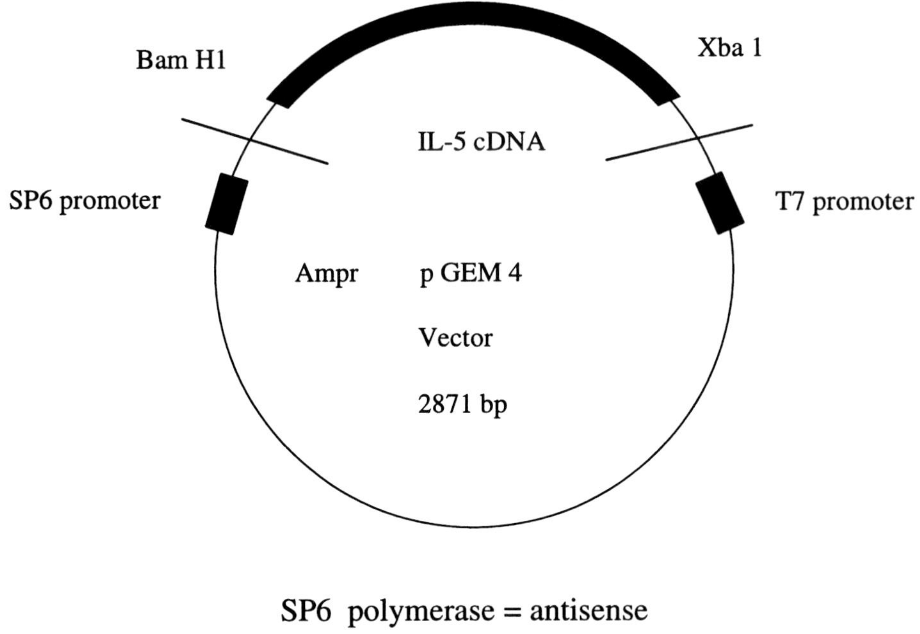

Fig. 2. Diagrammatic representation of cDNA subcloning into a pGEM vector.

probes have prompted the development of nonisotopic labeling of RNA probes. Biotin is one of the first nonisotopic labels to be used for RNA hybridization ***(14)***. Recently, a very sensitive and efficient label has been employed in labeling RNA probes: digoxigenin-11-uridine triphosphate (UTP) ***(15)***. RNA hybrids obtained by using nonradiolabeled probes are usually detected by immunocytochemical methods. A similar excellent resolution is obtained with the nonisotopic-labeled probe, and these probes have the advantage that their signals are developed in a very short time, compared to radiolabeled probes. The major limitation of nonisotopic methods is their relatively poor sensitivity for detection of low copy number of mRNA. Most of the cytokines are expressed in a very low copy number, and thus this method may not be optimal for use in ISH of cytokine mRNA (*see* **Note 2**).

2. Materials

2.1. In Vitro Transcription and Probe Labeling

All chemicals are of molecular biology grade.

1. 5X transcription buffer: 200 m*M* Tris-HCl, pH 7.5, 30 m*M* $MgCl_2$, 10 m*M* spermidine, 5 m*M* NaCl.

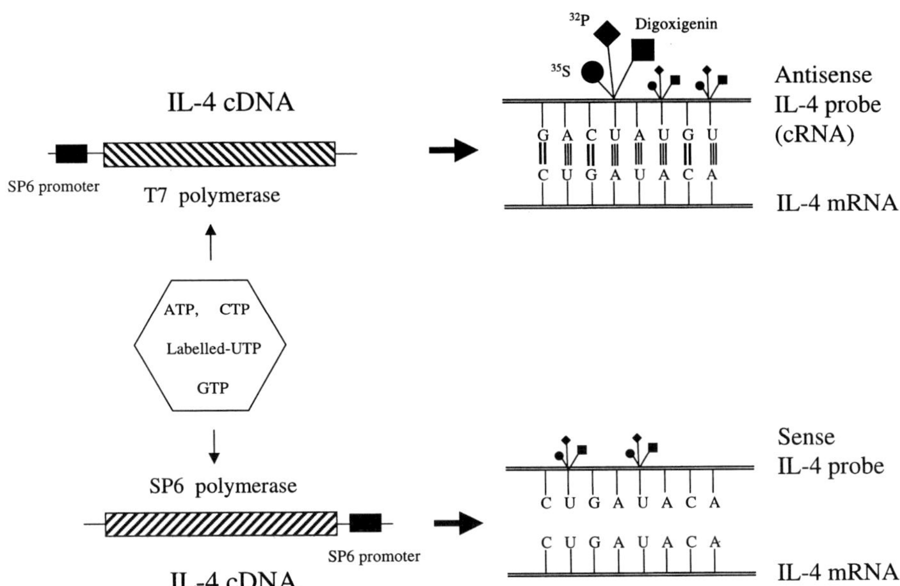

Fig. 3. Diagrammatic representation of ISH procedure. An IL-4 cRNA probe was generated after subcloning of IL-4 cDNA in a pGEM vector. After linearization, in vitro transcription was performed in the presence of GTP, CTP, labeled-UTP, and the appropriate RNA polymerases, to generate either antisense or sense probes.

2. 100 m*M* dithiothreitol (DTT).
3. RNasin: 25 U/µL human placental ribonuclease inhibitor.
4. Nucleotide mixture: 2.5 m*M* each of adenosine triphosphate (ATP), guanosine triphosphate (GTP), and UTP.
5. 100 µ*M* cytosine triphosphate (CTP).
6. Tris-ethlenediamine tetraacetic acid (EDTA) buffer (TE): 10 m*M* Tris-HCl, pH 8.0, 1 m*M* EDTA.
7. Linearized plasmid DNA (1 µg/µL) in water or distilled water.
8. 10 mCi/mL ^{32}P or ^{35}S CTP: ^{32}P or ^{35}S UTP can also be used, but the nucleotide mixture must be altered accordingly.
9. SP6, T3, or T7 polymerases, depending on the vector used (*see* **Note 3**).
10. RNase-free DNase.
11. Transfer RNA (tRNA, 10 µg/µL).
12. 4 *M* NaCl.
13. Phenol–chloroform (1:1, v/v).

2.2. Prehybridization Treatment of Cells and Tissues

1. Phosphate-buffered saline (PBS).
2. Proteinase K.

3. 100 m*M* Tris-HCl, pH 8.0, 50 m*M* EDTA.
4. 4% paraformaldehyde in PBS.
5. 0.25% acetic anhydride, 0.1 *M* triethanolamine, pH 8.0 (for ^{32}P-labeled probes).
6. 10 m*M* iodoacetamide.
7. 10 m*M* *N*-ethylmaleimide.
8. Deionized formamide.
9. 20X standard sodium citrate (SSC): 3 *M* NaCl, 0.3 *M* Na citrate, pH 7.0.

2.3. Hybridization of mRNA to cRNA Probes

1. Deionized formamide.
2. 100X Denhardt's solution: 2% (w/v) bovine serum albumin (BSA), 2% (w/v) Ficoll 400, 2% (w/v) polyvinylpyrrolidine (PVP) 360.
3. Salmon sperm DNA: 10 mg/mL, sheared by autoclaving or sonication.
4. 50% (w/v) dextran sulfate in diethyl pyrocarbonate (DEPC)-treated water.
5. Hybridization buffer: 50% deionized formamide, 5X Denhardt's solution, 10% dextran sulphate, 0.5% Na pyrophosphate, and 0.5% sodium dodecyl sulfate (SDS). Salmon sperm DNA should be denatured by boiling for 10 min, and added to 250 mg/mL prior to hybridization. DTT should be added to 100 m*M*, if ^{35}S-labeled probes are used.
6. Radiolabeled RNA probe.
7. Hybridization mixture: 9 vol hybridization buffer and 1 vol radiolabeled cRNA probe, to give $0.5–1 \times 10^6$ cpm/section. If required, the probe should be diluted in DEPC-treated water prior to addition to the hybridization buffer.
8. Dimethyldichlorosilane-coated cover slips.

2.4. Posthybridization Washing

1. 20X SSC: 3 *M* NaCl, 0.3 *M* Na citrate, pH 7.0.
2. Stock RNase: 10 mg/mL in distilled water. Store at –20°C.
3. RNase A solution: 20 mg/mL RNase A in 0.5 *M* NaCl, 10 m*M* Tris-HCl, pH 8.0, 1 m*M* EDTA.
4. 70, 90, and 100% ethanol containing 0.3 *M* ammonium acetate for 10 min each at room temperature (RT).
5. Air-dry the slides at RT for 1 h.

3. Methods

3.1. Labeling of RNA Probes by In Vitro Transcription

1. Add the following to a sterile microcentrifuge tube at RT in this order: 2 mL 5X transcription buffer: 200 m*M* Tris-HCl, pH 7.5, 30 m*M* $MgCl_2$, 10 m*M* spermidine, 5 m*M* NaCl; 1 µL DTT: 100 m*M* dithiothreitol); 0.4 µL RNasin: 25 U/mL human placental RNase inhibitor; 2 µL nucleotide mixture: 2.5 m*M* each of ATP, GTP, and UTP; 1 µL plasmid DNA (1 mg/mL): linearized plasmid DNA in distilled H_2O; 5 µL radiolabeled UTP (^{35}S) or CTP (^{32}P: 10 mCi/mL; 1 µL RNA polymerase: SP6, T3, or T7 polymerases, depending on the vector used.

2. Incubate the above mixture for a minimum of 1 h at 37°C, then add a further 0.5 µL RNA polymerase, to enhance the transcription, and incubate for a further 30 min.
3. To terminate the transcription, add 1 µL RNase-free DNase, and incubate for 10 min at 37°C to destroy the template.
4. Separate the probe from unincorporated nucleotides by adding the following: 1 µL tRNA; 175 µL DEPC-treated water; 5 µL 4 *M* NaCl; 200 µL phenol–chloroform (1:1) an equal volume.
5. Mix, spin for 5 min at 12,000*g* in a microcentrifuge, and remove the upper aqueous phase (200 mL). Extract again with an equal volume of chloroform, then mix by vortexing, and spin for 5 min at 12,000*g*.
6. Add 100 µL 7 *M* ammonium acetate (2.5 *M* final concentration) and 750 mL cold (from a –20°C freezer) absolute ethanol (approx 2.5 vol) to the upper aqueous phase, mix, and leave to precipitate overnight at –20°C or for 2 h at –80°C.
7. Spin in a microcentrifuge at 12,000*g* for 20 min, and discard the supernatant. Dry the RNA pellet under speed vacuum, and, when dry, dissolve it in 20 mL DEPC-treated water. Remove 1 mL for assessment of incorporation of radioactivity.
8. Store ^{32}P-labeled probes at –20°C and ^{35}S-labeled probes at –80°C.
9. Count the radioactivity of the probe using a β-counter, using scintillation fluid, if necessary, and calculate the specific activity of the probe.

3.2. Tissue Preparation

When performing ISH, it is essential to keep the tissue RNase-free. Because fingertips are a rich source of RNase, it is imperative to wear gloves whenever coming into contact with the tissue. The procedure of ISH begins with fixation of the involved tissue. The fixative must preserve the tissue in a morphologically intact state, while retaining the maximum accessible mRNA within the cells, particularly in the regular conditions used for ISH. One of the best fixatives commonly used for hybridization is 4% paraformaldehyde, which maintains morphological integrity while allowing efficient hybridization. Paraformaldehyde is a solid formaldehyde powder that can be solubilized by dissolving in PBS >60–90 min at a temperature not exceeding 58°C. Freshly prepared paraformaldehyde should be used before it breaks down into several substances, and thus lose its ability to retain maximum mRNA. The time of fixation differs according to the type of preparation. For endoscopic biopsies, a 2-h fixation is recommended, because overfixation can decrease the hybridization signal by masking the mRNA. After fixation, the tissue is rinsed with three changes of 15% PBS–sucrose (1 h each change, and the last change overnight). Once fixed, the tissue can be either blocked in paraffin or blocked with optimal cutting temperature (OCT) medium, and frozen in isopentane-cooled liquid nitrogen. Optimum morphological preservation in paraffin-embedded material may be accompanied by substantial reductions in the density of hybridization, compared to frozen-section material ***(13)***.

3.3. Slide Treatment

The pretreatment of slides is essential, because it serves to minimize nonspecific attachment of radiolabeled probes to slides, and to maximize retention of the tissue on the slides throughout the various rigorous treatments involved in *in situ* protocols. The authors recommend the following method:

3.3.1. Cleaning and Coating Slides with Poly-L-Lysine

1. Wash single-end frosted-glass slides in 1 *M* HCl for 20 min.
2. Rinse in deionized water.
3. Dip the slides in 100% ethanol for 20 min.
4. Dry at RT, and autoclave the slides to remove any trace of RNase activity.
5. Coat the slides with poly-L-lysine (PLL) (mol wt 150–30,000) prior to sectioning the tissue with the cryostat (do not use after 48 h).

3.4. Tissue Sectioning

Relatively thick sections are usually employed for ISH, and these are placed on PLL-precoated slides, allowed to dry, and then processed for hybridization.

1. Cut 10 mm thick sections, and mount them toward one end of the pretreated slide.
2. Put the slides in a clean rack, dry in fume hood.
3. Cover them loosely with foil, and bake them overnight at 37°C.
4. Use the sections the next day, or store them at –80°C for up to 12 mo.

3.5. Tissue Pretreatment

Before starting the hybridization procedure, the tissue preparation must be pretreated, to increase the efficiency of hybridization by rendering the target sequences more accessible to the probe. Most of the methods described are directed toward the permeabilization of the fixed cellular protein matrix, including the use of protease, acid, and detergents (*see* **Fig. 4**).

1. Rehydrate tissue sections in PBS (10 m*M* phosphate, 150 m*M* NaCl, pH 7.2) for 5 min.
2. Immerse in PBS containing 0.1 *M* glycine for 5 min, then PBS containing 0.3% Triton X-100 for 10 min.
3. Wash in two changes of PBS for 3 min each.
4. Incubate with 1 mg/mL proteinase K in 100 m*M* Tris-HCl, pH 8.0, 50 mM EDTA for 30 min at 37°C. This stage is critical: You may need to alter the concentration of proteinase K and the incubation time, according to the type of preparation.
5. Postfix in 4% paraformaldehyde in DEPC-treated PBS for 5 min.
6. Wash in two changes of PBS for 3 min each.
7. Immerse in 0.25% acetic anhydride, 0.1 *M* triethanolamine, pH 8.0, for 10 min, for ^{32}P-labeled probes. For ^{35}S-labeled probes, the slides should also be treated

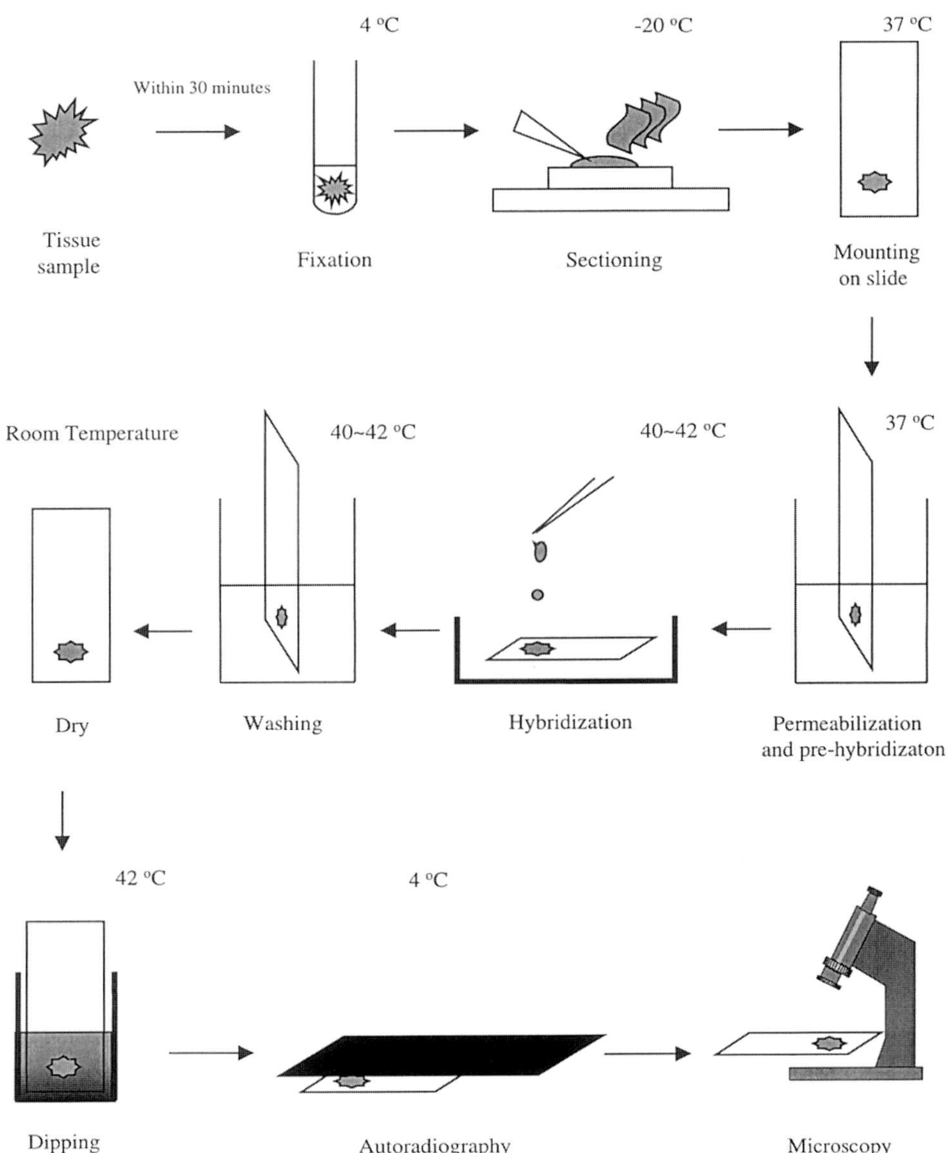

Fig. 4. Diagrammatic representation of ISH procedure.

with 10 m*M* iodoacetamide and 10 m*M* *N*-ethylmaleimide for 30 min to reduce nonspecific binding of the probe.

8. Prehybridize with 50% formamide, 2X SSC, pH 7.0, for at least 15 min at 37°C.

3.6. Hybridization

The conditions of hybridization vary, to allow the probe sufficient access to the cytoplasmic constituents, while allowing the appropriate stringency in tissue preservation. For the hybridization of cytokines, the probes should be incubated with the pretreated tissue within optimal incubation conditions, usually overnight, to allow the hybridization between the complementary RNA probe and the cytoplasmic mRNA.

3.6.1. Hybridization of mRNA to cRNA Probes

1. Drain the slides briefly (do not dry).
2. Apply 20 µL hybridization mixture (*see* **Subheading 3.6.2.**) preheated to 37°C.
3. Cover the section with suitably sized dimethyldichlorosilane-coated cover slips.
4. Incubate in a moist atmosphere at 37–43°C for 16 h (or overnight).

3.6.2. Hybridization Mixture

1. 9 vol hybridization buffer: 50% deionized formamide, 5X Denhardt's solution (2% BSA, 2% Ficoll 400, 2% PVP 360), 10% dextran sulfate, 0.5% Na pyrophosphate, and 0.5% SDS. Salmon sperm DNA should be denatured by boiling for 10 min, and added to 250 µg/mL prior to hybridization. DTT should be added to 100 m*M*, if ^{35}S-labeled probes are used.
2. 1 vol radiolabeled cRNA probe, to give 0.5–1 × 10^6 cpm/section. If required, the probe should be diluted in DEPC-treated water prior to addition to the hybridization buffer.

3.7. Posthybridization Washing

Not all the probes will be hybridized to the mRNA; thus, the preparation needs to be stringently washed to remove the background signal. The washing conditions determine the specificity of ISH and the degree of background staining, they should allow sufficient diffusion of material trapped in the section, and select for a good fit between probe and target mRNA. The availability of RNase to digest the unhybridized probe favors the use of RNA probes for cytokine *in situ* hybridization.

3.7.1. Posthybridization Washing Procedure

1. Remove the cover slips by immersion in 4X SSC.
2. Wash the slides in three changes of 4X SSC at 40–42°C for 20 min each, with gentle agitation.
3. Remove unhybridized, single-stranded cRNA probe by incubation in RNase solution for 20 min at 40–42°C (*see* **Note 4**).
4. Wash the slides in 2X SSC for 30 min at 40°C, then 0.1X SSC for 30 min at 40°C.
5. Dehydrate in 70 and 90%, then two changes of 100%, ethanol containing 0.3 *M* ammonium acetate for 10 min each at RT.
6. Air-dry the slides at RT for 1 h.

3.8. Detection of Hybridization

The hybridization signals are detected according to the label that has been incorporated into the probe. For nonradiolabeled probes, the RNA–RNA hybrid is usually detected by immunocytochemical methods, in which an antibody (i.e., antidigoxigenin) is used, and developed by chromogens ***(15,16)***. For radiolabeled probes, standard autoradiography is performed, and the slides are dipped in liquid emulsion ***(11)***. The incubation period will depend on the radiolabeled probe used, and should be standardized beforehand. Once developed, the signal will appear as dark silver granules overlaying the emulsion, which covers the cells or sections. When the morphology of the cell is difficult to identify, dark-field illumination can help.

3.8.1. Autoradiography of Slides

1. Place the dipping chamber and a vial of emulsion in a 45°C water bath for 10–15 min to warm, then pour the emulsion slowly down the side of the chamber, so that no bubbles form. (The emulsion used for ISH is Hypercoat LM; Amersham Pharmacia Biotech, Inc., Baie d'Urfé, Quebec, Canada). It is semisolid at RT, and becomes liquid when warmed with an equal part of distilled water at 42°C.)
2. Dip the slides and place them on end in a slide rack.
3. Allow the slides to dry for at least 3 h. A nonsparking fan can be used to reduce this time to 1 h.
4. Store the dried slides in light-tight plastic boxes, together with a small container of silica gel to maintain dryness. Seal the boxes with black electrical tape and store these light-proof containers at 4°C, for exposure to occur. Moisture will cause fading of the latent image, and, with very weak signals, the fading of the image can be nearly equal to its production. However, if the slides are kept very dry, even very weak signals can be detected after a long exposure. The autoradiographic exposure time may range from a few hours to many days. Therefore, it is necessary to have several replicated slides, so that test slides can be developed at intervals to determine the correct exposure time.
5. Although the exact temperature is not critical, it is best to develop the autoradiographs at 18–20°C. The lower the temperature, the smaller the grain size. However, it is more important that the slides and all of the developer and fixer solutions are at the same temperature, since temperature changes may produce wrinkles in the emulsion. The schedule for developing autoradiographs is:
   a. Kodak D19 developer: 2.5 min.
   b. Stop-bath (water): 30 s.
   c. Kodak rapid fixer: 5 min.
   d. Distilled water: 15 min wash. This step can be carried out in daylight.
   e. While the slides are in the developer, agitate them gently by rocking the dish back and forth for cycles of 6 s movement and 6 s rest. The movement ensures that the developer is mixed, and does not become depleted near areas of high grain density on the slides. Slides should also be agitated gently in the other

solutions from time to time. However, the amount of agitation is not as critical as during the incubation in the developer.

f. After the final rinse, counterstain the slides immediately in hematoxylin.

3.9. Controls and Specificity of ISH

Appropriate controls are necessary during every ISH experiment, in order to assess the specificity of the reagents and the procedures used. Proper positive and negative controls for tissue, probes, and reagents are essential.

3.9.1. Tissue

The tissue should be evaluated for specific mRNA content by Northern blot analysis, especially when studying the absence of specific hybridization or the change in message content under various physiological conditions. Northern blot analysis monitors mRNA levels within a large, often heterogeneous population of cells. In some cases, ISH reveals mRNA within such a small percentage of cells that a Northern blot analysis of tissue cannot detect it.

3.9.2. Probes

Northern blotting, however, is the most conclusive analysis of probe specificity. The probe must be able to hybridize to a specific mRNA population containing nucleic acids complementary to the probe. Furthermore, the accurate melting temperature of the probe and mRNA can be determined by Northern blot analysis, because these temperatures will reflect the stringency of hybridization required in subsequent experiments on tissue.

3.9.3. Hybridization Specificity

Controls for hybridization are also required to ensure that the autoradiographic signal is the result of specific nucleic acid interactions. Nonspecific interactions include edge artifacts and stickiness of probe to different tissue types. Weak specific interactions include the binding of probe to related sequences and to ribosomal RNA. The use of unrelated probes and sense probes on additional tissue sections addresses the contribution of these interactions. The specificity of hybridization must be assessed by estimating the melting temperature between the probe and signal. A specific signal will withstand increased stringency of hybridization, while non-specific or weak interactions will dissociate at elevated temperatures. RNase pretreatment is another method of demonstrating that the signals are bound to a digestible RNA species. Loss of signal by RNase pretreatment of slides shows only that the probe was interacting with digestible nucleic acids. For this type of control, treat the preparations with RNase (20 μg/mL) for 30 min prior to the prehybridization step, and then proceed. Histological controls are the least quantitative and the most important controls for ISH. The hybridization signal must conform to known anatomical structures. In addition, signals within a specific cell type should reflect the distribution of that cell type within the tissue. Adjacent histological cell types should be identified by a clear lack of signal, if possible.

3.10. Quantification and Interpretation of Results

Many factors must be carefully considered and controlled, if quantitative data are to be collected ***(18)***, including section thickness, nucleic acid retention, consistency of hybridization, length of exposure, and development conditions. The inclusion of a known standard and the construction of a standard curve are essential. However, even under optimal conditions, the quantification of cytokine mRNA at the ISH level is at best semiquantitative.

When interpreting ISH results, it is essential to be convinced that the autoradiographic signal is really specific. For example, a number of inflammatory cells, such as eosinophils and macrophages, have the capacity to bind probe nonspecifically, especially with ^{35}S-labeled probes ***(8)***. Caution must be exercised in the interpretation of autoradiographic signal at the edge of the section (edge artifact). It is also important to take into consideration other factors, such as the formation of imperfect duplexes with nonhomologous nucleic acids, electrostatic interactions among charged groups, and physical entrapment of probe in the three-dimensional lattice of the tissue section. A proper microscope with dark-field illumination and phase-contrast facilities is essential for correct interpretation of autoradiographic signals. It is essential to include a positive and negative control in each radioactive ISH experiment. Absence of autoradiographic hybridization signal does not necessarily indicate the absence of a particular mRNA and its translation product. mRNA could be expressed in low copy number, which is beyond the sensitivity of the technique. Moreover, ISH determines the steady-state amount of hybridizable specific mRNA; immunoreactive proteins are localized by immunocytochemistry. Despite the fact that the expression of the majority of genes is regulated by the amount of specific mRNA, conclusions drawn from double-staining experiments, such as estimation of secretory activity, must be considered carefully. In addition, several other factors at the posttranscriptional and posttranslational levels influence the amount and type of detectable gene expression products.

4. Notes

1. The diffusibility of the probe into the cell and its hybridization to the messenger sequences associated with ribosomes, and crosslinked with the cell matrix, are both influenced by the size of the probe fragment after transcription. Paraformaldehyde-fixed cells tolerate a broad range of probe sizes, which is consistent with the hypothesis that cells or tissue fixed with paraformaldehyde are less crosslinked, and hence more permeable. A reasonable result can be obtained with

probes of 100–400 bases. Probes of a length of more than 500 bases should be digested to an average of 150–200 bases using limited alkaline hydrolysis.

2. The choice of the probe is a trade-off between sensitivity and resolution. In general, high sensitivity implies the use of highly energetic, high-specific-activity labels, such as ^{32}P or ^{35}S. However, these radioisotopes produce the most energetic β particles on decay, which travel farther through autoradiographic emulsions and produce a wide scattering of silver grains. This leads to relatively poor resolution. In contrast, a low-energy radioisotope, such as ^{3}H, gives better resolution, but needs a long exposure time.
3. These enzymes (SP6, T3, and T7 polymerases) are very labile and should be kept out of the freezer for the minimum time posssible.
4. Nonspecific interactions can be greatly reduced, if the sections are exposed to an RNase that selectively degrades unhybridized RNA segments. Most specific hybridization is spared under these conditions, because the hybrids are double-stranded.

Acknowledgment

The authors would like to Sun Ying and the members of this molecular biology laboratory, who have contributed to the work done in this chapter. This work was supported by the Medical Research Council of Canada.

References

1. Robinson, D., Hamid, Q., Bentley, A., Ying, A., Kay, A. B., and Durham, S. R. (1993) Activation of CD4+ T cells and eosinophil recruitment in bronchoalveolar lavage after allergic allergen inhalation challenge in patients with atopic asthma. *J. Allergy Clin. Immunol.* **92,** 313–324.
2. Azzawi, M., Bradley, B., Jeffrey, P. K., Frew, A. J., Wardlaw, A., Assoufi, B., et al. (1990) Identification of activated T lymphocytes and eosinophils in bronchial biopsies in stable atopic asthma. *Am. Rev. Respir. Dis.* **142,** 1407–1413.
3. Bentley, A. M., Menz, G., Storz, C., Robinson, D. S., Bradley, B., Jeffrey, P. K., et al. (1992) Identification of T lymphocytes, macrophages, and activated eosinophils in the bronchial mucosa in intrinsic asthma. *Am. Rev. Respir. Dis.* **146,** 500–506.
4. Humbert, M., Durham, S. R., Ying, S., Kimmitt, P., Barkans, J., Assoufi, B., et al. (1996) IL-4 and IL-5 mRNA and protein expression in bronchial biopsies from patients with atopic and nonatopic asthma: evidence against "intrinsic" asthma being a distinct immunopathological entity. *Am. J. Respir. Crit. Care Med.* **154,** 1497–1504.
5. Ying, S., Durham, S. R., Corrigan, C.J., Hamid, Q., and Kay, A. B. (1995) Phenotype of cells expressing mRNA for Th2-type (Interleukin 4 and Interleukin 5) and Th1-type (Interleukin 2 and Interferon g) cytokines in bronchoalveolar lavage and bronchial biopsies from atopic asthmatic and normal control subjects. *Am. J. Respir. Cell Mol. Biol.* **12,** 477–487.

6. Kotsimbos, T. C., Ernst, P., and Hamid, Q. A. (1996) Interleukin-13 and interleukin-4 are coexpressed in atopic asthma. *Proc. Assoc. Am. Physicians* **108,** 368–373.
7. Hamid, Q. A., Azzawi, M., Jeffrey, P., and Kay, A. B. (1991) Expression of mRNA for interleukin-5 in mucosal bronchial biopsies from asthma. *J. Clin. Invest.* **87,** 154–159.
8. Kay, A. B., Ying, S., Varney, V., et al. (1991) Messenger RNA expression of the cytokine gene cluster IL-3, IL-4, IL-5 and GM-CSF in allergen-induced late-phase cutaneous reactions in atopic subjects. *J. Exp. Med.* **173,** 775–778.
9. Robinson, D., Hamid, Q. A., Ying, S., et al. (1992) Predominant Th2-type bronchoalveolar lavage T lymphocytes population in atopic asthma. *N. Engl. J. Med.* **326,** 298–304.
10. Pardue, M. L. and Gall, J. G. (1969) Molecular hybridization of radioactive DNA to the DNA of cytological preparations. *Proc. Natl. Acad. Sci. USA* **64,** 600–604.
11. Cox, K. H., DeLeon, D. V., Angerer, L. M., and Angerer, R. C. (1984) Detection of mRNAs in sea urchin embryos by *in situ* hybridization using RNA probes. *Dev. Biol.* **101,** 485–502.
12. Hofler, H., Childer, H., Montminy, M. R., Lachan, R. M., Goodman, R. H., and Wolfe, H. J. (1986) *In situ* hybridization methods for the detection of somatostatin mRNA in tissue sections using antisense RNA probes. *Histochem. J.* **18,** 597–662.
13. Hamid, Q., Wharton, J., Terenghhi, G., Hassall, C. J. S., Aimi, J., Taylor, K. M., et al. (1987) Localization of atrial natriuretic peptide mRNA and immunoreactivity in the rat heart and human atrial appendage. *Proc. Natl. Acad. Sci. USA* **84,** 6760–6764.
14. Giaid, A., Hamid, Q., Adams, C., Trenghi, G., and Polak, J. M. (1989) Non-isotopic RNA probes; comparison between different labels and detection systems. *Histochemistry* **93,** 191–196.
15. Ying, S., Durham, S. R., Jacobson, M., Masuyama, M., Kay, A. B., and Hamid, Q. (1994) Phenotype of cells expressing interleukin-4 (IL-4), IL-5, IL-2 and interferon-gamma (IFN-g) mRNA in the nasal mucosa following allergen provocation. *J. Allergy Clin. Immunol.* **93,** 270.
16. Ying, S., Durham, S. R., Barkans, J., et al. (1994) T lymphocytes and mast cells express messenger RNA for interleukin-4 in the nasal mucosa in allergen-induced rhinitis. *Immunology* **82,** 200.
17. Roger, A. W. (1979) *Techniques in Autoradiography*. Elsevier North Holland, Amsterdam.
18. Davenport, A. P. and Nunez, D. J. (1990) Quantification of hybridization signal. In: *In Situ Hybridization: Principles and Practice* (Polak, J. M. and McGee, J. O'D., eds.), Oxford University Press, Oxford, UK, pp. 173–281.

17

Immunohistochemical Analysis of Adhesion Molecules in Airway Biopsies

Susan J. Wilson and Stephen T. Holgate

1. Introduction

Adhesion molecules are receptors found on the surface of leukocytes and endothelial cells, which bind to their ligands, either on other cells or on the extracellular matrix. The function of adhesion molecules is to allow leukocytes to interact with other hemopoetic cells or with foreign antigens (Ags) in the blood, to transiently adhere to the vascular endothelium, to migrate between endothelial cells and through the basement membrane into the surrounding tissue, and to adhere to the epithelium. There are three main groups of adhesion molecules: the integrins, immunoglobulin (Ig) supergene family, and the selectins: These are summarized in **Table 1** *(1–7)*.

During the allergic inflammatory response, upregulation in the expression of several adhesion molecules under the influence of cytokines is a prerequisite for the increased recruitment of eosinophils, neutrophils, and lymphocytes into the mucosa. This is a dynamic series of events, and initially involves increased expression of E-selectin, induced by tumor necrosis factor-α (TNF-α) and interleukin-1β (IL-1β) *(8,9)*, and P-selectin by histamine *(10)*. Both of these selectins are involved in the margination and rolling of leukocytes along the endothelium *(10)* by interaction with the ligand, sialyl Lewis X, present on the cell surface *(11)*. A more permanent adhesion is then achieved with the upregulation of intercellular adhesion molecule-1 (ICAM-1) and vascular cell adhesion molecule-1 (VCAM-1) on the vascular endothelium *(12)*. The ligands for these are lymphocyte function-associated antigen 1 (LFA-1) and very late actuation-4 (VLA-4), respectively *(13)*; the

From: *Methods in Molecular Medicine, vol. 44: Asthma: Mechanisms and Protocols*
Edited by: K. F. Chung and I. Adcock © Humana Press Inc., Totowa, NJ

Table 1
Summary of Adhesion Molecules

Group	CD number	Name	Expressed on	Ligand
Integrins				
B1 very late antigens	CD 49a	VLA-1	T lymphocytes, fibroblasts, basement membrane	Laminin, collagen
	CD 49b	VLA-2	Activated T lymphocytes, platelets, fibroblasts, endothelium, epithelium	Collagen, laminin
	CD 49c	VLA-3	Epithelium, fibroblasts	Laminin, collagen, fibronectin
	CD 49d	VLA-4	Leukocytes, fibroblasts	VCAM-1, fibronectin
	CD 49e	VLA-5	Leukocytes, platelets, epithelium	Fibronectin
	CD 49f	VLA-6	T lymphocytes, platelets	Laminin
B2 leukocyte integrins	CD 11a	LFA-1	Leukocytes	ICAM-1, ICAM-2, ICAM-3
	CD 11b	Mac-1	Macrophages, monocytes, granulocytes	ICAM-1, fibrinogen, C3bi
	CD 11c	p150.95	Macrophages, monocytes, granulocytes	Fibrinogen, C3bi
IG Supergene family	CD 54	ICAM-1	Endothelium, leukocytes, epithelium	LFA-1 Mac-1
	CD 102	ICAM-2	Endothelium, leukocytes	LFA-1
	CD 106	VCAM-1	Endothelium, dendritic cells, tissue macrophages	VLA-4
Selectins	CD 62E	E selectin	Endothelium	Sialyl Lewis x
	CD 62P	P selectin	Platelets, endothelium	Sialyl Lewis x
	CD 62L	L selectin	Leukocytes	Mannose-6-P, fructose-6-P

former is involved in the recruitment of T-lymphocytes and neutrophils, and the latter in the selection of eosinophils ***(12,14)***. TNF-α and interferon-γ increase ICAM-1 expression, ***(15)*** and TNF-α in the presence of IL-4 upregulates and stabilizes VCAM-1 ***(13)***. Adhesion is followed by extravasation and diapedesis into the perivascular space, involving the platelet endothelial cell adhesion molecule ***(16)***.

Because of this important function of adhesion molecules in the airway mucosa in inflammation, the need has arisen to study and quantify their expression within tissue samples. The advent of immunohistochemistrry (IHC) procedures and availability of specific monoclonal antibodies (MAbs) directed to the different classes of adhesion molecules has made this possible (**Table 2**). Conventionally, IHC has been undertaken in frozen or paraffin-embedded samples ***(17,18)***. There are several disadvantages with these systems for the investigation of adhesion molecules: The morphological preservation of tissue in frozen sections is poor; there is diffusion of Ags; and the necessity for relatively thick sections, usually 7 µm, makes sequential sectioning through the same cell unlikely. The principle drawback of paraffin-embedded tissue is that the fixation regime of crosslinking fixatives; renders many surface Ags inaccessible. Although various Ag-retrieval techniques are now available, few of these facilitate the successful detection of adhesion molecules. For these reasons, the application of glycol methacrylate (GMA) embedding for airway biopsies and IHC has been developed ***(19)***, and offers several advantages over more conventional techniques: The processing technique employs gentle fixation, which preserves many of the Ag epitopes usually destroyed by standard fixation protocols; the use of a water-miscible resin means dehydration, and therefore tissue shrinkage is minimal, and thin sections (2 µm) can be cut, which itself has advantages beyond cryostat or other preparations; morphological preservation is excellent, thus allowing accurate quantification of results, sequential sections can be cut through one cell, which is essential for the study of adhesion molecules; and, finally, numerous sections can be obtained from one small biopsy. Therefore, this is the technique described in detail in this chapter.

In brief, airway biopsies are fixed in acetone containing protease inhibitors, overnight, and then embedded in GMA resin ***(19)***. Initially, 2-µm sections are cut and stained by a rapid toluidine blue method ***(20)*** to assess biopsy morphology. Subsequently, additional 2-µm sections are cut and stained immunohistochemically, using the streptavidin-biotin peroxidase detection system ***(17–19,21)*** and MAbs specific for the adhesion molecules, ICAM-1, VCAM-1, E- and P-selectin, LFA-1 and VLA-4. Adhesion molecule expression is then quantified in the stained sections.

Table 2
Adhesion Molecule Monoclonal Antibodies: Clones, Sources, and References

CD number	Antigen	Clone	Class	Source	Ref.
CD 11a	LFA-1	38	IgG2a	Cymbus Biotechnology Ltd. (Chandlers Ford, UK)	*22*
CD 54	ICAM-1	RR1.1.1	IgG1	Gift (*see* **Note 9**)	*23*
CD 49d	VLA-4	44H6	IgG1	Cymbus Biotechnology Ltd.	*24*
CD 62E	E selectin	1.2.B6	IgG1	Cymbus Biotechnology Ltd.	*25*
CD 62P	P selectin	CLB-Thromb/6	IgG1	Immunotech (Marseille, France)	*26*
CD 106	VCAM-1	1.4.C3	IgG1	Serotec (Kidlington, UK)	*25*
	Endothelium	EN4	IgG1	Monosan (Uden, Netherlands)	*27*

2. Materials

2.1. GMA Processing

Analar-grade reagents are used throughout unless otherwise stated.

1. Dry acetone: place molecular sieve 4A (Merck, Poole, Dorset, UK) in the bottom of 1-L storage bottle.
2. Protease inhibitors: iodoacetamide (Sigma, Poole, Dorset, UK), phenylmethylsulfonyl fluoride (PMSF) (Sigma).
3. Acetone fixative: 20 m*M* iodacetamide (370 mg/100 mL), 2 m*M* PMSF 35 mg/100 mL) in dry acetone. Gloves and face mask should be worn when handling dry protease inhibitors. Fixative can be made in advance and stored, aliquoted (5 mL), in glass vials at –20°C for up to 3 mo.
4. Methyl benzoate, GPR grade (Merck).
5. JB4 kit, includes monomer solution A, solution B, and benzoyl peroxide (Polysciences [Warrington, PA], cat. no. 0226). Monomer solution A (0226A) is available separately.
6. Glass vials with snap-on lids ~10 mL (e.g., G060, Taab, Reading, UK).
7. Polythene bottles: must be airtight and resin proof (recommend B053, Taab).
8. Taab 8-mm flat-bottomed polythene embedding capsules (cat. no. C094, Taab).
9. Rack for above capsules (cat. no. C054, Taab).
10. N-DEX blue nitrile gloves, disposable (Merck).
11. Airtight plastic storage boxes suitable for –20°C.
12. Silica gel (Merck).

2.2. GMA Cutting

1. Resin microtome with a binocular microscope head, and capable of sectioning at 2 µm.
2. Glass knives, 25-degree, made from 6-mm glass strips (Leica, Solms, Germany) using a glass knife maker (e.g., Leica).
3. Poly-L-lysine (PLL)-coated microscope slides: dilute PLL (Sigma) 1:10 with distilled water and place in a trough. Place glass microscope slides into a slide rack, and immerse in PLL for 5 min; allow to dry overnight, and replace into boxes, and store until required.
4. Ammonia.
5. Toludine blue stain: 1 g toluidine blue (Sigma), 1 g borax (Sigma) in 100 mL distilled water.
6. N-DEX blue nitrile gloves, disposable (Merck).

2.3. GMA Immunohistochemistry

1. Endogenous peroxidase inhibitor: 10 mL 0.1% aqueous sodium (Na) azide plus 100 µL 30% hydrogen peroxide. Prepare fresh before use. 0.1% aqueous sodium azide can be prepared as a stock solution and stored at room temperature (RT).
2. Culture-medium-blocking solution: 20% fetal calf serum (European standard), 1% bovine serum albumin in Dulbecco's modified essential medium (basic grade). This can be prepared in advance and stored, aliquoted (5 mL amounts), at –20°C.

3. Tris-buffered saline (TBS), pH 7.6: 80 g Na chloride, 6.05 g Tris, 38 mL 1 *M* hydrochloric acid. Dissolve and mix in 1 L distilled water and adjust to give final pH 7.6: This is a 10X stock, and should then be made up to 10 L. Store at RT for up to 1 wk.
4. Tris-HCl buffer, pH 7.6: 12 mL 0.2 *M* Tris (made as a stock solution and stored at 4°C), 19 mL 0.1 *M* HCl, 19 mL distilled water. Mix, and adjust pH to 7.6. Make fresh each day.
5. Acetate buffer, pH 5.2: 40 mL 0.1 *M* Na acetate (made as a stock solution and stored at RT), 10 mL 0.1 *M* acetic acid. Mix, and adjust pH to 5.2. Make fresh each day.
6. Aminoethylcarbazole (AEC) substrate solution: 1 mL 0.4% AEC (Sigma) in dimethylformamide (can be made as a stock solution and stored at 4°C), 15 μL 30% hydrogen peroxide, 14 mL acetate buffer. Prepare and filter immediately before use.
7. Mayer's hematoxylin.
8. Crystal mount (Biomedia Biogenesis, Poole, Dorset, UK).
9. Primary Abs: This is discussed in the **Subheading 3.3.1.**
10. Secondary Ab: biotinylated rabbit antimouse Fab_2 fragments (cat. no. E0413, Dako, Glostrup, Denmark).
11. Streptavidin-biotin peroxidase kit (cat. no. K377, Dako).

2.4. Analysis of Stained Sections

Light microscope with a grid eyepiece graticule and ×40 objective.

3. Methods

3.1. GMA Processing

CAUTION: Steps 4–7 of this procedure must be performed in a fume extraction hood, and N-DEX blue nitrile gloves should worn when handling resin components, because there is a risk of developing a contact hypersensitivity.

1. Place biopsy immediately into ice-cold acetone fixative (*see* **Note 1**).
2. Fix overnight at –20°C.
3. Replace fixative with acetone at RT, 15 min.
4. Methyl benzoate at RT, 15 min.
5. Infiltrate with processing solution: 5% methyl benzoate in GMA solution A at 4°C, 3 × 2 h (*see* **Note 2**).
6. Prepare embedding solution immediately before use: 10 mL GMA solution A, 250 μL GMA solution B, 45 mg benzoyl peroxide (*see* **Note 3**).
7. Embed specimens in freshly prepared embedding solution in Taab flat-bottomed capsules, placing biopsy in the bottom of the capsule, filling to the brim with resin, and closing lid to exclude air. A pencil-written label should also be placed in the capsule (*see* **Note 4**).
8. Polymerize overnight at 4°C.
9. Store in airtight boxes at –20°C (*see* **Note 5**).

3.2. GMA Cutting

3.2.1. Initial Assessment

1. Remove blocks from capsules (*see* **Note 6**).
2. Trim away excess resin to form a trapezium shape around the tissue (*see* **Note 7**).
3. Cut 2-μm sections, float out onto water, and pick up onto PLL slide.
4. Dry on hot plate, 10 min.
5. Stain with toluidine blue, 2 min.
6. Wash sections to remove excess stain.
7. Blot dry and mount in DPX (Merck).
8. Examine under light microscope to check biopsy quality.

3.2.2. Sectioning for IHC

1. Cut 2-μm sections, and float out onto ammonia water (1 mL ammonia in 500 mL distilled water) 1–1.5 min (*see* **Note 8**).
2. Pick sections up onto labeled PLL slides.
3. Dry for at least 1 h at RT.
4. Commence IHC staining the same day, or wrap slides back to back in aluminum foil and store at –20°C; use within 2 wk.

3.3. GMA Immunohistochemistry

3.3.1. Primary Abs

There is a wide range of companies producing Abs directed to adhesion molecules. These are all mouse antihuman monoclonal antibodies (*see* **Note 9**).

3.3.2. Titration of Abs

Before Abs can be used on test sections, the optimum working dilution needs to be established by titration. Initially, five double dilutions should be tried: If the concentration of the Ab is 1 mg/mL, this usually has a working dilution of approx 1:100; therefore, when titrating an Ab of this concentration, the following dilution series would be used: 1:25, 1:50, 1:100, 1:200, 1:400. Commercial Abs are usually very reliable, with little batch-to-batch variation, and, therefore, once a working dilution has been established, new batches only need checking by using the current working dilution and one either side.

When initially establishing an IHC system, the second- and third-stage Abs also require titration, and, for this purpose, checkerboard titrations are required, in which the concentration of two Abs are varied against each other ***(17,21)***.

3.3.3. Controls

The use of appropriate controls is essential in IHC. A positive control should be included to ensure that the technique is working, and negative controls, to ensure there is no nonspecific staining. When staining for adhesion molecules, the EN4 mAb serves as a positive control, because at least one, if not all, sections will contain endothelium. Two types of negative controls are routinely used: omission of the primary Ab, and isotype-matched IgGs (Sigma). These should be used at the same concentration, as the strongest test Ab in place of the primary Ab.

3.3.4. IHC Procedure

If sections have been stored at –20°C, they should be removed from the freezer, unwrapped, and laid out, to allow the condensation to evaporate. Prior to commencement of staining, sections should be circled with a diamond marker pen or a PAP pen (Dako), so that they can be visualized during the IHC procedure. Sections should not be allowed to dry out during the procedure and the staining tray should be covered during the blocking, Ab, and substrate stages.

1. Inhibit endogenous peroxidase with peroxidase inhibitor solution, 30 min.
2. Wash with TBS, 3 × 5 min.
3. Drain slides, and apply culture medium-blocking-solution, 30 min.
4. Drain slides, and apply primary Abs diluted in TBS, at appropriate dilutions, cover with cover slips, and incubate overnight (at least 16 h) at RT (*see* **Notes 10** and **11**).
5. Wash off cover slips with TBS.
6. Wash with TBS, 3 × 5 min.
7. Drain slides, and apply biotinylated second stage Ab, diluted in TBS, at appropriate dilution, for 2 h.
8. Wash with TBS, 3 × 5 min.
9. Drain slides, and apply Streptavidin-biotin peroxidase complexes, diluted in Tris-HCl buffer, at appropriate dilution, 2 h (*see* **Note 12**).
10. Wash with TBS, 3 × 5 min.
11. Drain slides, and apply AEC solution, 30 min at 37°C.
12. Rinse with TBS, place in staining racks, and wash in running tap water, 5 min.
13. Counterstain sections with Mayer's hematoxylin (approx 2 min, depending on age of solution) and blue in running tap water (*see* **Note 13**).
14. Drain slides, and apply Crystal mount (Biomedia) (one drop/section), and bake at 80°C for approx 10 min, until set.
15. Allow slides to cool and mount in DPX.

3.4. Analysis of Stained Sections

It is important, when analyzing a series of sections, that a repeatable method of quantification is employed that can be followed by all. To eliminate the interobserver viability, only one observer should analyze a study and this observer should count some sections several times to ensure that intraobserver viability is within acceptable limits (<5%).

Before commencing analysis, the parts of the submucosa and epithelium in which counting will be undertaken should be identified. Within the submucosa, areas to exclude are muscle, glands, damaged tissue, and holes. In the epithelium, counting is only undertaken in lengths of intact epithelium; lengths of tangentially cut or disrupted epithelium are excluded. It is helpful to make a sketch of the section identifying these features.

3.4.1. Cells

Both MAbs to LFA-1 and VLA-4 give a ring pattern of staining (*see* **Fig. 1**), which is red when AEC has been used as the substrate. Scoring of sections should be undertaken using the ×40 objective. Positive nucleated cells are counted in the whole section, except for the areas eliminated for reasons discussed above, a separate count should be made in the submucosa and the epithelium. The eyepiece graticule is used to assist in aligning the section, and a tally counter to record numbers. Both sections on each slide should be analyzed, and an average number of positive cells calculated. The area of the section is measured in square millimeters, and the length of intact epithelium in millimeters, using a computerized image analysis system (e.g., Colourvision or Open Lab, Improvision, Coventry, UK). Numbers of positive cells per square millimeter of submucosa and per millimeter length of epithelium are then calculated.

3.4.2. Vessels

As discussed in **Note 8**, the MAbs for endothelial adhesion molecules are cut in sequence with the endothelial marker, EN4, with these MAbs and AEC, as the substrate positive vessels will be stained red (*see* **Fig. 2**). Initially, the total number of vessels, positively stained with mAb EN4, are counted. The number of blood vessels immunoreactive for E-selectin, P-selectin, ICAM-1, and VCAM-1 are then counted and expressed as a percentage of the total number of vessels determined in the sequential EN4 section. Again, both sections on each slide should be analyzed, and an average result calculated.

3.5. Statistical Analysis of Data

Usually, the data generated in these types of studies are not normally distributed, and therefore should be analyzed using nonparametric statistics. The Mann-Whitney U-test is used to analyze nonmatched pairs and the Wilcoxon Rank Sign for matched pairs.

4. Notes

4.1. GMA Processing

1. When collecting airway biopsies for GMA processing, the acetone fixative must be kept cold on ice at all times, and the size of the biopsies must not be >2 mm^3.
2. Ten milliliters of processing solution should be allowed per pot to be processed.
3. One milliliter embedding solution should be allowed per biopsy to be embedded. The benzoyl peroxide takes approx 5 min to dissolve, and the bottle should be

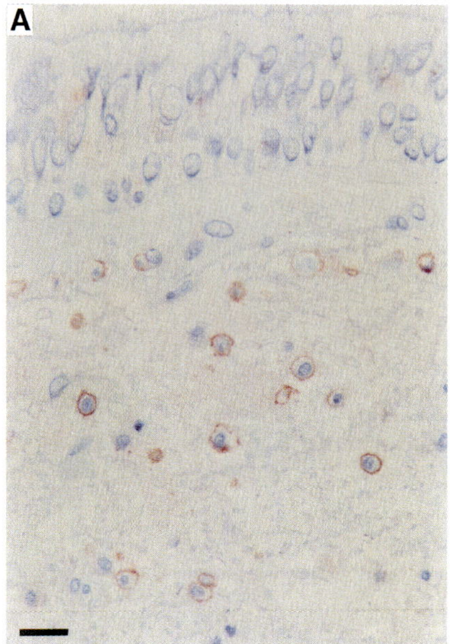

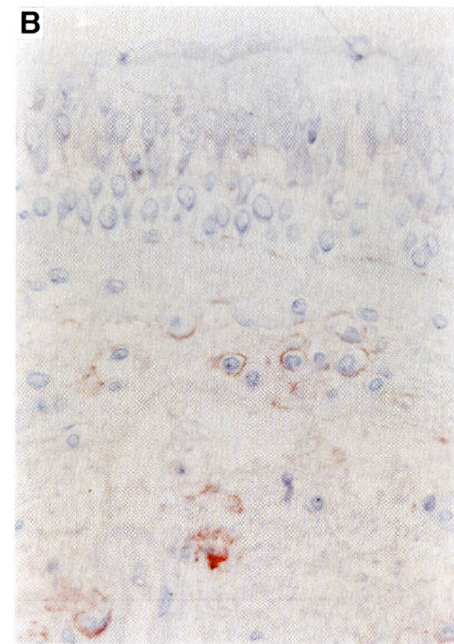

Fig. 1. Immunohistochemical staining of GMA-embedded nasal polyp for the adhesion molecule ligands LFA-1 **(A)** and VLA-4 **(B)**. Positive staining (red) is seen on the surface of the cells within the submucosa.

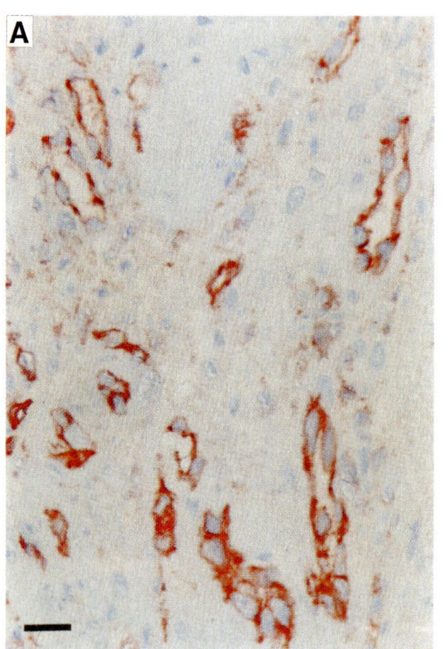

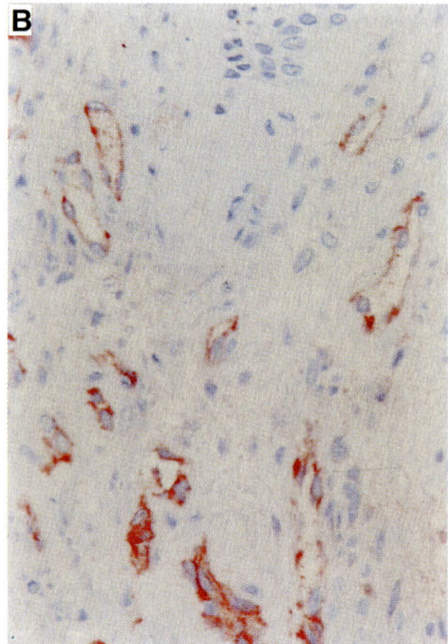

Fig. 2. IHC staining of GMA-embedded nasal polyp for the endothelial marker EN4 **(A)** and the adhesion molecules E-selectin **(B)**, *(continued on next page)*

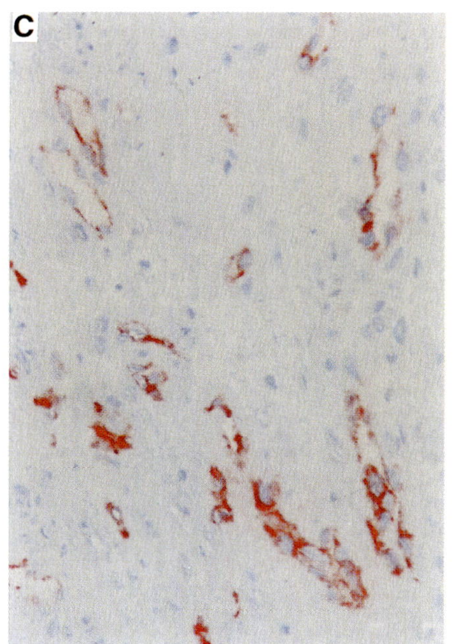

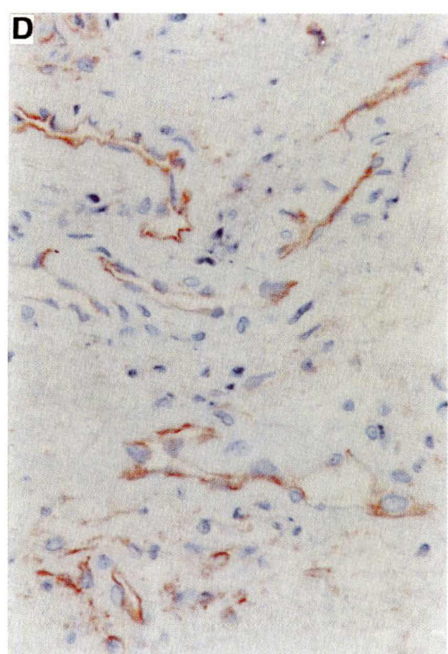

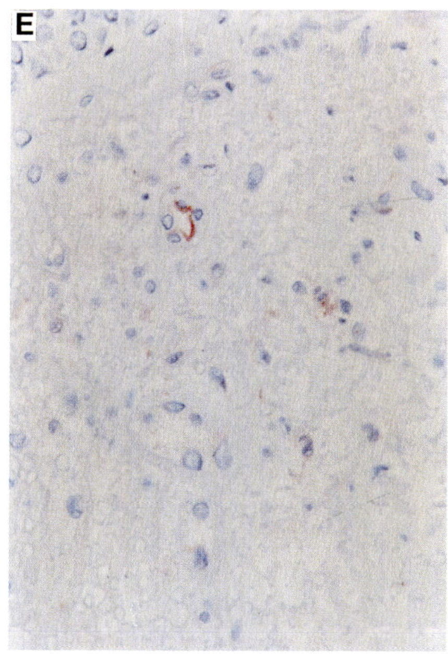

P-selectin **(C)**, ICAM-1 **(D)**, and VCAM-1 **(E)** (*see* **Note 13**). Positive staining (red) is seen on the surface of blood vessels. A, B, and C show sequential sections, and co-localization of positive staining can easily be observed. Scale bar = 20 μm.

shaken from side to side to keep the amount of air introduced into the solution to a minimum. While mixing, the color of the solution will change to a pale straw color; if agitated too much and for too long, the solution will turn brown, and should then be discarded, because it will not polymerize properly.

4. The label identifying the biopsy must be written in pencil; pen-written labels will run when in contact with the resin. The label is then coiled, writing outermost, and placed inside the Taab capsule, just above halfway. When the resin polymerizes, the label then becomes an integral part of the block.
5. Once the blocks are polymerized, there is usually a small amount of unpolymerized resin remaining in the very top of the capsule: This should be cleaned out with tissue (wearing the N-DEX blue nitrile gloves), before storing the blocks. The blocks still in their capsules are placed in small containers (e.g., empty cover slip boxes), which are then placed in larger, airtight, plastic storage boxes with silica gel at the bottom. This is then stored at –20°C.

4.2. GMA Cutting

6. **CAUTION:** N-DEX blue nitrile gloves should be worn when removing the blocks from the capsules, because any unpolymerized resin may cause a contact hypersensitivity.
7. When trimming the blocks, the trapezium should be close to the tissue on the sides and top, but approx 1–2 mm resin should be left at the bottom, to allow for picking up the sections with the forceps. The edges of the block face should be at an angle of about 45°; if too steep an angle, the block will be unstable, and could lead to cutting difficulties.
8. When cutting sections for adhesion molecule staining, sequential sections are required for assessment of vessel immunoreactivity. Sections should be cut in this sequence: 1. ICAM-1, 2. EN4, 3. VCAM-1, 4. E SEL, 5. EN4, 6. P SEL, 7. LFA-1, 8. VLA-4, 9. IgG1, 10. IgG2a, 11. TBS. Sections 1–3 and 4–6 need to be sequential. Two sections should be cut for each marker. Place one section on each of slides 1–11, then cut a second section and place it below the first on each slide, 1–11.

4.3. GMA Immunohistochemistry

9. The MAb directed to ICAM-1, clone RR1.1.1, is a gift from R. Rothlein (Boehringer-Ingelheim, Ridgefield). The commercially available clone 6.5.B5 (Dako or Serotec) does work satisfactorily in GMA sections.
10. 150 μL diluted Ab should be allowed per slide.
11. Cover slips are placed over the sections with the primary Abs, to prevent evaporation and to enable small quantities of Ab to be used.
12. The streptavidin-biotin peroxidase components need to be mixed at least 30 min in advance of use, to allow time for the complexes to form. These are mixed in Tris-HCl buffer for stability.
13. In areas where the water supply is not alkaline, Scotts tap water substitute *(28)* will be required to blue the hematoxylin.

References

1. Harlan, L. N. (1985) Leukocyte endothelial cell interactions. *Blood* **65,** 513–525.
2. Springer, T. A. (1990) Adhesion receptors of the immune system. *Nature* **346,** 425–434.
3. Albelda, S. M. (1991) Endothelial and epithelial cell adhesion molecules. *J. Am. Resp. Cell. Mol. Biol.* **4,** 195–203.
4. Montefort, S. and Holgate, S. T. (1991) Adhesion molecules and their role in inflammation. *Resp. Med.* **85,** 91–99.
5. Montefort, S., Holgate, S. T., and Howarth, P. H. (1993) Leukocyte adhesion molecules and their role in bronchial asthma and allergic rhinitis. *Eur. Resp. J.* **6,** 1044–1051.
6. Carlos, T. M. and Harlan, J. M. (1994) Leukocyte endothelial adhesion molecules. *Blood* **84,** 2068–2101.
7. Bevilacqua, M. P. (1993) Endothelial leukocyte adhesion molecules. *Ann. Rev. Immunol.* **11,** 767–804.
8. Bevilacqua, M. P., Pober, J. S., Mendrick, D. L., Cotran, R. S., and Gimborne, M. A. (1987) Identification of an inducible endothelial leukocyte adhesion molecule. *Proc. Natl. Acad. Sci. USA* **84,** 9238–9243.
9. Bevilacqua, M. P. and Nelson, R. M. (1993) Selectins. *J. Clin. Invest.* **91,** 379–387.
10. Tedder, T. F., Steeber, D. A., Chen, A., and Engel, P. (1995) Selectins, vascular adhesion molecules. *FASEB J.* **9,** 866–873.
11. von Andrian, U. H., Berger, E. M., Ramezani, L., Chambers, J. D., Ochs, H. D., Harlan, J. M., et al. (1993) *In vivo* behaviour of neutrophils from two patients with distinct inherited LAD syndromes. *J. Clin. Invest.* **91,** 2893–2897.
12. Zimmerman, G. A., Prescott, S. M., and McIntyre, T. M. (1992) Endothelial cell interactions with granulocytes: tethering and signalling molecules. *Immunol. Today* **13,** 93–99.
13. Shimizu, Y., Newman, W., Tanaka, Y., and Shaw, S. (1992) Lymphocyte interactions with endothelial cells. *Immunol Today* **13,** 106–112.
14. Ruegg, C., Postigo, A. A., Sikorski, E. E., Butcher, E. C., Pytela, R., and Erle, D. J. (1992) Role of integrin $\alpha 4\beta 7/\alpha 4\beta p$ in lymphocyte adherence to fibronectin and VCAM-1 and in homotypic cell clustering. *J. Cell. Biol.* **117,** 179–189.
15. Acevedo, A., de Poza, M. A., Arroyo, A. G., Sanchez-Mateos, P., and Gonzalez-Amaro, R., Sanchez-Madrid, F. (1993) Distribution of ICAM-3 bearing cells in normal human tissues. Expression of a novel counter-receptor for LFA-1 in epidermal langerhan cells. *J. Am. Pathol.* **143,** 774–783.
16. Mullër, A., Weigel, S. A., Deng, X., and Phillips, D. M. (1993). PECAM-1 is required for transendothelial migration of leukocytes. *J. Exp. Med.* **178,** 449–460.
17. Polak, J. M. and Van Noorden, S. (1997) *Introduction to Immunocytochemistry: Current Techniques and Problems.* Oxford Science, Oxford, UK.
18. Miller, K. (1996) Immunocytochemical techniques, in *Theory and Practice of Histological Techniques* (Bancroft, J. D. and Stevens, A., eds.), Churchill Livingstone, New York, pp. 435–470.

19. Britten, K. M., Howarth, P. H., and Roche, W. R. (1993) Immunohistochemistry on resin sections: a comparison of resin embedding techniques for small mucosal biopsies. *Biotech Histochem.* **68,** 271–280.
20. Lewis, P. R. and Knight, D. P. (1988) Staining methods for sectioned material, in *Practical Methods for Electron Microscopy* (Glauret, A. M., ed.), North Holland Publishing, Amsterdam, The Netherlands, pp. 25,26.
21. Nash, S. J., ed. (1989) *Immunohistochemical Staining Methods,* Dako Handbook. Dako, Carpinteria, CA
22. Dransfield, I. and Hogg, N. (1989) Regulated expression of Mg2+ binding epitope on leukocyte integrin alpha subunits. *EMBO J.* **8,** 3759–3765.
23. Rothlein, R., Dustin, M. L., Marlin, S. D., and Springer, T. A. (1986) Human ICAM-1 distinct from LFA-1. *J. Immunol.* **137,** 1270–1274.
24. Quackenbush, E. J. and Letarte, M. (1985) Identification of several cell surface proteins of non-T non-B acute lymphoblastic leukaemia by using monoclonal antibodies. *J. Immunol.* **134,** 1276–1285.
25. Wellicome, S. M., Thornhill, M. H., Pitzalia, C., Thomas, D. S., Lanchbury, J. S., Panayi, G. S., and Haskard, D. O. (1990) Monoclonal antibody that detects a novel antigen on endothelial cells that is induced by tumour necrosis factor, IL-1 or lipopolysaccharide. *J. Immunol.* **144,** 2558–2565.
26. Saunders, K. B., Kansas, G. S., and Tedder, T. F. (1993) Mapping of the selectin monoclonal antibodies. *Tissue Antigens* **42,** 494.
27. Jones, R. R., Spaull, J., Spry, C., and Jones, E. W. (1986) Histogenesis of Kaposi's sarcoma in patients with and without acquired deficiency syndrome (AIDS). *J. Clin. Pathol.* **39,** 742–749.
28. Bancroft, J. D. and Stevens, A. (1996) Appendix IV: preparation of useful solution, in *Theory and Practice of Histological Techniques,* Churchill Livingstone, New York, p. 732.

18

Site-Directed Mutagenesis in Investigation of β-Adrenoreceptor Exosite

Stuart A. Green

1. Introduction

β_2-adrenergic receptor agonists (β-agonists) are first-line agents for the treatment of acute bronchospasm. These drugs achieve bronchodilation primarily via activation of β_2-adrenergic receptors (β_2AR) located on airway smooth muscle cells. In addition, β-agonists may alleviate bronchospasm, and protect against airway hyperresponsiveness, by interacting with β_2AR expressed on other lung cells, resulting in such diverse actions as alterations in ion permeability, changes in mucocilliary beat frequency, and so on *(1)*. Most β-agonists in clinical use are structural derivatives of the endogenous β_2AR agonist, adrenaline, including substituted catecholamines, such as isoprenaline and isoetharine; resourcinols, such as metaproterenol, fenoterol, and terbutaline; and saligenins, such as salbutamol and salmeterol. Of these, salmeterol, a highly lipophilic derivative of the partial agonist, salbutamol, represents the latest long-acting generation of β-agonists, with a duration of activity in excess of 24 h *(2)*.

In addition to its markedly prolonged activity, salmeterol also exhibits an unusual propensity to reassert its actions following reversible blockade by βAR antagonists. This effect is highly β_2AR-specific, because it is not observed in β_1AR tissue preparations, even though salmeterol has some (albeit weak) affinity for the β_1AR. Such persistence of action, despite competition at the receptor-active binding site, ultimately led to the concept of a receptor exosite, i.e., an alternate receptor binding domain that could tether salmeterol near the active site, and thus facilitate the rapid reassertion of agonist activity following washout of an active site antagonist. Whether such an exosite was a truly distinct

From: *Methods in Molecular Medicine, vol. 44: Asthma: Mechanisms and Protocols*
Edited by: K. F. Chung and I. Adcock © Humana Press Inc., Totowa, NJ

domain of the receptor, or, rather, a localized membrane region in the vicinity of the receptor, was controversial. In either event, it became clear that the concept of receptor exosites represented a new and potentially groundbreaking aspect in the development of drug discovery and development.

1.1. Identification of Potential Exosite Domains

To approach this issue, it was desirable to identify candidate β_2AR domains that might function as exosites. Criteria for consideration included: The exosite should be accessible to salmeterol, and thus include residues either in the extracellular or transmembrane-spanning domains (TMDs); the exosite should be located in close proximity to amino acids known to comprise the receptor-active site, such as Ser204 and Ser207 in TMD5, and Asp113 in TMD3 *(3,4)*; the exosite should probably consist of residues that are specific to the β_2AR, because exosite activity was not observed in other, related receptors (particularly, β_1AR).

Because β_2AR agonists were known to interact primarily with amino acids of the lipophilic TMDs, and considering the highly lipophilic nature of the salmeterol side chain, the TMDs were selected as the most likely exosite candidate domains. Comparison of amino acid sequence between the β_2AR and the β_1AR reveals an overall ~85% homology within these regions, with virtually identical active site domains *(5)*. However, small regions of difference were noted, particularly in TMD4 and TMD7. Because TMD4 contained the largest variance between β_2AR and β_1AR, and because it clearly met the other criteria listed above, this domain was chosen for initial study as an exosite candidate domain. To accomplish this, chimeric receptors, consisting of β_2AR with small regions of the β_1AR TMD4 substituted for the analogous β_2AR residues, were constructed, and the pharmacological characteristics of salmeterol–chimera interactions were determined.

2. Materials

2.1. cDNA Vectors

1. M13mp18 phage.
2. β_2pBC12BI.
3. β_1pBC12BI.

2.2. Mutagenesis Reagents

1. 10X Oligonucleotide (oligo-NT) kinase buffer: 1 *M* Tris-HCl, pH 7.9, 100 m*M*, $MgCl_2$, and 50 m*M* dithiothreitol (DTT).
2. 10X Annealing buffer: 100 m*M* Tris-HCl, pH 7.9, 100 m*M* $MgCl_2$, and 500 m*M* NaCl.
3. 20X Reaction buffer: 200 m*M* Tris-HCl, pH 7.9, 100 m*M* $MgCl_2$, and 100 m*M* DTT.

4. Nucleoside triphosphate (NTP) mix: 3 m*M* each of deoxyadenosine triphosphate (dATP), deoxycytosine triphosphate (dCTP), deoxyguanosine triphosphate (dGTP), and deoxythymidine triphosphate (dTTP); 5 m*M* rATP.

2.3. Single-Stranded Phage Reagents

1. Polyethelene glycol (PEG)/sodium chloride (NaCl) solution: 2.5 *M* NaCl, 20% PEG 8000.
2. Phage extraction buffer (PEB): 0.3 *M* NaCl, 0.1 *M* Tris-HCl, pH 7.9, 1 m*M* ethylenediamine tetraacetic acid (EDTA), 0.2% sodium dodecyl sulfate.

2.4. Transfection Reagents

1. 2X Hank's balanced salt solution (HBSS): 280 m*M* NaCl, 50 m*M* HEPES, 1.5 m*M* Na_2HPO_4, pH to 7.13.
2. Na butyrate solution: Make a stock solution of 500 m*M*; dilute 1:100 fresh, immediately prior to use.
3. 2 YT broth: 16 g bacto-tryptone, 100 g yeast extract, 5 g NaCl in 1 L H_2O. Autoclave to sterilize.

3. Methods

3.1. Construction of Chimeras

Numerous methods have been developed to alter DNA sequences contained in various expression vectors. The central elements to each of these methods lie in the actual manner used to introduce the mutations (i.e., polymerase chain reaction (PCR), noncycling elongation) and the method used to select for the altered strand(s) of DNA. Although many of these methods have been touted for their ease of use and reliability, experience has shown that several factors may significantly reduce the effectiveness of the method chosen. Perhaps most important of these are the characteristics of the template DNA that is to undergo mutagenesis. Templates that feature unusual structural features, such as exceptionally high guanadine-cytosine (GC) content or a propensity to form loops and hairpins, are notoriously difficult to use in mutagenesis reactions. The β_1AR, in particular, and the β_2AR, to a lesser degree, exhibit considerable amounts of such structural features, and, as a result, several initial attempts at construction of the chimeras proved unsuccessful. The method that ultimately proved successful was (appropriately enough) one of the first such methods described, namely, oligo-NT-directed mutagenesis, using single-stranded M13-phage-based templates, as described by Kunkel *(7)*. This method uses T4 polymerase to perform second-strand synthesis on template DNA. Selection of the synthetic second strand (which contains the desired mutation encoded in an oligo-NT) is achieved by uracil-enriching the DNA template prior to mutagenesis. Most organisms contain proofreading enzymes that serve to ensure that uracil (normally present in RNA) is not present in DNA.

Because the synthetic second strand does not contain uracil, these proofreading enzymes degrade only the template DNA, and thus effectively select for the mutant second strand.

3.1.1. Preparation of Template DNA

3.1.1.1. Mutagenesis of TMD4 Region of β_2AR

The 328 bp KpnI/PstI fragment of the β_2AR cDNA *(5)* was subcloned into M13mp18 RF DNA. This allowed subsequent mutagenesis of a small region of the receptor, which could readily be verified by direct dideoxy sequencing of the entire *Kpn*I/*Pst*I fragment prior to further mutagenesis and/or subcloning (*see* **Note 1**).

3.1.1.2. Generation of Infectious Phage Stock

1. Transform competent DH$_5\alpha$F' *Escherichia coli* (i.e., Life Technologies [Baltimore, MD] catalog # 18264-010) by adding 2–5 µL ligation mixture to a prechilled 17 × 100 mm round-bottomed tube containing 100 µL cells on ice. Tap the tube gently to mix, then incubate on ice for 30 min.
2. Heat-shock the cells at 42°C for 45 s.
3. Incubate on ice for 2 min.
4. Add 3 mL melted (50–55°C) top agar and 100 µL noncompetent DH$_5\alpha$F' cells. If desired, add 30 µL 2% X-Gal and 10 µL isopropyl thiogalactose (IPTG) to allow blue/white screening. Pour the mixture evenly onto a 2X YT agar plate. Allow to set at room temperature (RT) (10 min), then invert, and incubate at 37°C overnight.
5. Insert a sterilized Pasteur pipet into a single, isolated plaque, and transfer the plaque, along with the underlying agar, to a sterile culture tube containing 3 mL 2X YT broth containing a 1:100 dilution of an overnight culture of DH$_5\alpha$F'. Vortex the tube to break apart the plug, and incubate at 37°C in a shaking incubator (~150–200 rpm) for 5–6 h.
6. Transfer the culture to two 1.5-mL microcentrifuge tubes, and centrifuge at 14,000*g* for 5 min.
7. Transfer the supernatant to two new tubes, and recentrifuge as above.
8. Store the resulting supernatant (infectious phage stock) at 4°C.

3.1.1.3. Preparation of Uracil-Enriched Template DNA

1. Prepare an overnight growth of a *Dut/Ung E. coli* strain, such as BW313.
2. Dilute the overnight culture 1:100 into 100 mL 2X YT broth. Add uridine (Sigma) to 0.25 µg/mL. Add 1 mL infectious phage stock, and incubate at 37°C in a shaking incubator for 5–6 h.
3. Centrifuge the culture at 14,000*g* for 15–20 min.
4. Add 20 mL PEG/NaCl, and incubate at 4°C overnight.
5. Centrifuge at 17,000*g* for 15 min. The resulting pellet may be difficult to locate, so it is advisable to mark the outside of the centrifuge tube prior to the spin.
6. Aspirate the supernatant, and invert several minutes on a towel.
7. Dissolve the pellet in 2 mL Tris-EDTA (TE) buffer, and transfer to two microcentrifuge tubes.

8. Centrifuge at 14,000*g* for 5 min, to pellet any insoluble debris, and transfer the supernatant to fresh tubes.
9. Add 200 µL PEG/NaCl to each tube, and incubate on ice for 30 min.
10. Pellet the phage for 5 min, 14,000*g* in a microcentrifuge. Aspirate all of the supernatant. Dry the pellets on the bench for a few minutes, then reaspirate any supernatant drops that may form. If necessary, respin the pellets for a few minutes, to ensure complete removal of the PEG solution, which may inhibit subsequent steps.
11. Dissolve and combine the pellets in 300 µL PEB buffer. It may be necessary to incubate at 68°C for a few minutes to ensure complete dissolution.
12. Add 300 µL Tris-saturated phenol, and vortex 15 s. Incubate at RT for 15 min, then revortex for 15 s.
13. Centrifuge for 2 min at 14,000*g* in a microcentrifuge, and collect the aqueous (upper) layer into a new tube.
14. Extract the aqueous layer with phenol–chloroform ($CHCl_3$) until the interface is clear (2–5×). Each time, vortex and centrifuge the mixture, then recollect the aqueous (upper) layer.
15. Extract the aqueous fraction with $CHCl_3$ once, and recentrifuge.
16. Precipitate the ssDNA from the final aqueous layer by adding 30 µL sodium acetate (NaOAc) and 600 µL ethyl alcohol (EtOH). Incubate at –20°C overnight.
17. Centrifuge at 14,000*g* for 30 min in a microcentrifuge, preferably at 4°C.
18. Dissolve the final pellet in 20–40 µL of TE buffer. The expected yield is 20–50 µg ssDNA.

*3.1.2. Preparation of Phosphorylated Oligo-NTs (see **Note 2**)*

1. Dissolve the original oligo in 150 µL TE buffer.
2. Extract the solubilized oligo 2–3× with phenol–$CHCl_3$, then once with $CHCl_3$ as described above.
3. Precipitate by adding 15 µL NaOAc and 300 µL EtOH, and incubating at –20°C for 2 h (or at –70°C for 15–20 min), and centrifuging at 14,000*g* for 30 min in a microcentrifuge, preferably at 4°C.
4. In a clean microcentrifuge tube, mix 200 pmol oligo with 3 µL, 10X kinase buffer and 3 µL 1 m*M* ATP.
5. Add H_2O to a final volume of 30 µL and add 5 U T4 poly-NT kinase.
6. Incubate at 37°C for 45 min, then at 68°C for 10 min (to inactivate the kinase and terminate the reaction).
7. Store the kinased oligo at –20°C.

3.1.3. Mutagenesis of Template DNA

3.1.3.1. Mutagenesis of Uracil-Enriched Template

This is accomplished by annealing the oligo (encoding the desired mutation) to the template, followed by second-strand synthesis and transformation of the resulting double-stranded DNA into *Dug/Ung*-competent *E. coli.*

3.1.3.2. Annealing of Oligo to Template

1. Add 7 µL of H_2O to 3 µL of kinased oligo.
2. In a screw-cap microcentrifuge tube, mix 0.1 pmol circular, uracil-enriched ssDNA template (volume) with 1 µL diluted oligo (~2 pmol kinased oligo).
3. Add 1 µL 10X annealing buffer, and H_2O to a final volume of 10 µL.
4. Heat the mixture to 95°C for 1 min, then allow to cool slowly (over at least 30 min) to <35°C.
5. Spin the mixture briefly to collect condensation, then place on ice.

3.1.3.3. Polymerization and Second-Strand Synthesis

1. To the solution from the annealing reaction above, add 1 µL 20X reaction buffer, 4 µL dNTP mix, and 5 µL H_2O (the solution volume should now be 20 µL).
2. Initiate the second-strand synthesis by adding 3 U T4 DNA polymerase and 2 U T4 DNA ligase.
3. Incubate 5 min on ice, 5 min at RT, then 2 h at 37°C.
4. Place the reaction on ice, and proceed immediately to transformation, or store at –20°C.

3.1.3.4. Transformation, Selection, and Sequencing of Reaction Products

1. Transformation is done exactly as described in **Subheading 3.1.1.2.**, using DH5αF's as host strain. Since the DH5αF' contain the normal complement of *Dut* and *Ung* enzymes, the uracil-enriched template strands are removed, but the synthetic second strands (containing the mutant oligo) are maintained. Following transformation, several (~6–10) plaques should be isolated, cultured, and ssDNA prepared for sequencing.
2. For each plaque, prepare 3 mL phage stock, as described in **Subheading 3.1.1.2., steps 5–7**. Save 1 mL phage stock at 4°C, and proceed with the remaining 2 mL (divided equally into two microcentrifuge tubes).
3. To each tube, add 200 µL PEG/NaCl, mix by inversion, and incubate at least 2 h at 4°C.
4. Centrifuge 5 min at 14,000*g* and aspirate the supernatant, again being sure to remove all traces of the PEG solution.
5. Resuspend the pellet in 50 µL PEB buffer. Vortex, and heat at 68°C to ensure complete resuspension.
6. Pool the contents of the two tubes, and add 50 µL Tris-saturated phenol. Vortex 15 s.
7. Incubate at RT 15 min.
8. Revortex 15 s, then centrifuge 3 min.
9. Transfer the aqueous (upper) layer to a new tube.
10. Add 10 µL NaOAc and 250 µL EtOH.
11. Incubate at –20°C overnight.
12. Centrifuge 30 min at 14,000*g* in a microcentrifuge, preferably at 4°C.
13. Aspirate the supernatant, dry briefly, and resuspend the pellet in 15 µL TE or H_2O. The expected yield is 1–3 µg ssDNA, suitable for automated sequencing.

3.1.4. Subcloning of Fragments to Mammalian Expression Vectors

3.1.4.1. Reintroducing New DNA Fragment

Following successful mutagenesis, it is necessary to reintroduce the new DNA fragment into a plasmid vector suitable for recombinant expression. This is most conveniently done by excising the cDNA fragment that was initially subcloned into the M13 mutagenesis vector (in this example, the *Kpn*I/*Pst*I fragment). Alternatively, a smaller fragment that encompasses the desired mutation may be utilized (*see* **Note 3**).

3.1.4.2. Preparation of Double-Stranded M13 Replicative Form (RF) DNA

1. Prepare an overnight growth of DH5αF' (4 mL).
2. Add 1 mL overnight culture to 100 mL 2X YT broth, and add 1 mL phage stock.
3. Incubate 5–6 h with shaking (~150 rpm) at 37°C.
4. Pellet the growth by centrifuging 14,000*g* for 5 min.
5. Aspirate the media. (**Note:** This differs from previous steps, in which the supernatant was saved. Alternatively, the supernatant may be collected and prepared as infectious phage stock for future use, if desired).
6. Prepare double-stranded DNA by alkaline lysis, as described for plasmids in standard texts (e.g., *see* **ref.** ***8***). Several commercial kits have been developed that facilitate this process, and generally improve both the quantity and the quality of the resulting DNA.
7. Digest both the double-stranded M13 and target plasmid vector with the appropriate restriction enzymes, and resolve the fragments on agarose gels. Virtually all preparations of dsM13 DNA are contaminated with ssDNA, resulting in the appearance of extra bands on the gel, which have no effect on subsequent ligations or transformations, but may cause some confusion in selecting DNA fragments for subsequent cloning steps.
8. Purify the appropriate fragments from the agarose. In the author's experience, the best results have been obtained using a kit developed for this purpose (Qiagen Valencia, CA). Other methods have been described that may be equally suitable, however, including DNA isolation and ligation directly in the agarose gel slices.
9. Ligate the fragments with T4 DNA ligase, transform a suitable strain of *E. coli,* and screen recombinant colonies for the desired mutation.

3.2. Recombinant Expression

Two methods of recombinant expression are described: transient expression in COS-7 cells, and stable expression in fibroblasts. The transient method is utilized because of its rapidity (generally 48–72 h) and relatively high level of recombinant protein expression (often 10-fold more than that seen in stably transfected cells). However, the cells most commonly utilized for these experiments (COS-7, HEK293) also contain an endogenous β_2AR, making some studies, particularly functional measures of signal transduction pathways, problematic, because of background noise. In addition, only a fraction (generally 10–30%) of the transient cells in fact express the recombinant protein, which further contributes to the background noise arising from the nonexpressing cells. Thus, although the transient systems are simple and useful for many basic studies, it is often necessary to perform stable transfections, as well, especially when subtle differences in functional assessments are being sought.

3.2.1. Transient Transfection in COS-7 Cells

COS-7 monkey kidney cells are widely utilized in recombinant expression studies. These cells have been transformed with SV40 virus to express the SV40 large-T antigen. Plasmids that contain an SV40 promoter sequence will undergo high-level transcription and translation when the large-T antigen is present. Many common plasmid vectors contain an SV40 origin of replication (promoter sequence).

1. Grow COS-7 cells to ~70% confluence in 150-cm^2 tissue culture dishes or flasks.
2. Wash the plate twice with 20 mL HBSS. Remove the final wash.
3. Add plasmid DNA (1–10 µg) to 5 mL diethylaminoethyl–dextran solution. Add to the COS cells, and incubate at 37°C for 45 min in a 5% CO_2 incubator.
4. Add 40 mL chloroquine–Delbecco's modified Eagle's medium (DMEM) to the plate. Mix gently, and incubate at 37°C for 3 h.
5. Aspirate the media, and wash once with HBSS, as above.
6. Add 10 mL 10% dimethylsulfoxide (DMSO)/DMEM and incubate for 2 min at RT.
7. Aspirate the DMSO solution, and wash twice with HBSS.
8. Add 30 mL normal media, and incubate at 37°C in a 5% CO_2 incubator until confluent, generally 48–72 h. Cells may be detached and replated after 24 h as necessary. It may also be necessary to replace the media with fresh media during the incubation.

3.2.2. Stable Transfection in Chinese Hamster Fibroblasts (CHW Cells)

CHW-1102 cells were chosen for study, since they do not express an endogenous adrenergic receptor. They do, however, contain elements of the βAR signal transduction cascade, such as Gs and adenylyl cyclase.

1. On the day prior to transfection, pass cells to 3×10^{-5} cells/25 cm^2 flask at ~40–50% confluency. Use two flasks per transfection. Incubate overnight.
2. Add sterile H_2O to 30 µg plasmid DNA, to yield a total volume of 100 µL.
3. Add 500 µL 2X HBSS to a sterile microcentrifuge tube (tube 1).
4. To a second sterile microcentrifuge tube (tube 2), add 125 µL $CaCl_2$, 275 µL sterile H_2O, and the 100 µL DNA solution.
5. Add the contents of tube 2 to tube 1 dropwise, while continuously bubbling the contents of tube 1. This is most conveniently done using an automated tissue culture pipet with a 1-mL pipet.

6. Incubate at RT for 30 min.
7. Rinse the CHW cells with HBSS, and add 5 mL serum-free media to each flask.
8. Add 500 µL of the mixture to each flask, and incubate at 37°C for 4 h.
9. Remove the media, and add 5 mL media + fetal calf serum (FCS) to each flask.
10. Add 3 mL 15% glycerol to each flask, and incubate 2 min at 37°C.
11. Remove the glycerol solution, and wash twice with media + FCS.
12. Add 6 mL media + Na butyrate, and incubate at 37°C overnight.
13. Remove the Na butyrate/media, wash once, and replace with fresh normal media + FCS. Incubate overnight.
14. Detach the cells with trypsin and dilute into 100-mm^2 plates. Add selection agent (i.e., Geneticin [G418], Life Technologies cat. no. 11811-023) at this point.
15. Change media every 3–4 d. When clones begin to appear, separate using cloning rings, detach, and replate into multiwell dishes.
16. When confluent, divide into two dishes. Use one for screening of recombinant proteins. Reserve the other for subsequent passes.

3.3. Functional Assessment of Salmeterol Interactions with Recombinant Receptors

The ability of salmeterol to interact with each recombinant receptor was assessed in two ways: by equilibrium binding, and by persistent binding under conditions that would otherwise be expected to remove the ligand from the receptor (i.e., exosite-type binding). Equilibrium binding is performed in crude membranes, using the radioligand [^{125}I]cyanopindolol (ICYP). Initially, binding studies were performed in transiently transfected COS or HEK cells, but final characterizations were done in stably transfected CHW cells, to avoid any signal errors from the endogenous β_2AR in the COS and HEK cells.

3.3.1. Preparation of Crude Membrane Fractions

1. Plate transfected CHW cells in 75 cm^2 tissue culture flasks, and grow to 95% confluency.
2. Rinse plates twice with 10 mL cold (4°C) phosphate-buffered saline. This step removes media and serum, as well as nonadherent cells.
3. Add 10 mL cold hypotonic lysis buffer (5 m*M* Tris, 2 m*M* EDTA, pH 7.4, at 4°C). Mechanically detach the cells using a rubber policeman, and transfer the suspension to a centrifuge tube on ice.
4. Collect the membrane fraction by centrifugation at 40,000*g* for 10 min at 4°C.
5. Aspirate the supernatant, add 2 mL lysis buffer, and homogenize the pellet on ice, using a polytron-type tissue homogenizer (two 5-s bursts at ~75% power).
6. Add 10 mL lysis buffer, mix briefly, and recentrifuge as in **step 4**.
7. Aspirate the supernatant and suspend the pellet in assay buffer (75 m*M* Tris, 12.5 m*M* $MgCl_2$, 2 m*M* EDTA, pH 7.4, at RT) at a final protein concentration of ~ 1 mg/mL. Keep on ice until ready to assay; alternatively, membranes can be frozen in liquid N_2 and stored at –80°C for several months without loss of binding activity.

3.3.2. Analysis of Radioligand Affinity by Saturation Binding

Saturation binding was originally analyzed by the method of Scatchard *(8)*. Today, the availability of computer software capable of performing nonlinear regressions has allowed the more reliable analysis of untransformed data.

1. Prepare serial dilutions of ICYP. Because the expected affinity of ICYP is ~30–50 p*M*, a series of dilutions of ~400, 200, 100, 50, 25, 12.5, 6.25, and 3.125 p*M* is usually adequate to establish a reliable curve. The concentration of ICYP is determined by its specific activity (2200 Ci/mmol) and the volume of the assay; for a 250-μL assay, and assuming a 75% counter efficiency, the specific activity translates to 915 cpm/p*M*. Thus, 400 p*M* is roughly estimated by ~400,000 cpm. Each tube will need 25 μL diluted ICYP (*see* **step 5**); assuming duplicate total, nonspecific, and standard measurements, this translates into a minimum 6 × 25 μL = 150 μL ICYP per concentration.
2. Add GTP or GppNHp (a nonhydrolyzable GTP analog) to the membranes, to yield a concentration of 1×10^{-4} *M* (*see* **Note 4**).
3. Prepare a competitor ligand to define the presence of nonspecific binding. Usually this is done with either propranolol or alprenolol, although, classically, an agonist, such as isoprenaline, is used. The drugs should be made at 10X concentration (1X concentration for alprenolol and propranolol = 1 μ*M*, 1X concentration of isoprenaline = 100 μ*M*). If isoprenaline is used, ascorbic acid at a final concentration of 100 μ*M* should also be added, to retard oxidative degradation of the catecholamine.
4. Aliquot 25 μL of each ICYP dilation into glass tubes, and set aside to be counted as known concentrations.
5. Set up duplicate or triplicate reactions for each ICYP concentration as follows: 175 μL buffer, 25 μL membrane, 25 μL competitor, 25 μL ICYP, total of 250 μL (*see* **Note 5**).
6. For each concentration, the specific binding = total binding (obtained in the absence of competitor) minus nonspecific binding (obtained in the presence of competitor). Nonlinear analysis of a plot of specific ICYP counts vs ICYP added (using commercially available software) will allow determination of binding affinity (K_d), as well as maximum binding sites (Bmax).

3.3.3. Exosite Analysis

Exosite activity is defined by the persistence of ligand binding, despite conditions that would otherwise be expected to remove such binding. In vitro, this was translated as persistent binding under washout conditions. Normally, the affinity of a βAR agonist for the receptor is such that continuous dilution (such as occurs during persistent washing of the receptor preparation) shifts the binding equilibrium away from the receptor, and thus removes the ligand from the preparation. Thus, an effective measure of exosite binding activity is the persistent occupation of receptors by a drug under washout conditions, compared to that exhibited by a drug having no such exosite activity. Receptors that are bound by drug are not as readily available for binding to a radioligand such as ICYP; thus, the presence of retained ligand is manifested as an apparent reduction in *B*max (determined by saturation binding, as described above). In the author's hands, perfusion of cells in 100-mm^2 tissue culture dishes for 30 min at 20 mL/min with PBS was optimal for identifying the retention of salmeterol to β_2AR, vs the negligible retention of the prototypical agonist, isoprenaline. This retention was lost when mutated receptors containing a short (five-amino-acid) domain of the β_1AR was substituted into the proximal TMD4 domain of the β_2AR; conversely, retention was observed when the β_2AR short domain was substituted into the β_1AR, but not into the wild-type β_1AR. Thus, the short TMD4 domain confers the ability of salmeterol to persist at the β_2AR, and therefore represents an exosite domain in the receptor.

4. Notes

1. Sequencing after each round of mutagenesis is recommended, in order to detect any unwanted mutations, such as might arise because of poor primer specificity or random incorporation events.
2. It is generally not necessary to gel-purify oligo-NTs prior to mutagenesis; the products of most standard oligo-NT synthesizers are sufficient. However, it is necessary to add a terminal phosphate group to the oligo, in order to allow for efficient polymeration and incorporation into the circular second strand of DNA.
3. It is important that, whatever the fragment selected, any DNA that has been carried through a mutagenesis reaction should be examined by sequencing, in order to verify that no untoward mutations were inadvertently generated. Because it is generally easier to sequence ssDNA than dsDNA, this sequencing is usually done in the ssDNA stage, prior to subcloning. If the sequencing reveals any questionable data, then it should be repeated in the dsDNA stage as well.
4. Agonist binding to G-protein-coupled receptors is guanine-NT dependent. Although saturation binding is often performed using antagonists (which do not require guanine NTs), guanine NTs are usually added to the reaction anyway.
5. For each ICYP concentration, one set of tubes is prepared with competitor, as described above, and one set with 25 µL buffer substituted for the competitor; the former are referred to as nonspecific and the latter as total.

References

1. Green, S. A. and Liggett, S. B. (1996) G protein coupled receptor signalling in the lung, in *The Genetics of Asthma* (Liggett, S. and Meyers, E., eds.), Dekker, New York, pp. 67–90.
2. Johnson, M. (1995) Salmeterol. *Med. Res. Rev.* **15,** 225–227.
3. Strader, C. D., et al. (1989) Identification of two serine residues involved in agonist activation of the β-adrenergic receptor. *J. Biol. Chem.* **264,** 13,572–13,578.

4. Strader, C. D., et al. (1988) Conserved aspartic acid residues 79 and 113 of the β-adrenergic receptor have different roles in receptor function. *J. Biol. Chem.* **263,** 10,267–10,271.
5. Kobilka, B. K., et al. (1987) cDNA for the human β_2-adrenergic receptor: a protein with multiple membrane-spanning domains and encoded by a gene whose chromosomal location is shared with that of the receptor for platelet-derived growth factor. *Proc. Natl. Acad. Sci. USA* **84,** 46–50.
6. Green, S. A., et al. (1996) Sustained activation of a G protein coupled receptor via "anchored" agonist binding: molecular localization of the salmeterol exosite within the β_2-adrenergic receptor. *J. Biol. Chem.* **271,** 24,029–24,035.
7. Kunkel, T. A. (1985) Rapid and efficient site-specific mutagenesis without phenotypic selection. *Proc. Natl. Acad. Sci. USA* **82,** 488–492.
8. Scatchard, G. (1949) The attractions of proteins for small molecules and ions. *Ann. NY Acad. Sci.* **51,** 660–672.

19

Methods for Determining β_2-Adrenoceptor Genotype

Jane C. Dewar, Amanda P. Wheatley, and Ian P. Hall

1. Introduction

Polymorphisms of the β_2-adrenoceptor (β_2AR) have been the focus of much interest as part of the search to elucidate the genetic basis of asthma and allergic disease. More recently, these polymorphisms have also been implicated in the genetic etiology of essential hypertension *(1,2)* and obesity *(3,4)*. This chapter describes in detail the method of allele-specific-oligonucleotide hybridization (ASO), a technique that has been used extensively by the authors' group to determine β_2AR genotype. This method should prove useful not only to those intending to analyze β_2AR polymorphisms, but also for the analysis of other candidate genes, given that this technique can be adapted and applied to any known single-base mutation.

The basic principles involved, necessary materials, detailed methodology, and methodological problems are outlined here. For completeness, other techniques that have been effectively utilized by different groups, to determine β_2AR genotype, are described briefly. The relative advantages and disadvantages of these techniques, compared with ASO, are then presented.

First, in order to place these methods in context, a brief overview of β_2AR polymorphisms is given.

1.1. β_2AR Polymorphisms

The gene encoding the β_2AR is an intronless gene located on the short arm of chromosome 5q (5q31–33), and was first cloned in 1987 *(5)*. Subsequently, in 1993, Reishaus et al. *(6)* screened the open-reading frame of the β_2AR gene for polymorphisms, using the technique of temperature gradient gel electrophoresis (TGGE). Nine polymorphisms were identified, five of which were degenerate. Four, however, resulted in a single amino acid (AA) change in the

From: *Methods in Molecular Medicine, vol. 44: Asthma: Mechanisms and Protocols*
Edited by: K. F. Chung and I. Adcock © Humana Press Inc., Totowa, NJ

receptor, corresponding to nucleic acid residues 46 (A-G), 79 (C-G), 100 (G-A), 491 (C-T). These result in the substitution of glycine for arginine at AA position 16 (Arg-Gly 16), glutamate for glutamine at AA position 27 (Gln-Glu 27), methionine for valine at AA position 34 (Val-Met 34), and isoleucine for threonine at AA position 164 (Thr-Ile 164) respectively, as shown in **Fig. 1**.

In vitro physiological studies have shown that the Val-Met 34 polymorphism has no effect on receptor function, and, as such, it has not been further characterized ***(6,7)***. The Thr-Ile 164 polymorphism significantly decreases ligand-binding affinity, and also uncouples the receptor from its effector system. However, this polymorphism is rare (3% in the general population) ***(8)***, occurring mainly in a heterozygote form, and it has therefore not been possible to determine the clinical effects of this mutation.

The *N*-terminal polymorphisms at codons 16 and 27 occur commonly in equal numbers in both asthmatic and nonasthmatic subjects ***(6)***. These polymophisms have significant effects on receptor downregulation ***(6,7)***, and have been shown to both modulate the asthmatic phenotype ***(9)***, and to determine in part the responsiveness to β_2-agonist therapy ***(10,11)***. These polymorphisms are in significant linkage disequilibrium with one another ***(8)***. The physiological and clinical effects of β_2AR polymorphisms are summarized in **Table 1**.

2. Materials

The following is a comprehensive list of materials and reagents required to perform ASO:

2.1. DNA Extraction

1. Nucleon Genomic DNA Extraction Kit (Anachem Scot-lab, Bedfordshire, UK).
2. 1.5-mL microcentrifuge tubes.
3. Deionized H_2O (ddH_2O).

2.2. Polymerase Chain Reaction

1. Sterile 0.5-mL microcentrifuge tubes.
2. *Taq* DNA polymerase (Promega, Southampton, UK). Store 4°C.
3. 50 ng genomic DNA template. Store 4°C.
4. β_2AR upstream (5') and downstream (3') primer.
5. Each of the four deoxynucleotides, deoxycytosine triphosphate, deoxyguanosine triphosphate, deoxadenosine triphosphate (dATP), and deoxythymidine triphosphate (Promega). Stored at 4°C.
6. Polymerase chain reaction (PCR) 10X buffer (Promega). Store 4°C.
7. $MgCl_2$ solution (Promega). Store 4°C.
8. ddH_2O.

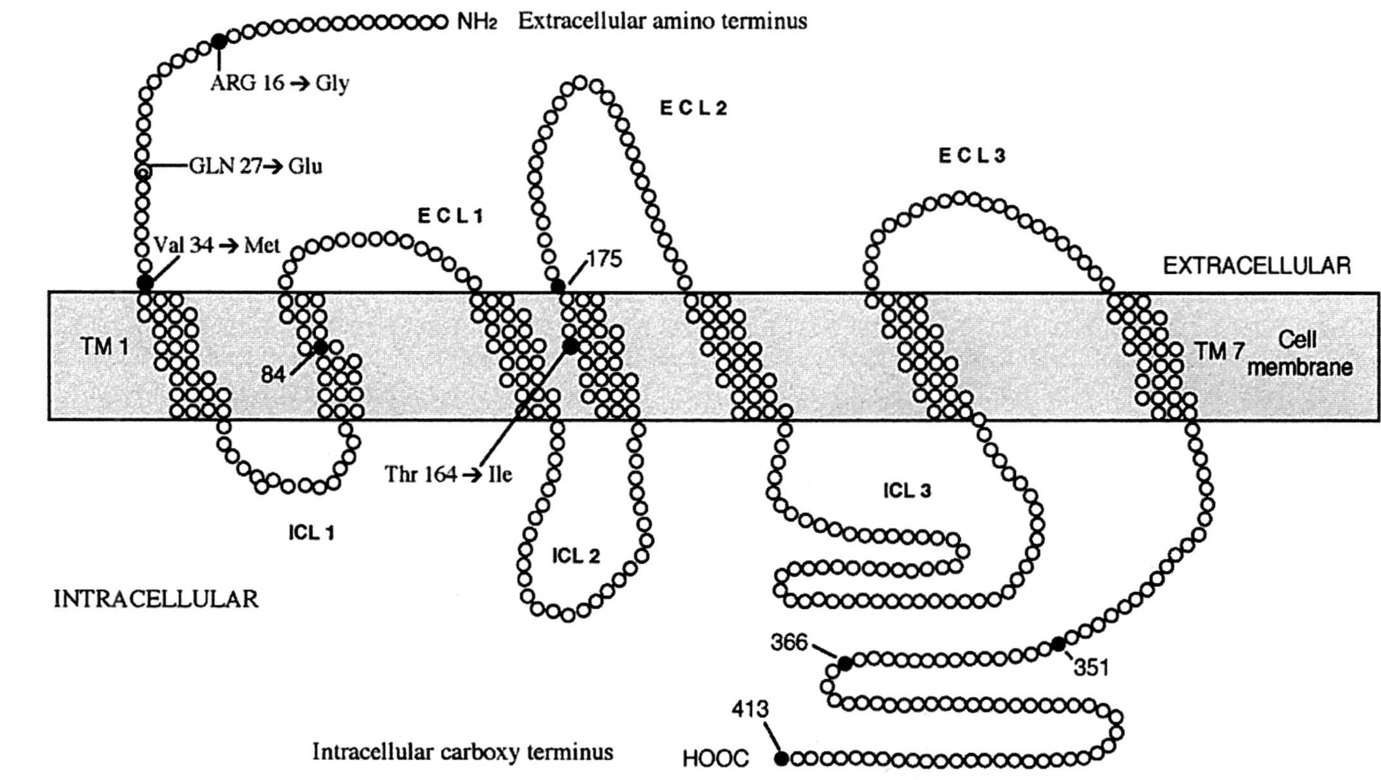

Fig. 1. Structure of the β_2AR showing identified polymorphisms.

Table 1
Physiological and Clinical Effects of β_2AR Polymorphisms

Amino acid position:	Nucleotide position & domain	*In vitro* effects	Potential mechanism of effect	Clinical effects of mutant receptor	Authors
Arg- Gly 16	• 46 A→G • Extracellular N-terminus	• Enhanced Gly 16 receptor downregulation in response to agonist exposure	• Altered receptor degradation	• ↑ severity of asthma • Associated with nocturnal asthma • Tachyphylaxis to β_2 agonists • Decreased responsiveness to Albuterol	• Reishaus *et al*, 1993 (6) • Turki *et al*, 1995 (19) • Tan *et al*, 1997 (10) • Martinez *et al*, 1997 (11)
Gln-Glu 27	• 79 C→G • Extracellular N-terminus	• Attenuated receptor downregulation in response to agonist exposure	• Altered receptor degradation	• ↓ bronchial hyperreactivity to methacholine • ↓ serum total IgE • Decreased childhood self-reported asthma	• Hall *et al*, 1995 (18) • Dewar *et al*, 1997 (9) • Hopes *et al*, 1997 (14)
Thr-Ile 164	• 491 C→T • TMD IV	• ↓ ligand binding • Uncoupling from intracellular effector systems • ↓ exosite binding of salmeterol • ↓receptor internalisation	• Perturbation of the Ser [165] residue & and its interaction with catecholamines	• Too rare to characterise	• Green *et al*, 1998 (32)
Codon 175	• 523 Degenerate			• Coincides with Ban-1 RFLP, associated with airway responsiveness and asthma • In linkage disequilibrium with amino acid 27	• Ohe *et al*, 1995 (22)

2.3. Gel Electrophoresis

1. Blue/orange 6X loading dye (Promega).
2. DNA size marker *Hae*III Φ× 174 (Kramel Biotech International Ltd, Northumberland, UK).
3. 1X (TAE) buffer.
4. 1% agarose gel: 2 mL 50X TAE buffer, 98 mL ddH_2O, 10 μL ethodium bromide, 1 g agarose. 50X TAE: 242 g Tris-base, 57.1 mL glacial acetic acid, 100 mL 0.5 *M* ethylenediamine tetraacetic acid (EDTA), pH 8.0.

2.4. ASO Hybridization

2.4.1. Preparation of Filters

1. Bromophenol blue.
2. 0.4 *M* NaOH solution.
3. 4X (SSC) solution.
4. 2X SSC solution.
5. Sterile 1.5 mL microcentrifuge tubes.
6. Hybond N+ plus filter (Amersham Pharmacia, Amersham, UK).
7. Blotting paper.
8. Dot-blot apparatus (e.g., Hybri-Dot model, Gibco Life Technologies, Paisley, UK).
9. Gauze.
10. Biometra hybridization chambers.
11. 5X (SSPE), 1% sodium dodecyl sulfate (SDS) solution.
12. 5X SSPE, 0.1% SDS solution.
13. 2X SSPE, 0.1% SDS solution.
14. 20X SSPE solution.
15. 20X SCC solution.

2.4.2. Labeling of Oligonucleotide Probes

1. Oligonucleotide (oligo-NT) probe. Stored 4°C.
2. ddH_2O.
3. 10X polynucleotide kinase (PNK) buffer (Strategene). Store 4°C.
4. PNK (Amersham, Buckinghamshire, UK). Store 4°C. Always keep on ice.
5. (γ^{32}P) dATP (9.25 Mbq, 10.0 mCi/mL, Amersham). Store 4°C.

2.4.3. Solutions

1. 5X SSPE, 1% SDS: 250 mL 20X SSPE, 10 g SDS, 750 mL ddH_2O. Store at room temperature (RT).
2. 5X SSPE, 0.1% SDS: 250 mL 20X SSPE, 1 g SDS, 750 mL ddH_2O. Store at RT.
3. 2X SSPE, 0.1% SDS: 100 mL 20X SSPE, 1 g SDS, 900 mL ddH_2O. Store at RT.
4. 20X SSPE: 175.3 g Na Cl, 27.6 g $NaH_2\ PO_4^-\ H_2O$, 7.4 g EDTA, 800 mL ddH_2O. Adjust pH to 7.4 with NaOH; adjust volume to 1 L with H_2O. Store at RT.
5. 20X SCC: 175.3 g Na Cl, 88.2 g Na citrate, 800 mL ddH_2O. Adjust pH to 7.0 with NaOH, and then adjust volume to 1 L with ddH_2O. Sterilize with autoclaving. Store at RT.

3. Methods

3.1. Determining β_2AR Genotype

Several different techniques have been used to determine β_2AR genotype. The principles behind these methods, and their relative merits, are discussed in **Note 1**, and are summarized in **Table 4**. Many other currently available methods could also be applied to these polymorphisms, and these are outlined in **Note 2**. From this array of methods, the technique of ASO hybridization was chosen for use by the authors' group because of its rapidity, sensitivity, and simplicity.

3.2. ASO

3.2.1. Theoretical Background

ASO hybridization is a modified technique developed by Gunneberg et al. ***(12)***, based on the use of ASOs for the detection of single-point mutations ***(13)***. An oligo-NT is a short segment of synthetic DNA (approx 20 nucleotides in length), which is designed to be complementary to a region of DNA containing a specific polymorphism. A single base mismatch between an oligo-NT probe and template DNA will substantially decrease its annealing affinity, thus allowing discrimination between different alleles. ASO is a competitive assay, in which amplified DNA products are applied to duplicate filters (e.g., A and B) with a dot-blot apparatus. **Figure 2** shows a schematic representation of the technique: In brief, filter A is incubated initially with unlabeled (cold) oligo-NT probe homologous to the wild-type form of receptor, and filter B with cold (unlabeled) oligo-NT probe homologous to the mutant form of receptor. Each filter is then hybridized with hot (^{32}P-labeled) probes in the opposite order, so that filter A is exposed to probe homologous to the mutant form of receptor, and filter B to probe homologous to the wild-type form of receptor. The two filters are read in parallel: Filter A thus displays signal for mutant homozygotes, and heterozygotes; filter B displays signal for wild-type homozygotes and heterozygotes. The heterozygote signal is intermediate to the homozygote signal, and interpretation is aided by the application of control samples with known genotypes to the filters. This also verifies that filters have been appropriately labeled and probes added in the correct order.

3.2.2. Specific Methodology

The general protocol for ASO is as follows: Genomic DNA is extracted from appropriate samples. Whole blood is commonly used, although β_2AR genotype has been successfully determined using buccal cells, following washing with normal saline ***(14)***. The PCR is then used to generate fragments of DNA spanning the region of interest. This PCR product is next applied to filters, using a dot-blot apparatus. The filters are then competitively hybridized with labeled/unlabeled mutant and wild-type oligo-NT probes. The filters are exposed to autoradiographic film overnight at –20°C, and the results read in parallel the following day. The separate stages of this protocol are now outlined in detail.

3.2.3. Genomic DNA Extraction

Genomic DNA is extracted from whole blood samples collected in Na EDTA tubes, using a Nucleon Genomic DNA Extraction Kit (Anachem, Scot-lab) (or equivalent). The protocol recommended by the manufacturers is followed, as summarized below.

3.2.3.1. Cell Preparation

1. 3–10 mL whole blood is added to a 50-mL propylene centrifuge tube and 4 × the volume of reagent A (10 m*M* Tris-HCl, 320 m*M* sucrose, 5 m*M* $MgCl_2$, 15 Triton X-100, pH adjusted to 8.0 with 40% NaOH).
2. The sample is rotary-mixed for 4 min at RT, and then centrifuged at 1300*g* for 4 min.
3. The supernatant is discarded without disturbing the pellet.

3.2.3.2. Cell Lysis

1. 2 mL reagent B (400 m*M* Tris-HCl, 60 m*M* EDTA, 150 m*M* NaCl, 1% SDS, pH adjusted to 8.0 with 40% NaOH) is then added to the pellet.
2. This is followed by a brief vortex, in order to resuspend the pellet.

3.2.3.3. Deproteinization

1. 500 µL Na percholate solution is next added.
2. The solution is mixed by inverting at least 7× by hand.

3.2.3.4. DNA Extraction

1. 2 mL chloroform is added, and then mixed by inverting at least 7× by hand, in order to emulsify the phases.
2. 300 µL Nucleon resin is added, and the solution centrifuged at 1300*g* for 3 min without remixing the phases.

3.2.3.5. DNA Precipitation

1. The upper phase is then transferred to a clean tube, without disturbing the Nucleon resin layer. If any resin is inadvertently transferred, the solution is again briefly centrifuged at a minimum of 1300*g* to pellet the resin, and the supernatant is transferred to a new tube.
2. Two volumes of cold absolute (100%) ethanol are added and the solution inverted several times until the DNA precipitates.

3.2.3.6. DNA Washing

1. The solution is centrifuged at 4000*g* (minimum) for 5 min in order to pellet the DNA, and the supernatant is then discarded.
2. 2 mL cold 70% ethanol is added, and inverted several times, followed by recentrifugation.

A

Filter A: 'Mutant'
Filter B: 'Wildtype'

B

Filter A: 'Mutant'
Filter B: 'Wildtype'
W-T HOM
HET
MT HOM

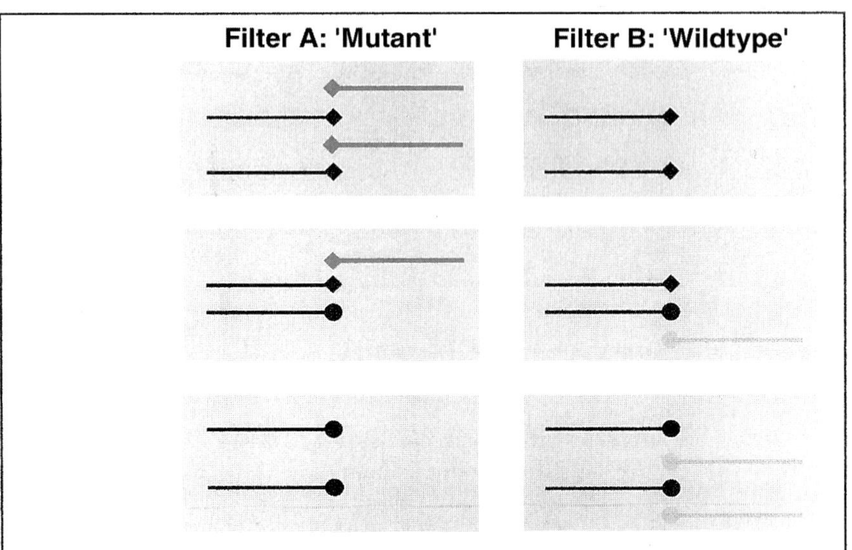

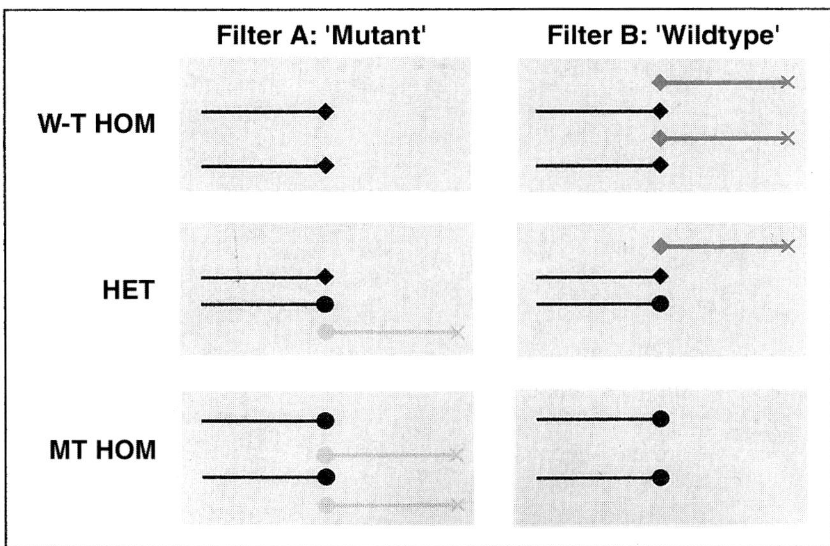

C

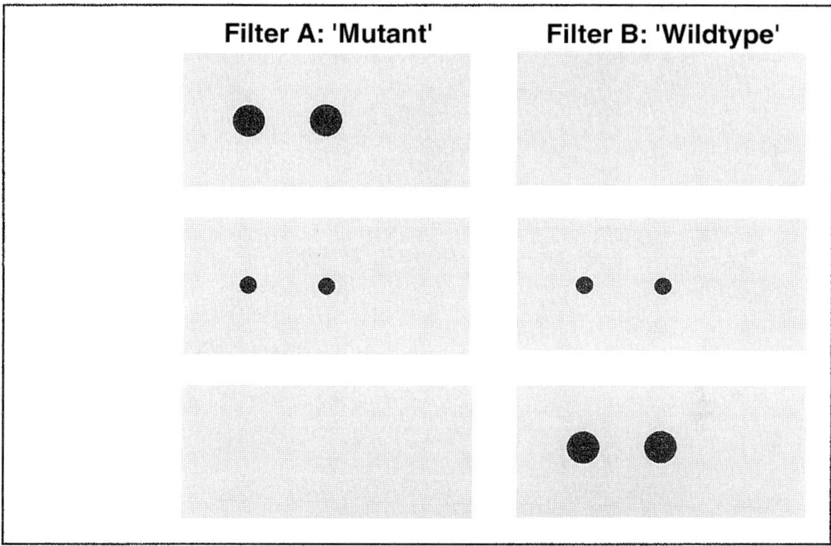

Fig. 2. Schematic representation of allele-specific oligonucleotide hybridization. The PCR product is shown on the left of each filter, and the oligonucleotide probe on the right. The wild-type probe is shown as gray diamonds, and the mutant probe is shown as gray circles. Unlabeled wild-type probe is hybridized to the filter labeled "mutant," and the unlabeled mutant probe is hybridized to the filter labeled "wild-type." The subsequent hybridization between probe and PCR product for different genotypes is shown. W-T HOM: wild-type homozygote; HET: heterozygote; MT HOM: mutant homozygote. **(A)** Hybridization with cold (unlabeled) "opposite probe. **(B)** Hybridization with hot "same" probe. Labeled "hot" mutant probe is hybridized to the filter labeled "mutant," and the labeled wild-type probe is hybridized to the filter labeled "wild-type"**(C)** Schematic representation of autoradiograph of filters (A) and (B) following the hybridizations illustrated above. Note that the filters are read in conjunction with one another, and the heterozygote signal is intermediate to that of the homozygote samples.

3. The supernatant is discarded, and the step repeated as necessary.
4. Finally, the DNA pellet is air-dried for 15 min, then the DNA is resuspended in 1 mL ddH_2O, aided by rotary mixing, if necessary.
5. Samples are subsequently stored at –80°C. Repeated freeze-thawing is to be avoided. Reagents A and B, Na percholate solution, and resin are all supplied by Nucleon.

3.2.4. Polymerase Chain Reaction

The PCR was first described in 1985 ***(15)***. It is a rapid method of producing large amounts of specific DNA sequence. PCR amplification involves succes-

Table 2
PCR Conditions for AA Residues 16, 27, 164, and 523 β_2AR Polymorphisms

Amino acid	5' Primer	3' primer	Fragment size	Annealing temperature	Cycles
Arg-Gly 16 & Gln-Glu 27	CCC AGC CAG TGC GCT TAC CT	CCG TCT GCA GAC GCT CGA AC.	234	60	36
Thr-Ile 164 & Nucleic acid residue 523	CC AGC CAG TGC GCT TAC CT	GAC ATG GAA GCG GCC CTC AG	761	64	30

sive cycles of DNA heat denaturation, oligo-NT primer annealing to their complementary strands flanking the DNA segment to be generated, and subsequent DNA extension with a thermostable DNA polymerase, resulting in the generation of an exponential amount of DNA relative to the quantity of template. The thermostable DNA polymerase used is generally *Taq* polymerase, which is produced by the thermophilic bacterium, *Thermus aquaticus* ***(16)***. The PCR and its applications are comprehensively reviewed by Ma et al. ***(17)***. The aspects of this method relevant to genotyping the β_2AR gene are next outlined.

3.2.4.1. Primer Design

Oligo-NT primers are designed to span the region of DNA of interest. The rules for primer design, which should ideally be adhered to are detailed in **Note 3**. The authors' group uses oligo-NT primers synthesized by Oswell (Southampton, UK) and these are high-pressure liquid chromatography (HPLC) purified.

3.2.4.2. PCR Amplification

The four nondegenerate β_2AR polymorphisms at AA positions 16, 27, 164, and nucleic acid residue 523, have been analyzed using the technique of ASO *(8)*; the PCR conditions for each are summarized in **Table 2**. In general, the gene encoding the β_2AR is readily amplified using PCR. Strategies that may be employed if PCR is problematic are described in **Note 3**.

3.2.4.2.1. Codon 16 and 27

PCR is used to generate a 234-bp fragment from the 5' end of the β_2AR spanning the two polymorphisms of interest. The primer sequences are as follows: upstream, CCC AGC CAG TGC GCT TAC CT; and downstream, CCG TCT GCA GAC GCT CGA AC. The authors use hot-start PCR to help reduce false priming: An initial period of 5 min at 94°C is used for the first cycle, followed by 1 min at 60°C, after which 1 U *Taq* polymerase is added to each reaction. Each reaction is ended with a 10-min extension period at 72°C. Samples should be paused, and stored at 4°C. The details for each step are as follows:

1. A 50-μL PCR reaction is performed using 50 ng genomic DNA, 34 μL sterile H_2O, 200 μ*M* of each deoxynucleotide, 5 μL PCR 10X buffer, 1.5 m*M* MgCl, and 2 μ*M* of each primer.
2. Reagents are thoroughly mixed by microcentrifuging at 10,000*g* for 1–2 min.
3. A drop of mineral oil is added to each reaction.
4. A negative control sample is run with each batch, to ensure that DNA contamination between samples has not occurred.
5. Samples are then placed on a Biometra Trio-Thermoblock (Anachem, Bedfordshire, UK). The PCR reaction employed consists of 36 cycles, and the conditions for each step are as follows:
   a. An initial period of 5 min at 94°C is used in the first cycle, followed by 1 min at 60°C, after which 1 U *Taq* polymerase is added to each reaction.
   b. This is followed by 36 cycles of melting temperature 94°C, 90 s; annealing temperature 60°C, 90 s; and extension temperature 72°C, 90 s.
   c. At the end of the reaction, a 10-min extension period at 72°C is employed.
   d. Samples are paused at 4°C.
   e. Samples are stored at 4°C, until required for analysis.
   f. Repeated freeze-thawing of samples should be avoided.

3.2.4.2.2. Codon 164 and Nucleic Acid Residue 523

The primers used are CC AGC CAG TGC GCT TAC CT upstream, and downstream GAC ATG GAA GCG GCC CTC AG, yielding a 761-bp fragment. The PCR reaction is as described above, but with 20 cycles, and an annealing temperature of 64°C (*see* **Table 2**).

3.2.4.3. Agarose Gel Electrophoresis

In order to ensure that the PCR has generated adequate product that is the right size, PCR products are resolved by electrophoresis through a 1% agarose gel (*see* **Subheading 2.3.**) with a DNA marker.

1. 10 μL PCR sample is loaded with 1 μL blue/orange 6X loading dye (Promega).
2. Electrophoresis is carried out in a 1X TAE buffer.
3. The DNA size marker *Hae*III ΦX 174 (Kramel Biotech) is electrophoresed with

samples, in order to ensure appropriate strand size, 1 µL 6X loading dye diluted with 5 µL ddH_2O. This restriction enzyme digests DNA into 11 fragments of the following sizes: 1353, 1078, 872, 603, 310, 281, 271, 234, 194, 118, and 72 bp.
4. PCR fragments are separated with 4.25–5.75 V/cm for approx 30 min.
5. Gels are visualized with a short-wave (302 nm) UV transilluminator, and photographed.

3.2.4.4. Preparation of Filters

Two identical filters are required for each bi-allelic polymorphism:

1. For the preparation of two filters, 2 µL PCR product is mixed well by pipeting with 200 µL 0.4 *M* NaOH, 200 µL 4X SSC, and 20 µL bromophenol blue in 1.5-mL microcentrifuge tubes.
2. 100 µL of this solution is then applied to duplicate wells for two Hybond N+ filters per polymorphism, using a dot-blot apparatus (e.g., Hybri-Dot model, Bethseda Research).
3. For each filter, two pieces of blotting paper and one piece of Hybond N+ membrane are cut to size and soakcd in 20 mL 2X SSC.
4. These are then secured on the dot-blot filter block, with the Hybond N+ plus membrane being uppermost, and suction is applied via a manifold pump.
5. 100 µL PCR solution, prepared as above, is applied to each well in duplicates (i.e., two wells per sample).
6. Suction is applied until all of the solution has disappeared from each well.
7. The filters are then clearly labeled and allowed to air-dry.
8. Each filter should have several samples applied at a recorded position that has a known genotype, in order to act as controls. This also aids interpretation of the filters.

This stage is generally unproblematic, and mistakes usually arise because of lapses of concentration while applying samples to the dot-blot apparatus. Problems during this stage can, however, lead to poor-quality filters: These are discussed in **Note 4**.

3.2.4.5. Labeling of Oligo-NT Probes

The sequences for the ASO probes used are shown in **Table 3**. The position of each polymorphism is underlined. ASO probes are labeled thus:

1. 1 µL (0.05 nmols) of oligo-NT probe is added to 5.5 µL H_2O, 1 µL 10X PNK buffer (Stratagene), 5 U polynucleotide kinase (PNK) (Stratagene), and 2 µL (γ^{32}P) dATP (9.25 Mbq, 10.0 mCi/mL, Amersham), and mixed well by pipeting.
2. The mixture is incubated at 37°C for 1 h in a water bath.
3. It is then heated for 5 min at 70°C, in order to inactivate the PNK enzyme.
4. The labeled probe is stored at 4°C. Probe should be used within a few days of preparation.

Table 3
β_2AR ASO Hybridization Probes

Amino Acid	Oligonucleotide Probe Sequence
• Gln27	• CAC GCA GGA AAG GGA CGG AG
• Glu27	• CAC GCA GCA AAG GGA CGA G
• Arg16	• GCA CCC AAT AGA AGC CAT G
• Gly16	• GCA CCC AAT GGA AGC CAT G
• Thr 164	• CAG GCC TTA CCT CCT TCT T
• Ile 164	• CAG GCC TTA TCT CCT TCT T
• 523 wild-type	• CAC TGG TAC CGG GCC ACC C
• 523 mutant	• CAC TGG TAC AGG GCC ACC C

3.2.4.6. Hybridization

To determine genotype, one filter is hybridized, as appropriate, with cold (unlabeled) ASO probe homologous with the wild-type form of the receptor, followed by hot (^{32}P-labeled) ASO probe homologous with the mutant form of the receptor. The duplicate filter is treated in an identical fashion, but using probes in the reverse order. The authors perform hybridization in a Biometra OV2 hybridization oven. The exact methodology for genotyping the *N*-terminal β_2 adrenoceptor polymorphisms is outlined below:

1. The four filters are rolled separately in gauze (gauze outermost, sample-side of filter innermost), and placed in Biometra hybridization chambers, so that the gauze is closely approximated to the edge of the chamber.
2. Each chamber is clearly labeled for each genotype (i.e., mutant/wild-type, corresponding to the filter label).
3. The hybridization conditions employed are as follows:
   a. 10 µL of cold (unlabeled) Arg-Gly 16 probe is added to the opposite labeled filter (e.g., mutant (Gly) probe to wild-type (Arg) filter, and vice versa).
   b. 30 µL cold (unlabeled) Gln-Glu 27 probe is added to the opposite labeled filter (e.g., mutant (Glu) probe to wild-type (Gln) filter, and vice versa).
   c. Filters are then hybridized in 20 mL 5X SSPE, 1% SDS solution, at 52°C, 60 min for each probe.

d. 1 µL labeled (hot) Arg-Gly 16 probe is added to the same labeled filter (e.g., mutant (Gly) probe to mutant (Gly) filter, and vice versa).
e. 1 µL labeled (hot) Gln-Glu 27 probe is added to the same labeled filter (e.g., mutant (Glu) probe to mutant (Glu) filter, and vice versa).
f. Filters are then hybridized in 20 mL 5X SSPE, 1% SDS solution, at 52°C, 60 min for each probe.
g. The filters are next washed with 20 mL 2X SSPE, 0.1% SDS solution, at room temperature, 2× for 30 min. Solution is replaced after each wash.
h. This is followed finally by two washes with 20 mL 5X SSPE, 0.1% SDS solution, 52°C, for 15 min.
i. Probed filters are then exposed to autoradiographic film with intensifying screens, overnight at –80°C.
j. Filters are read in conjunction after correct control genotype is confirmed in control samples.

Protocols for genotyping the AA 164 and nucleic acid residue 523 polymorphisms are identical, except that equal quantities of labeled and unlabeled probe are used (e.g., 1 µL [0.05 nmol]) for each hybridization. Problems encountered during this stage, and strategies to avoid them, are outlined in **Note 4.**

4. Conclusion

ASO is a reliable and rapid technique that has been successfully used in several studies ***(8–10,14,18)*** to genotype the nondegenerate β_2AR polymorphisms. It is a sensitive technique, and compares well with other techniques (*see* **Note 4**). It can be applied to any known single-point mutation, and hence, once acquired, will prove to be an useful tool in the field of molecular genetics.

5. Notes

1. Other methods also utilized to determine β_2AR genotype: The N-terminal β_2AR polymorphisms have been the focus of much current interest, and a number of groups have studied their clinical effects, employing methods other than ASO for determining genotype. For example, Martinez et al. ***(10)*** used a primer-induced restriction assay to determine genotype at locus 16, and a restriction fragment assay for locus 27. Green et al. ***(7)***, Turki et al. ***(19)*** and Hancox et al. ***(20)*** have all used an Amplification Refractory Mutation System (ARMS)-based technique, called allele-specific PCR ***(21)***, to determine β_2AR genotype. Finally, Ohe et al. ***(22)*** have analyzed a known restriction-length fragment polymorphism within the β_2AR gene ***(23)***, in a Japanese population. This assay employs a more complicated technique than the ones described so far, and does not involve the PCR: High-mol wt DNA is digested with the restriction endonuclease *Ban*I, and is then electrophoresed in a 0.7% agarose gel for 24 h. The digest products are then transferred to a nylon membrane by Southern blot. A 2.6-kb radiolabeled DNA probe homologous to the whole of the open-reading frame of the 1.2-kb β_2AR

gene, extending 1.0 kb upstream and 0.4 kb downstream of the gene, is then used to detect the receptor gene among the genomic *Ban*I fragments ***(23)***. Using this method, two different-sized alleles (2.3 and 2.1 kb) have been detected, and the 2.1-kb allele was found to be associated with decreased airway responsiveness to β_2-agonists, and an increased incidence of asthma. The chief disadvantage of this method is that the actual polymorphic site involved cannot be specifically identified. Although the restriction fragment length polymorphism (RFLP) may be located outside of the β_2AR coding block, the authors considered it highly likely that the site analyzed corresponds to the degenerate β_2AR polymorphism at nucleic acid position 523, given that a *Ban*I site coincides with this region, and could therefore similarly alter restriction fragment lengths. The authors therefore defined the site of the 2.1–2.3 kb *Ban*I polymorphism by direct sequencing, and confirmed that it arises because of the nucleic acid residue 523 polymorphism ***(8)***. Furthermore, the authors have recently shown that this polymorphism is in linkage disequilibrium with the AA 27 polymorphism (analyzed by ASO, as described in **Subheading 3.2.4.6.**) ***(8)***, and this phenomenon may therefore explain the *Ban*I 2.1 kb allelic association with airway responsiveness and asthma.

All of the assays described above, other than that employed by Ohe et al. ***(22)***, have the advantage of not involving the use of radioactivity. In general, they are relatively easy to perform and only those techniques involving PCR or restriction digest will give rapid results. There are some problems inherent in these techniques, however:

a. Allele-specific PCR is very sensitive to error: Mismatch between the primer and allele may not always occur, resulting in template DNA of the wrong genotype, which is then exponentially amplified. Problems with this method may indeed account for the inability of several groups, including the authors' own ***(24–27)***, to detect the Iso-181-Leu substitution in the high-affinity immunoglobulin E receptor gene (FCεR1β). This polymorphism was initially reported to be associated with atopy and elevated total immunoglobulin E ***(28,29)*** with evidence for maternal inheritance, but doubts now exist as to whether the polymorphism actually occurs, or whether it is merely the result of a methodological artifact.
b. RFLP can sometimes pose problems as a result of incomplete digestion by certain restriction enzymes, leading to an appearance identical with heterozygotes on resolution by agarose gel electrophoresis. These false heterozygotes are misgenotyped, leading to an inaccurate estimation of allelic distribution. Both the ARMS and RFLP assays use agarose gel electrophoresis, which is sometimes not powerful enough to separate DNA fragments of a similar size. The relative merits of these assays are summarized in **Table 4**.
c. Finally, none of these techniques, including ASO, are 100% sensitive in detecting polymorphism, and the gold standard for the analysis of any mutation is therefore direct sequencing. This can be very time-consuming if done manually, although the use of T-tracking, in which all identical dideoxynucleotide reactions for different samples are run out together (i.e., all Ts), allows easy visualization of any polymorphism. The use of automated sequencing obviously expedites results, but can be very expensive.

Table 4
Techniques Used to Genotype β_2AR Polymorphisms

Polymorphism	Technique	Advantages	Disadvantages	Authors
Arg- Gly 16	Primer - induced restriction assay	• Non-radioactive • Quick	• Difficulty resolving small PCR fragments	• Martinez *et al*, 1997 (11)
Gln-Glu 27	Restriction fragment assay	• Non-radioactive • Simple • Quick	• Incomplete digest results in 'false heterozygotes'	• Martinez *et al*, 1997 (11)
Arg- Gly 16 & Gln-Glu 27	Allele Specific oligonucleotide hybridisation (ASO)	• Rapid • Sensitive • Simple	• Radioactive • Genotype can sometimes be ambiguous	• Hall *et al*, 1995 (18) • Dewar *et al*, 1997, 1998 (7)
Thr-Ile 164	Amplification refractory mutation system - allele-specific PCR	• Non-radioactive • Quick	• Sensitive to error	• Turki *et al*, 1995 (19)
Codon 175	Restriction fragment length polymorphism assay (RFLP)	• Clear determination of genotype	• Radioactive • Site of polymorphism undefined	• Ohe *et al*, 1995 (22)

2. Alternative methods of detecting polymorphisms: There are many other methods available for the analysis of polymorphisms (reviewed in **ref. *30***), some of which are more appropriate for the detection of novel polymorphisms, such as TGGE, denaturing-gradient gel electrophoresis, chemical cleavage, heteroduplex analysis, and RNase protection assay. The technique of single-strand conformational polymorphism (SSCP) can be used either to detect novel mutations, or as a screening method for a known mutation ***(31)***.
3. Polymerase chain reaction: In the authors' hands, the open-reading frame of the β_2AR gene is readily amenable to PCR. Problems do occur from time to time with PCR in general, and the following strategies can be useful:
   a. Check that the DNA has not degraded, e.g., electrophoresis.
   b. If PCR repeatedly fails after having worked for some time, change all reagents, including primers and *Taq* polymerase.
   c. If a band is generated in the negative control, contamination has occurred. Reagents should all be changed, and pipets thoroughly cleaned.
   d. Multiple bands can be eliminated by performing MgCl titrations between 1.5 and 4.0 m*M*, adding 10% dimethyl sulfoxide, reducing the number of cycles, and optimizing the annealing temperature. If the temperature is too high, no annealing occurs; if too low, nonspecific annealing occurs.
   e. Primer-dimer formation indicates that there are complementary base pairs within the two primers, leading to base pairing between the 3' ends. These will be seen as very small products on gel electrophoresis.

   Primer design:

   a. Oligo-NT primers should be designed to incorporate a G-C content of 40–50%, with no internal palindromes or homology between primer pairs of more than three G–Cs, or of a total length of more than 4 bp.
   b. The theoretical annealing temperature of the primers is calculated in the following way: Melting temperature = 4 (G + C) + 2 (A + T), according to the rule that G/C = 4°C, A/T = 2°C, with the annealing temperature being within ±7°C of the melting temperature.
   c. Primers should generally be approx 20 bp in length, and have similar annealing temperatures (within 10°C). They should be stored at 4°C, and not be subjected to repeated freeze-thawing, which results in DNA degradation.
4. ASO hybridization: The authors have successfully used ASO to determine β_2AR genotype in several studies ***(8,9,18)***. It is a relatively simple molecular technique that can be quickly acquired, and is invaluable as a rapid screening technique for known single-point mutations. Preparation of filters takes only about 2 h; hybridization takes 4 h. Thus, approx 40 subjects can be genotyped within 24 h. Several filters can be hybridized together to increase this yield. However, in the authors' hands, this has usually resulted in filters of a poorer quality.

   Validation of assay:

   a. When setting up an ASO assay, it is obviously important to validate the method initially by jointly sequencing and hybridizing several samples, and ensuring that results concur. It may also sometimes be necessary to sequence samples in whom genotype is ambiguous.

b. ASO is a competitive assay, and probe stringencies will differ. If ASO is applied to other polymorphisms, the optimal probe concentrations will need to be determined by performing the assay with different ratios of probe pairs.
c. Because of these differing probe annealing stringencies, for the Arg-Gly polymorphism, a 10-fold excess of cold probe is used in the initial part of the hybridization procedure; a 30-fold excess of cold probe is used for the Gln-Glu polymorphism, thus allowing the standardization and optimization of respective signals.

Sensitivity of the assay:

In the authors' experience, ASO displays >95% sensitivity in detecting the correct genotype when confirmed by sequencing. This compares very favorably with other techniques, such as SSCP, which are reviewed by Marian et al. ***(30)***.

Preparation of filters:

a. Filters must be clearly labeled with a permanent waterproof marker, in order to avoid incorrect genotyping.
b. Cut a corner off the filter, so that it can be orientated correctly after probing: The blue dots often disappear during washes. Failure to do this will lead to incorrect genotyping.
c. Samples should be thoroughly mixed by pipeting before application to each filter. This is crucial in ensuring that an equal concentration of PCR product is applied to each well.
d. The dot-blot apparatus must be applied with even pressure to the filters to ensure uniform suction.
e. All the sample must have been drained before filters are removed. The time for this can vary from 15 min to over 1 h. If one or two samples have not drained, gently touching the membrane a few times with a clean pipet can aid this.

Hybridization:

a. The hybridization ovens will need assistance to cool down rapidly between washes, which can be achieved by fanning with the door. The nearer to the recommended temperature, the better.
b. Check that the filters do not unroll/loosen from the hybridization chamber wall during washes, because this will result in poor-quality filters. This problem is often ameliorated by orientating all the chambers in the same direction.
c. Check that the right filters are in the right hybridization chamber.

Interpretation of filters:

a. Interpretation of filters is greatly facilitated by the application of samples that are known to have each of the different possible genotypes at each locus. These act as controls and allow wrongly labeled filters/probes, or probes applied in the incorrect order, to be detected.
b. The control samples allow the signal from other samples to be accurately

interpreted: It is not unusual for ghost signals to be seen in homozygote samples, e.g., very weak signal occurs on the filter, which should have no signal. These samples can be difficult to interpret, because heterozygotes will have signal on both filters, also. However, heterozygote samples will give equal signal on both filters, and can be readily interpreted by referral to the control heterozygote sample. Likewise, referral to the homozygote control samples will facilitate correct interpretation of genotype.

c. Filters may sometimes give smeary or speckled results, which cannot be interpreted. Smeary filters generally occur because samples have run, indicating that the dot-block apparatus was not applied tightly enough. Speckled filters occur as a result of nonspecific radioactive uptake, indicating that the dot-blot apparatus, nylon membrane, gauze, or the chambers were not clean. Regular replacement of the gauze is recommended, and the chambers should be cleaned thoroughly after each use.
d. Individual dots (in separate pairs of samples) may sometimes differ in intensity of signal. This indicates either that samples have not been thoroughly mixed, or that there has been incomplete drainage during preparation.
e. Sometimes, none of the samples are readable, indicating that ASO has not worked. Ensure that all reagents are fresh, and that PCR product is present, and repeat. If ASO consistently fails, renew probes.
f. ASO is generally unproblematic, but genotype can sometimes be ambiguous because of insufficient PCR product binding to the filter. In these instances, genotype can usually be determined by repeating hybridization after preparing new filters, or by direct sequencing.
g. Finally, ASO is only useful for detecting known single-point mutations, and is therefore not appropriate for the screening of genes for novel polymorphisms.

References

1. Svetky, L. P., Timmons, P. Z., Emovon, O., Anderson, N. B., Preis, L., and Chen, Y. T. (1996) Association of hypertension with beta-2 and alpha-2c10-adrenergic receptor genotype. *Hypertension* **27,** 1210–1215.
2. Kotanko, P., Binder, A., and Tasker, J. (1997) Essential hypertension in African-Caribbeans associates with a variant of the beta-2-adrenoceptor. *Hypertension* **30,** 773–776.
3. Large, V., Hellstrom, L., and Reynisdottir, S. (1997) Human beta-2-adrenoceptor gene polymorphisms are highly frequent in obesity and associated with altered adipocyte beta-2-adrenoceptor function. *J. Clin. Invest.* **100,** 3005–3013.
4. Meirhaeghe, A., Helbecque, N., Cottel, D., and Amuoyel, P. (1999) β_2-Adrenoceptor gene polymorphism, body weight, and physical activity. *Lancet* **353,** 896.
5. Kobilka, B. K., Dixon, R. A. F., Frielle, T., Dohlman, H. G., Bolanowski, M. A., Sigal, I. S., et al. (1987) cDNA for the human β_2-adrenergic receptor: a protein with multiple membrane-spanning domains and encoded by a gene whose chromosomal location is shared with that of the receptor for platelet-derived growth factor. *Proc. Natl. Acad. Sci. USA* **84,** 46–50.

6. Reishaus, E., Innis, M., MacIntyre, N., and Liggett, S. B. (1993) Mutations in the gene coding for the β_2 adrenergic receptor in normal and asthmatic subjects. *Am. J. Respir. Cell. Mol. Biol.* **8,** 334–339.
7. Green, S. A., Turki, J., Bejarano, P., Hall, I. P., and Liggett, S. B. (1995) Influence of β_2 adrenergic receptor genotypes on signal transduction in human airway smooth muscle cells. *Am. J. Respir. Cell. Mol. Biol.* **13,** 25–33.
8. Dewar, J. C., Wheatley, A. P., Venn, A., Morrison, J. F. J., Britton, J. R., and Hall, I. P. (1998) β_2 adrenoceptor polymorphisms are in linkage disequilibrium but are not associated with asthma in an adult population. *Clin. Exp. Allergy* **28,** 442–448.
9. Dewar, J. C., Wilkinson, J., Wheatley, A. P., Thomas, N. S., Doull, I., Morton, N. E., et al. (1997) The glutamine 27 β_2 adrenoceptor polymorphism is associated with elevated IgE levels in families with asthma. *J. Allergy Clin. Immunol.* **100,** 261–265.
10. Tan, K. S., Hall, I. P., Dewar, J. C., Dow, E., and Lipworth, B. J. (1997) β_2-adrenoceptor (β_2-AR) polymorphism determines susceptibility to bronchodilator desensitisation in asthmatics. *Lancet* **350,** 995–999.
11. Martinez, F. D., Graves, P. E., Baldini, M., Solomon, S., and Erickson, R. (1997) Association between genetic polymorphisms of the β_2-adrenoceptor and response to albuterol in children with and without a history of wheezing. *J. Clin. Invest.* **12,** 3184–3188.
12. Gunneberg, A., Scobie, G., Hayes, K., and Kalsheker, N. (1993) Competitive assay to improve the specificity of detection of single point mutations in alpha-1-antitrypsin deficiency. *Clin. Chem.* **39,** 2157–2162.
13. Connor, B. J., Reyes, A. A., Morin, C., Itakaru, K., Teplitz, R. L., and Wallace, R. B. (1983) Detection of sickle cell beta-globin allele by hybridization with synthetic oligonucleotides. *Proc. Natl. Acad. Sci. USA* **80,** 278–282.
14. Hopes, E., McDougall, C., Christie, G., Dewar, J. C., Wheatley, A. P., Hall, I. P., and Helms, P. (1998) Association of the Glutamate 27 β_2 adrenoceptor polymorphism with reported childhood asthma. *Br. Med. J.* **316,** 664.
15. Saiki, R. K., Scharf, S., Faloona, F., Mullis, K. B., Horn, G. T., and Erlich, H. A. (1985) Enzymatic amplification of β-globin genomic sequences and restriction site analysis for diagnosis of sickle cell anaemia. *Science* **230,** 1350–1354.
16. Saiki, R. K., Gelfand, D. H., Stoffel, S., Scharf, S., Higuchi, R., Horn, G. T., Mullis, K. B., and Erlich, H. A. (1988) Primer-directed enzymatic amplification of DNA with a thermostable DNA polymerase. *Science* **239,** 487–491.
17. Ma, T. (1995) Applications and limitations of polymerase chain reaction amplification, *Chest* **108,** 1393–1404.
18. Hall, I. P., Wheatley, A., Wilding, P., and Liggett, S. B. (1995) Association of the Glu 27 β_2 adrenoceptor polymorphism with lower airway reactivity in asthmatic subjects. *Lancet* **345,** 1213, 1214.
19. Turki, J., Pak, J., Green, S. A., Martin, R. J., and Liggett, S. B. (1995) Genetic polymorphisms of the β_2-adrenergic receptor in nocturnal and non-nocturnal asthma. *J. Clin. Invest.* **95,** 1635–1641.
20. Hancox, R. J., Sears, M. R., and Taylor, D. R. (1998) Polymorphism of the β_2 adrenoceptor and the response to long-term β_2 agonist therapy in asthma. *Eur. Respir. J.* **11,** 589–593.

21. Newton, C. R., Graham, A., Heptinstall, I. E., Powell, S. J., Summers, C., and Kalsheker, N. (1989) Analysis of any point mutations in DNA. The amplification refractory system. *Nucleic Acid Res.* **17,** 2503–2515.
22. Ohe, M., Munakata, M., Hizawa, N., Itoh, A., Doi, I., Yamaguchi, E., Homma, Y., and Kawakami, Y. (1995) $Beta_2$ adrenergic receptor gene restriction length polymorphism and bronchial asthma. *Thorax* **50,** 353–359.
23. Lentes, K. U., Berrettini, W. H., Hoehe, M. R., Chung, F. Z., and Gershon, E. S. (1988) A bi-allelic DNA polymorphism of the human beta-2-adrenergic receptor detected by Ban I-Adrbr-2. *Nucleic Acid Res.* **16,** 2369.
24. Duffy, D. L., Healey, S. C., Chenevix-Trench, G., Martin, N. G., Weger, J., and Lichter, J. (1995) Atopy in Australia. *Nature Genet.* **10,** 260.
25. Hall, I. P., Wheatley, A., Dewar, J., Wilkinson, J., and Morrison, J. (1996) FcεRI-beta polymorphisms unlikely to contribute substantially to genetic risk of allergic disease. *Br. Med. J.* **312,** 311.
26. Martinati, L. C., Trabetti, E., Casartelli, A., Boner, A. L., and Pignatti, P. F. (1996) Affected sib-pair and mutation analysis of the high affinity IgE receptor beta chain locus in Italian families with atopic asthmatic children. *Am. J. Respir. Crit. Care. Med.* **153,** 5.
27. Shirakawa, T., Mao, X.-Q., Sasaki, S., Enomoto, T., Kawai, M., Morimoto, K., and Hopkin, J. (1996) Association between atopic asthma and a coding variant of FCεR1β in a Japanese population. *Hum. Mol. Genet.* **5,** 1129, 1130.
28. Hill, M. R., James, A. L., Faux, J. A., Ryan, G. F., and Cookson, W. O. C. M. (1995) FCεR1β polymorphism and risk of atopy in a general population sample. *B. Med. J.* **311,** 776–779.
29. Shirakawa, T., Hashimoto, T., Furuyama, J., and Morimoto, K. (1994) Linkage between severe atopy and chromosome 11q in Japanese families. *Clin. Genet.* **46,** 228–232.
30. Marian, A. J. (1995) Molecular approaches for screening of genetic disease. *Chest* **108,** 255–265.
31. Orita, M., Suzuki, Y., Sekiya. T., and Hayashi, K. (1989) Rapid and sensitive detection of point mutations and DNA polymorphisms using the polymerase chain reaction. *Genomics* **5,** 874–879.
32. Green, S. A., Rathz, D. A., and Liggett, S. B. (1998) Genetic basis of atypical responses to salmeterol and other β agonists. *Am. J. Respir. Crit. Care Med.* **157,** A657.

20

Modulation of β-Adrenoceptor Expression

Judith C. W. Mak

1. Introduction

β-Adrenoceptors (βAR) are members of the G-protein-coupled receptor superfamily, consisting of three subtypes: β_1, β_2, and β_3 *(1)*. cDNAs and genes encoding three subtypes have been cloned from several species, including human. There are only β_1- and β_2ARs to be found in lung *(2)*, which regulate many aspects of lung function. In addition to desensitization and downregulation at the cell surface membrane, the number of βARs expressed is modulated by regulation of steady-state levels of mRNA and the rate of gene transcription *(3)*. Regulation of β_1- and β_2AR mRNAs and gene transcription in lung may occur after exposure to receptor agonists or drug treatments *(4–6)*. Thus, this could represent a mechanism for long-term modulation of βAR expression.

The levels of βAR mRNA and gene transcription rate are regulated by complex, intracellular signal transduction pathways, which can lead to regulation of mRNA by two general mechanisms. First, the level of receptor mRNA can be modulated by regulation of its stability. Mechanisms that control mRNA stability appear to involve the presence of RNA-binding proteins that influence mRNA degradation *(7–10)*. These proteins recognize and bind to specific RNA sequences that are usually localized in the 3' noncoding region of mRNA. Second, the level of receptor mRNA is dependent on the rate of mRNA synthesis, or rate of gene transcription. Gene transcription is regulated by factors that bind to specific DNA sequences, which are usually, but not always, localized in the promoter region of the gene. These gene transcription factors can be regulated by phosphorylation, such as cAMP response element-binding protein *(11)*.

Radioligand binding is a straightforward technique that measures the binding of a labeled antagonist to its receptor in membranes from tissues. Radioligand binding allows the affinity of drugs for their receptors to be determined very

From: *Methods in Molecular Medicine, vol. 44: Asthma: Mechanisms and Protocols*
Edited by: K. F. Chung and I. Adcock © Humana Press Inc., Totowa, NJ

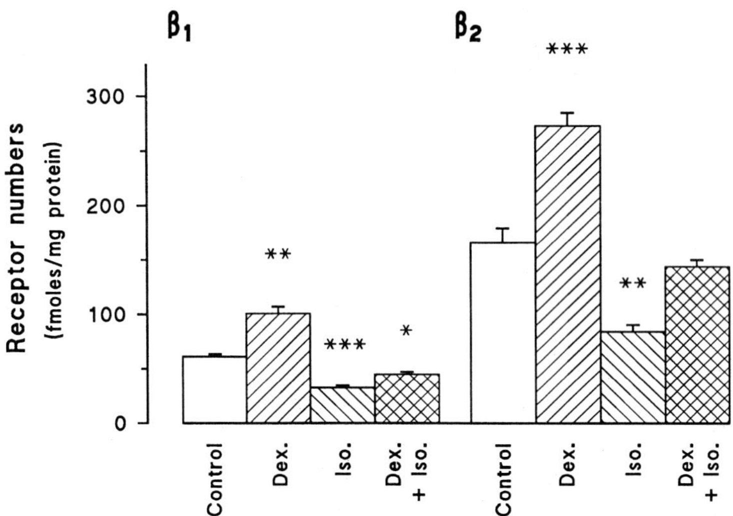

Fig. 1. Effects of treatment with dexamethasone (Dex) and/or isoproterenol (Iso) on βAR subtypes in rat lung membranes. Control, Dex, Iso, and combination of Dex and Iso groups are shown. The density of β_1- and β_2AR subtypes were analyzed by ICYP saturation binding in the presence of either 0.1 μ*M* ICI 118,551 or 0.1 μ*M* CGP 20712A, respectively. Significance of difference from the control value, $*P < 0.05$, $**P < 0.01$, $***P < 0.001$ ($n = 7$). Reprinted with permission from **ref. *5***.

readily, and it also allows the number of receptors in a tissue to be quantified. Several methods are also available for analysis of receptor mRNA and gene transcription. Steady-state levels of receptor mRNA can be determined by Northern blot analysis, which provides a determination of the levels of a specific receptor mRNA species in total RNA that has been extracted from tissues by an adaptation of the method described by Chomczynski and Sacchi ***(12)***. The success and reproducibility of this technique are dependent on the quality of the extracted RNA.

Isolation of poly(A)$^+$ RNA from extracted total RNA is preferred for receptors that are expressed at relatively low levels in tissues. This method involves the probing of blots with a cDNA that is specific for the receptor of interest, labeled to high specific activity by random primer labeling ***(13)***. To determine the stability of mRNA, the half-life can be determined from the rate of mRNA decay in the presence of gene transcription inhibitor, such as actinomycin D ***(14)***. Finally, the rate of gene transcription can be determined by nuclear run-on assay, a procedure that measures newly transcribed, radiolabeled RNA transcripts in isolated cell nuclei.

This chapter describes the detailed protocols required to determine the number of β_1- and β_2ARs (**Fig. 1**) and steady-state levels of mRNAs (**Figs. 2** and **3**), and therefore to determine if the expression of a particular receptor is regulated at the

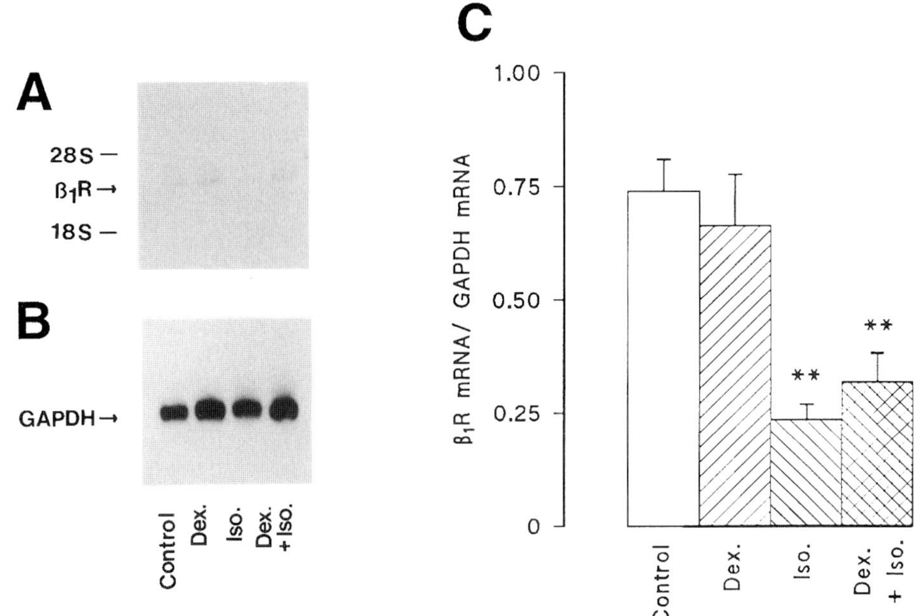

Fig. 2. Effects of treatment with Dex and/or Iso on β_1AR mRNA in rat lung. Representative autoradiograms from Northern blot of rat β_1AR mRNA **(A)** and rat GAPDH mRNA **(B)** using β_1AR and GAPDH cDNA probes. The size of mRNA was estimated from 18S and 28S rRNA markers. Densitometric measurement **(C)** of β_1AR mRNA, which was normalized to that for GAPDH mRNA from control, Dex-treated, Iso-treated, and Dex + Iso-treated rat lungs ($n = 7$ in each group). Significance of difference from the control value. ** $P < 0.01$. Reprinted with permission from **ref. *5***.

level of its mRNA. To determine if the changes in levels of receptor mRNA result from regulation of the stability of mRNA or rate of gene transcription, mRNA half-life and nuclear run-on analyses are carried out. These studies are performed in rat lung tissues from an in vivo model ***(4,5)***, and in human lung tissues in vitro after removal from surgery ***(6)***. These approaches will provide information regarding the molecular mechanisms underlying the regulation of receptor mRNA.

2. Materials

2.1. Radioligand Binding Assay

1. Rat lung membranes: Prepare as described in **Subheading 3.1.1.**
2. 50-mL Nalgene centrifuge tubes (Marathon Laboratory Supplies, London, UK).

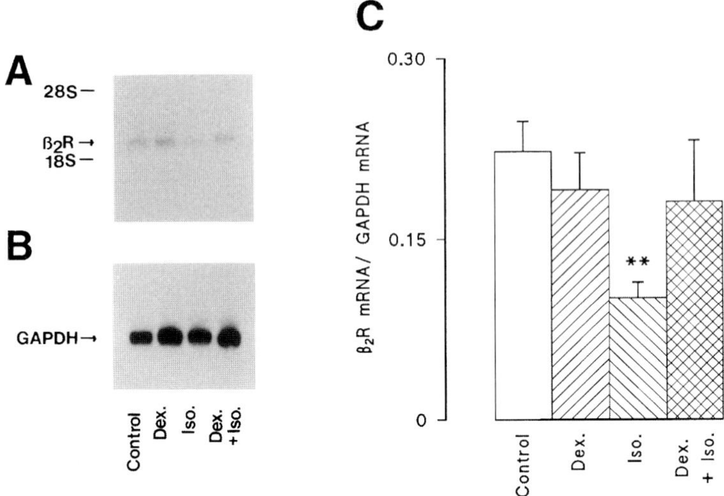

Fig. 3. Effects of treatment with Dex and/or Iso on β_2AR mRNA in rat lung. Representative autoradiograms from Northern blot of rat β_2AR mRNA **(A)** and rat GAPDH mRNA **(B)** using β_2AR and GAPDH cDNA probes. The same membrane as used in **Fig. 2**. The size of mRNA was estimated from 18S and 28S rRNA markers. Densitometric measurement **(C)** of β_2AR mRNA, which was normalized to that for GAPDH mRNA from control, Dex-treated, Iso-treated, and Dex + Iso-treated rat lungs ($n = 7$ in each group). Significance of difference from the control value. ** $P < 0.01$. Reprinted with permission from **ref. 5**.

3. Homogenizing buffer: 25 m*M* Tris-HCl, pH 7.4, 0.32 *M* sucrose at 4°C. **Note: Items 2** and **3** may all be prepared in liter quantities and stored at 4°C until required.
4. Wash buffer: 25 m*M* Tris-HCl, pH 7.4, at 4°C.
5. Assay buffer: 25 m*M* Tris-HCl, 132 m*M* NaCl, 1.1 m*M* ascorbic acid (to prevent oxidation of isoproterenol [ISO]), pH 7.4, at 37°C. This buffer should be prepared on the day of the experiment.
6. [^{125}I]iodocyanopindolol (ICYP) may be obtained from Amersham Pharmacia, Amersham, UK. The stock should be stored at –20°C, and diluted in assay buffer on the day of the experiment.
7. 5-mL Borosilicate (Marathon Laboratory Supplies) tubes and SARSTEDT tubes (SARSTEDT Ltd., Leicester, UK).
8. Cell harvester and filters: 24-place Brandel cell harvester and Whatman GF/C glass-fiber filters were used in the experiments presented here. Both cell harvester and filters may be obtained through Semat Technical, St. Albans, UK.
9. Curve-fitting programs: EBDA, followed by Ligand, Graphpad, or Prism (GraphPad Software, Inc.), may be used for analyzing binding data.

2.2. Northern Blot Analysis

2.2.1. RNA Isolation

1. Diethyl pyrocarbonate (DEPC): All solutions that will come into contact with RNA must be treated with 0.1% (v/v) DEPC. The DEPC-treated distilled H_2O must be shaken vigorously, placed in a 37°C incubator overnight and autoclaved.
2. Solution D: 4.0 *M* guanidinium thiocyanate, 25 m*M* Na citrate, pH 7.0, 0.5% sarcosyl solution, and 0.1 *M* 2-mercaptoethanol (ME), which is added immediately prior to use. To a fresh 500-g guanidinium thiocyanate bottle (Sigma, Poole, UK), add 586 mL DEPC-treated H_2O, 35.2 mL 0.75 *M* Na citrate, pH 7.0, and 52.8 mL 10% sarcosyl solution. This solution keeps for several months at room temperature (RT). Complete solution D is made by adding 0.36 mL 2-ME to 50 mL prior to use.
3. 2 *M* Na acetate, pH 4.0, autoclaved.
4. H_2O-saturated phenol (not neutralized), stored at 4°C.
5. Chloroform:isoamyl alcohol (49:1).
6. Isopropanol stored at 4°C.
7. 75 and 100% ethanol, stored at 4°C.
8. Autoclaved RNase-free Oakridge tubes, pipet tips, and microcentrifuge tubes (Marathon Laboratory Supplies).
9. Oven-baked RNase-free Corex tubes.
10. Spectrophotometer.

2.2.2. Random Primer Labeling of DNA

1. Midiprepped plasmid DNA containing full-length or fragment of target sequence.
2. Restriction enzymes that cut out fragment of interest, with complete removal of vector DNA.
3. Multiprime DNA labeling system (Amersham International, Amersham, UK), which includes deoxynucleotide triphosphates (dNTPs), reaction mixture containing hexanucleotide primers, and Klenow fragment. All of these reagents can be purchased separately.
4. [α-^{32}P] deoxycytosine triphosphate (dCTP) (3000 Ci/mmol, Amersham).
5. 1 *M* Tris-HCl, pH 7.5, autoclaved.
6. 0.5 *M* ethylenediamine tetra-acetic acid (EDTA), pH 8.0, autoclaved.
7. 10% sodium dodecyl sulfate (SDS) in DEPC-treated H_2O.
8. Sephadex G-50 in 10 m*M* Tris-HCl, pH 7.5, 1 m*M* EDTA, pH 8.0, and 0.1% SDS.
9. Tris-EDTA (TE) buffer: 10 m*M* Tris-HCl, pH 7.5, and 1 m*M* EDTA, pH 8.0.
10. Oven-baked RNase-free glass pipets.

2.2.3. RNA Formaldehyde Gel

1. Suitable RNase-free agarose (1.0%) (Promega, Southampton, UK).
2. 3-*N*-morpholine-propanesulfonic acid (MOPS) 20X buffer: 400 m*M* MOPS, 100 m*M* Na acetate, 20 m*M* EDTA. Autoclaved.

3. Gel loading buffer: 75% formamide, 1.5X MOPS, 10% formaldehyde. Store in aliquots at –20°C.
4. 20X standard sodium citrate (SSC): 3 *M* NaCl, 0.3 *M* Na citrate, pH 7.0. Autoclaved.
5. Ethidium bromide: generally available in a 10 mg/mL stock.
6. Orange G dye: 0.4% orange G, 50% glycerol, 1 m*M* EDTA. Autoclaved.
7. Formaldehyde: 37% solution.

2.2.4. Capillary Transfer of RNA to Solid Support

1. Whatman 3MM filter paper.
2. Nylon membranes commonly used include Magna (Genetic Research Instruments, Telsted Dunmow, UK) and Hybond-N (Amersham).
3. Plastic sandwich box, glass plates, sponge, weights.
4. UV Stratalinker-2400 (Stratagene, Cambridge, UK).

2.2.5. Hybridization

1. Hybridization buffer: 50% formamide, 4X SSC, 50 m*M* Tris-HCl, pH 7.5, 5X Denhardt's solution, 0.1% SDS, 5 m*M* EDTA, and 250 µg/mL denatured salmon sperm DNA.
   a. 100% deionized formamide.
   b. 20X SSC.
   c. 1 *M* Tris-HCl, pH 7.5.
   d. 50X Denhardt's solution: 1% bovine serum albumin, 1% polyvinyl pyrrolidone (PVP-360), 1% Ficoll 400.
   e. 10% SDS.
   f. 0.5 *M* EDTA, pH 8.0.
   g. 10 mg/mL denatured salmon sperm DNA (Sigma).
2. Hybridization oven (Techne, Cambridge, UK).

2.2.6. Posthybridization Washes

1. 20X SSC.
2. 10% SDS.
3. Saran Wrap (Genetic Research Instruments).
4. Cassettes, X-OMAT-S films (Kodak, Hemel Hempstead, UK).

2.3. Half-Life Studies

Actinomycin D (Sigma).

2.4. Nuclear Run-On Assay

2.4.1. Preparation of Plasmid(s) Containing cDNA(s) of Interest

1. Plasmid Midi-Prep kit (Qiagen, Ltd., Crawley, UK).
2. Restriction enzymes.
3. 50X TAE buffer (for 1 L); 242 g Tris-base, 57 mL glacial acetic acid, 100 mL 0.5 *M* EDTA, pH 8.0).

2.4.2. Preparation of Plasmid DNA(s) Slot Blot

1. DEPC-treated H_2O.
2. 2 *M* NaOH. Autoclaved.
3. 3 *M* Na acetate, pH 5.2. Autoclaved.
4. TE buffer: 10 m*M* Tris-HCl, 1 m*M* EDTA, pH 7.4.
5. 20X and 15X SSC.
6. Bio-Rad Bio-Dot SF Microfiltration apparatus (Bio-Rad, Hemel Hempstead, UK).

2.4.3. Prehybridization of Slot Blots

1. Prehybridization buffer: 50% formamide, 5X SSC, 0.1% SDS, 1 m*M* EDTA, 10 m*M* Tris-HCl, pH 7.5, 5X Denhardt's solution, 50 μg/mL yeast tRNA, 100 μg/mL salmon sperm DNA, 0.02 μg poly(A), and 0.02 μg poly(G).
2. Rotating hybridization oven.

2.4.4. Preparation of Nuclei for Nuclear Run-On

1. Buffer I: 10 m*M* HEPES, pH 7.4, 5 m*M* KCl, 10 m*M* $MgCl_2$, and 0.32 *M* sucrose. Autoclaved.
2. Triton X-100 (Sigma).
3. Buffer II: 10 m*M* HEPES, pH 7.4, 5 m*M* KCl, 10 m*M* $MgCl_2$, and 2.2 *M* sucrose. Autoclaved.
4. Buffer III: 10 m*M* HEPES, pH 7.4, 5 m*M* KCl, and 10 m*M* $MgCl_2$. Autoclaved.
5. Keller storage buffer: 10 m*M* Tris-HCl, pH 7.5, 5 m*M* $MgCl_2$, 0.5 *M* sorbitol, 2.5% Ficoll (400,000), 0.008% spermidine, 1 m*M* dithiothreitol, and 50% glycerol.
6. Hemocytometer.
7. 10-mL ultracentrifuge tubes. Autoclaved.
8. SORVALL refrigerated ultracentrifuge with swinging rotor (SORVALL Ltd., Stevenage, UK).

2.4.5. Nuclear Run-On

1. 2-mL screw-capped Eppendorf tubes. Autoclaved.
2. [α-^{32}P] uridine triphosphate (UTP) (specific activity 800 Ci/mmol; New England Nuclear, Boston, MA).
3. 1 *M* Tris-HCl, pH 8.3. Autoclaved.
4. 1 *M* NH_4Cl. Autoclaved.
5. 1 *M* $MgCl_2$. Autoclaved.
6. 10 m*M* adenosine triphosphate (ATP), CTP, and guanosine triphosphate (GTP) (Promega, UK).
7. Recombinant RNasin (Promega).
8. RNase-free DNase (Promega).
9. Extraction buffer: 10 m*M* Tris-HCl, pH 7.4, 15 m*M* EDTA, 3% SDS, 1 mg/mL proteinase K, and 3 mg/mL heparin.
10. Saturated phenol solution.
11. Phenol–chloroform (1:1) solution.
12. 5 *M* ammonium acetate. Autoclaved.
13. Benchtop microcentrifuge.

14. 75% ethanol.
15. Wash buffer A: 300 mM NaCl, 10 mM Tris-HCl, pH 7.4, 2 mM EDTA, and 0.1% SDS.
16. Wash buffer B: 10 mM NaCl, 10 mM Tris-HCl, pH 7.4, 2 mM EDTA, and 0.4% SDS.
17. Saran Wrap.
18. Cassettes, X-OMAT-S films (Kodak).

3. Methods

3.1. Radioligand Binding Assay

3.1.1. Preparation of Rat Lung Membranes

1. Grind frozen rat lung tissues under liquid nitrogen, with a prechilled mortar and pestle.
2. Resuspend the powder in approx 10 vol of ice-cold 0.32 M sucrose in 25 mM Tris-HCl, pH 7.4.
3. Homogenize with a Polytron homogenizer (Philip Harris Scientific, London, UK) at setting 6 for 30-s bursts.
4. Centrifuge the homogenate at 1000g for 10 min at 4°C, to remove debris.
5. Filter the supernatant through two layers of cheesecloth. Discard the pellet.
6. Centrifuge the supernatant at 40,000g for 20 min at 4°C. Discard the supernatant, and resuspend the pellet in a convenient volume of ice-cold wash buffer.
7. Repeat step 3 twice.
8. Centrifuge at 40,000g for 20 min at 4°C. Resuspend the final pellet in assay buffer to a concentration of approx 5–10 mg protein/mL. Freeze the final suspension in 1-mL aliquots at –70°C, until required.
9. On the day of the binding assay, thaw the frozen membranes, and dilute with assay buffer a few minutes before starting the binding assay, so that the membrane suspension just has time to come up to RT before pipeting (*see* **Note 1**).

3.1.2. Saturation Binding

This type of assay measures the equilibrium binding of a range of concentrations of the radioligand. It is necessary to determine the nonspecific binding of each concentration of radioligand by the inclusion of a saturating concentration of an unlabeled ligand (*see* **Note 2**). Specific binding can then be calculated as the difference between total and nonspecific binding.

1. Prepare appropriate dilutions of [^{125}I]ICYP (3–100 pM) (*see* **Notes 3** and **4**) in assay buffer. Each concentration is prepared in the absence (total binding) and presence of 0.1 μM ICI-118,551 (a selective β_2AR antagonist), 0.1 μM CGP-20712A (a selective β_1AR antagonist), or 200 μM (–)Iso to define β_1- and β_2AR binding and nonspecific binding, respectively (*see* **Note 5**), with each determination being performed in triplicate.
2. Pipet the assay components into glass tubes, as follows: 100 μL assay buffer, 25 μL drug or assay buffer, 25 μL [^{125}I]ICYP, and 100 μL membranes (*see* **Note 6**).
3. Following the addition of the membranes, mix each sample well, and incubate at 37°C for 2 h, for equilibrium to be achieved (*see* **Note 7**). Reserve leftover

membranes for protein determination, and dilutions of radioligand for counting (*see* **step 6**).

4. At the end of the incubation period, separate bound ligand from free ligand. In this case, filter the samples onto GF/C glass-fiber filters that have been presoaked in ice-cold wash buffer using a Brandel cell harvester, and rapidly rinse the filters with 3 × 5 mL ice-cold wash buffer (*see* **Note 8**).
5. Place the filters in 5-mL SARSTEDT tubes.
6. Prepare radioligand standards: Pipet 25 μL of each radioligand dilution into 5-mL plastic tubes. These provide an accurate estimate of the actual amount of radioligand added to each sample.
7. Count the samples and standards in an Auto Gamma Counting System (COBRA™ II, Packard Instrument, Pangbourne, UK) at an efficiency of 80%.

3.2. Northern Blot Analysis

Northern blot analysis identifies a full-length specific mRNA species, using radiolabeled probes that contain the complementary sequence to that of the mRNA. Total RNA or poly(A)$^+$ selected RNA is size-fractionated on an agarose gel and then transferred to a solid filter. The filter is then hybridized with the radiolabeled probe, and the specific RNA band is visualized by autoradiography.

3.2.1. RNA Isolation

1. For preparation of RNA from tissue: The tissue should be removed quickly from the animal and frozen immediately in liquid nitrogen (*see* **Note 9**).
2. Pulverize larger frozen tissue with a prechilled mortar and pestle, before homogenizing in 1 vol denaturing solution D with a Polytron.
3. Add 1/10 vol 2 *M* Na acetate, pH 4.0, to each sample, and mix.
4. Add 1 vol H_2O-saturated phenol to each sample, and mix.
5. Add 1/5 vol chloroform–isoamyl alcohol mixture to each sample, mix vigorously for 15 s, and leave on ice for 15 min.
6. Spin for 15 min at 12,000*g* at 4°C.
7. Take off aqueous (i.e., RNA) phase to a Corex tube. Add 1 vol ice-cold isopropanol, vortex, and either place on dry ice for 60 min or precipitate overnight at –20°C.
8. Spin for 20–30 min at 17,000*g* at 4°C.
9. Remove supernatant, and resuspend pellet in 75% ethanol.
10. Spin RNA for 15 min at 17,000*g* at 4°C.
11. Decant supernatant, freeze-dry the RNA pellet, and thoroughly resuspend in small volume of DEPC-treated water by repeat pipeting (*see* **Note 10**).
12. Carefully transfer RNA to microcentrifuge tube, and keep on ice.
13. Quantitate RNA at optical density 260 (OD_{260}) (OD_{260} 1 = 40 μg/mL) (*see* **Notes 11** and **12**).
14. Store RNA at –70°C.

15. If required, isolate poly(A)$^+$ RNA from total cellular RNA using PolyATtract mRNA Isolation System (Promega), according to the manufacturer's protocol.

3.2.2. Random Primer Labeling of DNA

1. DNA fragment to be random primed labeled must be gel purified. There are numerous kits to accomplish this. The JETsorb DNA Gel Extraction Kit (Genomed, UK) is recommended.
2. The DNA (50–100 ng) dissolved in distilled H_2O must be denatured at 100°C for 3–5 min, followed by quick-cooling on ice.
3. Other components are added to the tube to give a final volume of 25 or 50 µL, according to the manufacturer's protocol.
4. Add 3–5 µL [α-^{32}P]dCTP, and mix.
5. Add Klenow fragment (1 µL) to the tube.
6. Mix gently by pipeting up and down. Spin for a few seconds in a microcentrifuge.
7. Incubate reaction at 37°C for 45–60 min.
8. Stop reaction by addition of TE buffer.
9. Purify the probe from unincorporated radiolabel by Sephadex G-50 column, using TE buffer as the eluent.
10. Count an aliquot of the probe to determine the amount of incorporated radioactivity in a liquid scintillation counter.

3.2.3. RNA Formaldehyde Gel

1. Preparation of gel (*see* **Notes 13–15**): Microwave 1.0% agarose in 1X MOPS at medium setting, until the agarose is in solution. When the flask is cool enough to grasp, add a final concentration of 6.6% formaldehyde (27 mL of a 37% formaldehyde solution, to a total volume of 150 mL. In a fume hood, pour mixture into casting tray with combs, and allow to solidity (>45 min).
2. Aliquot RNA (containing 20 µg total RNA) into RNase-free microcentrifuge tubes, or resuspend lyophilized poly(A)$^+$ RNA pellets in 10 µL DEPC-H_2O.
3. Add 2 vol of gel-loading buffer and 1 µL 400 µg/mL ethidium bromide, heat to 65°C for 5 min, then chill on ice. Pulse-spin tubes in microcentrifuge.
4. Place gel in electrophoresis tank filled with 1X MOPS, and load the RNA samples into the gel wells (*see* **Note 16**).
5. Run the gel at 60–100 V (approx 100 mA), until the orange dye runs off the edge (*see* **Note 17**).
6. Place the gel onto Saran Wrap (*see* **Note 10**) and photograph on UV transilluminator, to visualize the ribosomal RNA (28S, 18S, which correspond to approx 5 and 2 kb, respectively. This will also demonstrate the quality of the RNA (i.e., if degradation has occurred).

3.2.4. Capillary Transfer of RNA to Solid Support

1. Cut nylon membrane and four Whatman 3MM filters the same size as the gel.
2. Set up gel capillary transfer apparatus (i.e., the sandwich box) as follows (*see* **Note 18**): Fill reservoir with 20X SSC; place wick (i.e., the sponge) on a platform

suspended above reservoir, and submerge both ends of the wick in reservoir; prewet four Whatman filter papers in 20X SSC, and place two of them on top of the wick; place gel on top of the Whatman filter papers, with the open side of the wells facing down; place nylon membrane on top of the gel; place another prewetted Whatman filter paper on top of the nylon membrane; add 8–10 absorbent filters (available from Sigma) and a stack of paper towels; place glass plate on top of transfer apparatus; on top of plate, place heavy objects, such as one 500-mL bottle, with 400 mL H_2O in it.
3. Transfer for approx 14–18 h.
4. Dismantle transfer apparatus, and view nylon membrane on transilluminator. With a pencil, mark the orientation of gel and location of ribosomal bands on the side of the nylon membrane.
5. UV crosslink the nylon membrane.
6. Store blot in Saran Wrap in the refrigerator at 4°C, or use immediately.

3.2.5. Hybridization

1. For hybridization in oven (*see* **Note 19**): Place blot in hybridization tube, and add 5–6 mL hybridization buffer. Place in preheated rotating oven.
2. Prehybridization: 4–6 h at 42°C for cDNA probes.
3. Denaturation of probe: Heat cDNA probes at 95–100°C for 5 min. It should immediately be quick-cooled on ice before use.
4. Hybridization: Add probes to hybridization buffer without additional buffer (*see* **Notes 20** and **21**). Hybridization reaction should proceed overnight.

3.2.6. Posthybridization Washes

1. If washes are in hybridization oven, then pour buffer out of the tube into radioactive sink. Add 4X SSC, 0.1% SDS, heated to hybridization temperature (*see* **Note 22**) to the tube, and place back in the rotating oven for 30 min.
2. Additional washes (*see* **Note 23**): The remaining washes are in increasingly stringent conditions (i.e., increasing temperature and reducing salt in the presence of 0.1% SDS) in the rotating oven. Wash hybridized blots in 2X SSC, 0.1% SDS at 50°C, 1X SSC, 0.1% SDS 50°C, 0.5X SSC, 0.1% SDS at 55°C, and 0.1X SSC, 0.1% SDS at 55°C for 30 min and check radioactivity remaining on blots after each wash, with a hand-held Geiger counter.
3. Cover blots with Saran Wrap and expose to film. After exposure, strip blot in 50% formamide, 10 m*M* NaH_2PO_4, pH 6.8, at 65°C for 30–60 min. Rinse blot in 2X SSC, 0.1% SDS at RT. Store blot in Saran Wrap for hybridization with additional probes.
4. The method of quantitation depends on the equipment available in the laboratory. Quantitate using the Protein and DNA Imageware systems by laser densitometry (Discovery Series, NY) and normalize the signal from the cDNA of interest with the control cDNA, such as glyceraldehyde-3-phosphate dehydrogenase (GAPDH).

3.3. Half-Life Studies

The half-life of mRNA in tissues can be determined by measuring the decay of the mRNA in the presence of a RNA synthesis inhibitor. The mRNA can be measured by Northern blot analysis (*see* **Fig. 4**).

1. Pretreat the human lung tissues with drug of interest (dexamethasone [Dex], in this case) for time period that shows maximum effect.
2. Add actinomycin D (10 μg/mL) to the treated tissues, as well as to control tissues, freeze at 1, 2, 3, 4, and 6 h after addition of the transcription inhibitor.
3. Perform Northern blot analysis (*see* **Subheading 3.2.**) on RNA isolated from these samples, as well as from control and drug-treated tissues not treated with actinomycin D.
4. Compare the rate of decay of the mRNA species of interest in control and drug-treated tissues (*see* **Note 24**).

3.4. Nuclear Run-On

The nuclear run-on assay gives a measure of the rate of gene transcription. Nuclei are isolated from tissues and then incubated with [α-^{32}P]UTP and unlabeled NTPs, in order to label nascent RNA transcripts. [α-^{32}P]-labeled RNA is then purified and specific RNA transcripts are detected by hybridization to cDNA that is immobilized on nylon membranes. The level of hybridization to the cDNA is a measure of the transcription rate. This technique provides important information on the regulation of transcription rate (*see* **Fig. 5**).

3.4.1. Preparation of Plasmid(s) Containing cDNA(s) of Interest

1. Isolate at least 100 μg of the plasmid(s) containing cDNA(s) of interest, using the Qiagen Midi-Prep kit.
2. Incubate plasmid at 37°C, with appropriate restriction enzymes to check the cDNA of interest from the vector.

3.4.2. Preparation of Plasmid DNA(s) Slot Blot

1. Dilute the plasmid DNA (20 μg) containing cDNA of interest to a final volume of 152 μL in a 1.5-mL Eppendorf tube.
2. Add 8 μL 2 *M* NaOH.
3. Heat for 5 min at 100°C.
4. Add 15 μL 3 *M* Na acetate, pH 5.2, and mix well.
5. Precipitate with 3 vol 100% ethanol.
6. Resuspend in 200 μL TE buffer, pH 7.4.
7. Heat for 5 min at 100°C, and place on ice.
8. Add 600 μL 20X SSC, and mix well.
9. Assemble a Bio-Rad Bio-Dot SF Microfiltration apparatus with four pieces of filter paper (prewetted with DEPC-treated H_2O), with one piece of nylon membrane on top (*see* **Note 25**).

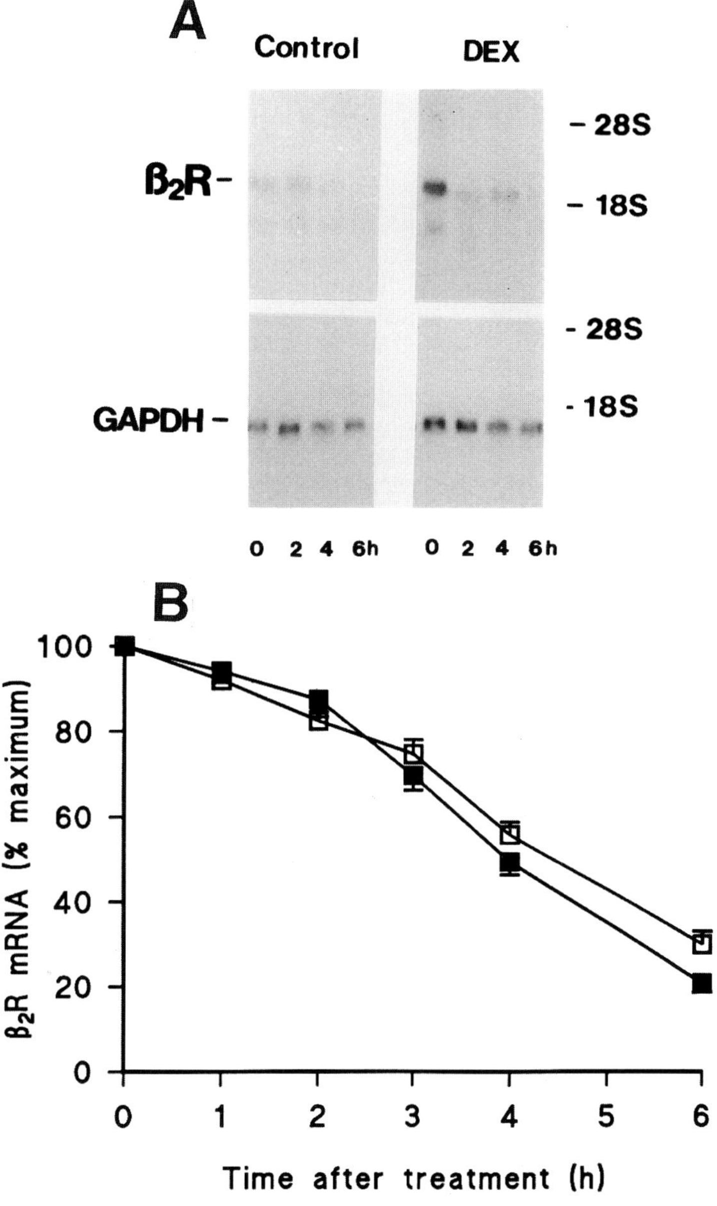

Fig. 4. Effect of dexamethasone (DEX) on stability of β_2AR mRNA in human lung in vitro. **(A)** Northern blot analysis. Actinomycin D, 10 μg/mL, was added at 0 min to lung tissues pretreated for 2 h with vehicle (control) or 10^{-6} *M* Dex. At indicated time-points, RNA was isolated as described. **(B)** densitometric measurements of half-life of β_2AR mRNA from four separate experiments. ■, control; □, Dex. Reprinted with permission from **ref. *6***.

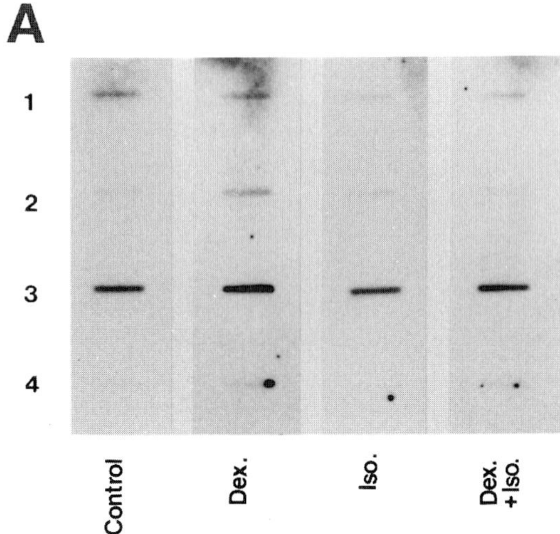

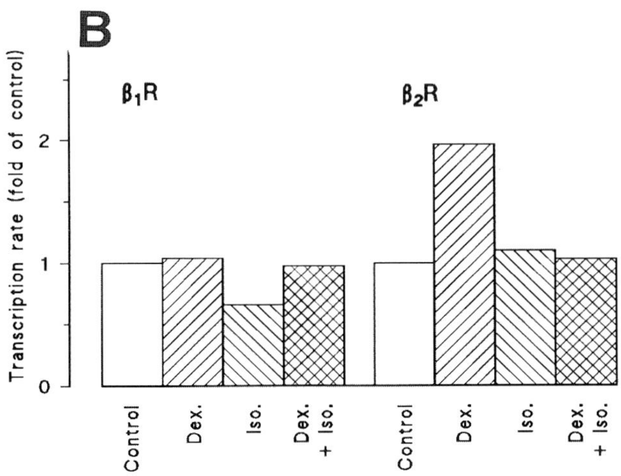

Fig. 5. Effects of treatment with Dex and/or Iso on the transcription rates of β_1- and β_2AR gene in rat lung. **(A)** Representative autoradiograms from nuclear run-on transcription assays on β_1AR and β_2AR genes in control, Dex-treated, Iso-treated, and Dex + Iso-treated rat lung. Labeled RNA isolated was hybridized either to plasmid (10 µg/slot) containing β_1AR cDNA *(1)*, β_2AR cDNA *(2)*, GAPDH cDNA *(3)*, or to the plasmid lacking the cDNA insert (pGEM-3Z; 4) as control. **(B)** Densitometric measurement of β_1AR and β_2AR transcription rates from control, Dex-treated, Iso-treated, and Dex + Iso-treated rat lungs. The transcription rate was calculated as the ratio of β_1AR and β_2AR cDNA signal relative to the GAPDH cDNA signal. Average values from two separate experiments are shown. Reprinted with permission from **ref. 5**.

10. Attach the apparatus to a vacuum, and apply 400 μL 15X SSC through each slot, to equilibrate.
11. Apply 400 μL plasmid DNA to each slot (*see* **Note 26**). It is necessary to use at least 10 μg of each plasmid DNA.
12. Wash the slots twice with 15X SSC.
13. Mark the locations of those slots containing DNA.
14. Remove the nylon membrane, and immediately UV-crosslink.
15. Cut the membrane into strips, each containing cDNA of interest and the control(s) cDNA. The blots are now ready for prehybridization.

3.4.3. Prehybridization of the DNA Slot Blots

1. Place each strip into a separate screw-capped hybridization tube, and add 5 mL prehybridization buffer.
2. Prehybridize at 42°C for at least 4 h in a rotating hybridization oven. The blots are now ready for hybridization with the newly transcribed RNA from **Subheading 3.4.5.**

3.4.4. Preparation of Nuclei for Nuclear Run-On

1. Pulverize frozen lung tissue in liquid nitrogen, with a mortar and pestle.
2. Homogenize tissue in buffer I (after addition of 5 m*M* 2-ME, 0.1% Triton X-100, 0.1 m*M* phenylmethylsulfony fluoride, and 20 U/mL RNasin) with a Polytron homogenizer for 30 s at setting 6.
3. Filter the homogenate through gauze filter.
4. Centrifuge at 2000*g* for 10 min.
5. Resuspend the pellet in buffer II (after addition of 5 m*M* 2-ME and 20 U/mL RNasin).
6. Centrifuge at 100,000*g* for 90 min.
7. Resuspend the nuclear pellet in a small volume of buffer III (after addition of 5 m*M* 2-ME and 2 U/mL RNasin).
8. Count the number of nuclei isolated, using a hemocytometer.
9. Recentrifuge the nuclei suspension at 9000*g* for 5 min in a microcentrifuge.
10. Resuspend the pellet in 100 μL Keller storage buffer to give ~5×10^7 nuclei (*see* **Note 27**); freeze in liquid nitrogen, and store at –80°C until needed.

3.4.5. Nuclear Run-On

1. Thaw the nuclei in a 2-mL Eppendorf tube (*see* **Note 28**); add 40 m*M* Tris-HCl (pH 8.3), 150 m*M* NH_4Cl, 7.5 m*M* $MgCl_2$, 0.625 m*M* ATP, 0.313 m*M* GTP, 0.313 mM CTP, 120 U/mL RNasin and RNase-free water, followed by 25 μL (250 μCi) of [α-^{32}P]UTP, to a final volume of 400 μL.
2. Incubate for 30 min at 27°C.
3. Add 1 μL RNasin (40 U/μL), followed by 75 μL RQ-1 RNase-free DNase (1 U/μL), and incubate for a further 15 min at 27°C.
4. Add 160 μL extraction buffer, and incubate for 3 h at 42°C, with occasional vortexing.

5. Add 210 μL TE, pH 7.4, followed by extraction with phenol (equal volume-to-reaction mixture), phenol–chloroform mixture, and chloroform, respectively.
6. After centrifugation at RT, carefully transfer the final aqueous layer to another new 2-mL Eppendorf tube.
7. Add 290 μL 5 *M* ammonium acetate and an equal volume of isopropanol.
8. Reprecipitate the pellet 3× with 3 vol of 100% ethanol in the presence of 1.33 *M* ammonium acetate.
9. After final centrifugation, remove the supernatant carefully, and wash with 75% ethanol.
10. Air-dry the pellet, and resuspend in 100 μL TE, pH 7.4.
11. Count 1 μL in triplicate from each sample.
12. Heat the samples to 95°C for 5 min, and place on ice.
13. Add an equal number of radioactive counts to each of the prehybridized blots from **Subheading 3.4.3.** (*see* **Note 29**).
14. Hybridize for 72 h at 42°C in a rotating hybridization oven.
15. Wash blots in wash buffer A or B at increasing temperatures (i.e., RT to 55°C), with a 30-min RNase A (1 μg/mL) and RNase T_1 (10 U/mL) treatment in buffer A at 37°C (*see* **Note 30**).
16. Cover the blots with Saran Wrap, and expose to film.
17. Quantitate using image analysis, and normalize the signal from the cDNA of interest with the control cDNA.

4. Notes

1. Cold membrane suspensions tend to clump together, making accurate pipeting difficult. The suspension will be more homogeneous if warmed to RT before pipeting. However, the membranes will deteriorate if kept at RT for too long.
2. In order to define nonspecific binding, it is best to use an unlabeled ligand that is different from the radioligand, and, ideally, one that is as structurally distinct as possible. This minimizes the risk of displaceable nonreceptor binding. The unlabeled ligand needs to be used at concentration sufficient to occupy all the available receptors, even when competing with the highest concentration of radioligand.
3. The choice of radioligand: high-affinity ligands are generally preferred; they can be used at lower concentrations, which tends to reduce the level of nonspecific binding, and they are less likely to dissociate from the receptor during the separation procedure. However, the level of nonspecific binding for different ligands in different tissues may vary enormously; the only way to find the most appropriate ligand may be by trial and error. Antagonist ligands, such as [^{125}I]ICYP, are generally preferred to agonists, partly because antagonists often exhibit higher affinity than agonists, and partly because the binding of agonists tends to be more sensitive to the assay conditions. If the radioligand is nonselective, such as [^{125}I]ICYP, it may be possible to suppress binding to unwanted receptors by including a saturating concentration of an unlabeled ligand that is highly selective for that receptor. In this case, CGP-20712A (a selective β_1AR antagonist) and ICI-118,551 (a selective β_2AR antagonist), are used to define β_1- and β_2AR binding, respectively.

4. The choice of radioligand concentrations in a saturation experiment depends partly on the separation method to be used, and partly on the question to be addressed. In this case, the different concentrations of [^{125}I]-ICYP (3–100 p*M*) have been chosen to span the expected affinity of [^{125}I]-ICYP: ~20 p*M*. If the affinity of the radioligand is unknown, it may be necessary to perform range-finding experiments, with fewer concentrations over a wider range.
5. Choice of assay buffer. Radioligand binding can usually be performed in very simple buffer systems. The choice depends on the preparation, and on the ligand. The precise conditions of the binding assay (temperature, ionic composition of buffers, and so on) can affect binding affinity; it is important to consider this when comparing data from different laboratories.
6. One of the largest sources of error in radioligand binding experiments is poor pipeting technique. It is important to add low concentrations of ligands before high ones, to ensure that all additions reach the bottom of the assay tube, and to mix everything thoroughly.
7. Sufficient time needs to be followed for equilibrium to be achieved.
8. The rapid removal of free ligand during filtration necessarily disrupts the equilibrium and promotes dissociation of ligand from the receptor. In all cases, filtering and rinsing the membranes as rapidly and reproducibly as possible, using ice-cold buffers throughout, should minimize the impact of dissociation.
9. In order not to overload, a maximum of 2 g lung tissue per 15 mL solution D. The tissue must be homogenized as quickly as possible, to avoid degradation of RNA.
10. The volume in which the final RNA pellet is resuspended depends on the amount of RNA expected. It is better to make concentrated samples, which can be diluted following quantitation, than to make samples that are too dilute to be useful. These latter samples would have to be lyophilized or reprecipitated.
11. A large quantity of RNA should be diluted into several aliquots, to avoid freeze–thawing unnecessarily.
12. To check the quality of the RNA, an $OD_{260/280}$ ratio of >1.7 is acceptable. Values of <1.7 may indicate protein contamination.
13. Wash flasks, gel casters, combs, and gel apparatus in DEPC-treated water, to ensure that they are RNase free prior to use.
14. If feasible, a gel apparatus and tank should be dedicated solely for RNA gels.
15. RNA sample amounts: The amount of RNA necessary for message detection is dependent on the relative abundance of the target mRNA. Rare messages may require the isolation of poly(A)$^+$ RNA, in order to detect a signal.
16. The outermost lanes on either side of the gel should not be used if at all possible. RNA in these lanes tend not to transfer as well.
17. Running the gel too fast may heat the agarose and distort the lanes of migrating RNA.
18. Prior to removing the gel from the tank, it is advisable to cut off a righthand corner of the gel for orientation purposes.
19. It is important to remove all air bubbles between layers of materials being added to the capillary transfer apparatus. Air bubbles will prevent even transfer of RNA to nylon membrane. A disposable 10-mL serological pipet works well to roll out the bubbles.

20. If using hybridization tubes, be sure that the blots are covered evenly by hybridization buffer. Check this during the prehybridization step.
21. The amount of labeled probe added to the hybridization buffer depends on the relative abundance of the target RNA. A good starting point is $0.5–1 \times 10^6$ cpm/mL buffer for abundant clones and 2×10^6 cpm/mL for rare messages.
22. Internal standards: Quantitation by Northern blot analysis may require the use of an internal standard to normalize results caused by uneven RNA loading or transfer. If the size of the internal standard transcript is different from the target RNA, it is more efficient to hybridize both probes at once. It is important to remember that often the level of RNA encoding the commonly used internal standards far exceeds the level of the target RNA.
23. It is important to preheat the wash buffers to temperature prior to addition to the blot. This will ensure that the appropriate wash conditions have been reached. The wash protocol outlined here is only a starting point. Additional or longer washes may be necessary.
24. Plot time (*x*-axis) against % of maximum for both control and drug-treated tissues. The half-life (50% of maximum) can be derived by extrapolating from the graph (*see* **Fig. 4**).
25. Handle the nylon membrane with blunt forceps and gloved hands.
26. It is a good idea to have an internal standard that can be used to normalize the results. This should be a gene that is ubiquitous, and which is unaffected by the experimental conditions under observation. GAPDH is commonly used. Vector without the insert of the cDNA of interest serves as a useful negative control.
27. The pellet can be hard to resuspend; however, it is necessary that the nuclear suspension is as homogeneous as possible in the nuclear run-on assay. Therefore, take time to resuspend the pellet well by flicking the tube, and pipeting the pellet up and down.
28. Use 2-mL Eppendorf tubes with screw caps and O-rings, to reduce radioactive contamination.
29. On average, add at least 1×10^6 cpm/mL radiolabeled RNA into each hybridization tube. The more radiolabeled RNA added, the better the hybridization.
30. Check the blots (using a Geiger counter) after several washes to prevent overwashing.

References

1. Bylund, D. B., Eikenberg, D. C., Hieble, J. P., Langer, S. Z., Lefkowitz, R. J., Minneman, K. P., et al. (1994) International union of pharmacology nomenclature of adrenoceptors. *Pharmacol. Rev.* **46,** 121–136.
2. Mak, J. C. W., Nishikawa, M., Haddad, E.-B., Kwon, O.-J., Hirst, S. J., Twort, C. H., and Barnes, P. J. (1996) Localization and expression of beta-adrenoceptor subtype mRNAs in human lung. *Eur. J. Pharmacol.* **302,** 215–221.
3. Barnes, P. J. (1995) β-adrenergic receptors and their regulation. *Am. J. Respir. Crit. Care Med.* **152,** 838–860.
4. Nishikawa, M., Mak, J. C. W., Shirasaki, H., and Barnes, P. J. (1993) Differential down-regulation of pulmonary β_1- and β_2-adrenoceptor messenger RNA with pro-

longed *in vivo* infusion of isoprenaline. *Eur. J. Pharmacol. (Mol. Pharmacol. Section)* **247,** 131–138.

5. Mak, J. C. W., Nishikawa, M., Shirasaki, H., Miyayasu, K., and Barnes, P. J. (1995) Protective effects of a glucocorticoid on down-regulation of pulmonary β_2-adrenergic receptor *in vivo*. *J. Clin. Invest.* **96,** 99–106.
6. Mak, J. C. W., Nishikawa, M., and Barnes, P. J. (1995) Glucocorticosteroids increase β_2-adrenergic receptor transcription in human lung. *Am. J. Physiol.* **268,** L41–L46.
7. Port, J. D., Huang, L.-Y., and Molbon, C. C. (1992) β-adrenergic agonists that down-regulate receptor mRNA up-regulate a Mr 35,000 protein(s) that selectively binds to β-adrenergic receptor mRNAs. *J. Biol. Chem.* **267,** 24103–24108.
8. Pende, A., Tremmel, K. D., DeMaria, C. T., Blaxall, B. C., Minobe, W. A., Sherman, J. A., et al. (1996) Regulation of the mRNA-binding protein AUF1 by activation of the β-adrenergic receptor signal transduction pathway. *J. Biol. Chem.* **271,** 8493–8501.
9. Tholanikunnel, B. G. and Malbon, C. C. (1997) 20-nucleotide (A + U)-rich element of β_2-adrenergic receptor (β_2AR) mRNA mediates binding to β_2AR-binding protein and is obligate for agonist-induced destabilization of receptor mRNA. *J. Biol. Chem.* **272,** 11,471–11,478.
10. Danner, S., Frank, M., and Lohse, M. (1998) Agonist regulation of human β_2-adrenergic receptor mRNA stability occurs via a specific AU-rich element. *J. Biol. Chem.* **273,** 3223–3229.
11. Collins, S., Altschmied, J., Herbsman, O., Caron, M. G., Mellon, P. L., and Lefkowitz, R. J. (1990) cAMP element in the β_2-adrenergic receptor gene confers autoregulation by cAMP. *J. Biol. Chem.* **265,** 19,330–19,335.
12. Chomczynski, P. and Sacchi, N. (1987) Single-step method of RNA isolation by acid guanidinium thiocyanate-phenol-chloroform extraction. *Anal. Biochem.* **162,** 156–159.
13. Feinberg, A. P. and Vogelstein, B. (1983) A technique for radiolabeling DNA restriction endonuclease fragments to high specific activity. *Anal. Biochem.* **132,** 6–13.
14. Rodgers, J. R., Johnson, M. L., and Rosen, J. M. (1985) Measurement of mRNA concentration and mRNA half-life as a function of hormonal treatment. *Methods Enzymol.* **109,** 572–592.

21

Chemical Mutational Analysis of Human Glucocorticoid Receptor in Bronchial Asthma

Stephen J. Lane and Tak H. Lee

1. Introduction

This chapter describes a chemical method for mutational analysis of the human glucocorticoid receptor (hGR) cDNA. Corticosteroid-resistant (CR) asthma is associated with in vitro and in vivo defects in mononuclear cell function *(1)*. In addition, molecular studies using these cells have revealed that there is reduced binding of the hGR to its DNA recognition site, the glucocorticoid response element, compared to corticosteroid-sensitive (CS) controls *(2)*. The authors therefore postulated that a point mutation of the primary structure of the GR was responsible for this functional defect, necessitating a method that would be sensitive enough to detect single-base-pair (bp) mismatches.

Chemical mutational analysis (CMA) has advantages beyond other techniques that are currently being actively used for screening of mutations, in that its sensitivity approaches 100%, and it allows screening of long stretches of DNA without the need for specialized apparatus *(3)*. Its chief disadvantage is the number of steps involved. It compares very favorably with single-strand conformation polymorphism, which, although a relatively uncomplicated procedure, allows screening of only short lengths of DNA and at only 80–90% detection rate *(4)*. G-C-clamped denaturing gradient gel electrophoresis has a similar sensitivity to CMA, but allows screening only of short sequences of DNA, and requires specialized apparatus *(5)*. RNase protection is limited, because its sensitivity is only about 70% *(6)*.

CMA is now currently widely applied in screening for mutations in inherited diseases and in cancer *(7–10)*. In this method, overlapping fragments of the entire coding region of the wild-type hGR cDNA were amplified by the

From: *Methods in Molecular Medicine, vol. 44: Asthma: Mechanisms and Protocols*
Edited by: K. F. Chung and I. Adcock © Humana Press Inc., Totowa, NJ

polymerase chain reaction (PCR) (DNA Thermal Cycler 180, Perkin-Elmer, Norwalk, CT), radioactively labeled and hybridized to corresponding fragments of unlabeled patient hGR cDNA fragments derived from monocytes from six CS and six CR asthmatic subjects by reverse transcription-PCR (RT-PCR) ***(11)***. The heteroduplex hybrids were chemically modified in order to render them susceptible to cleavage by piperidine at sites of non-Watson-Crick bp mismatches. The regions containing sites of mutations are detectable by autoradiography, and so can direct sequencing to these areas, obviating the need for sequencing the entire cDNA of interest. In order to control for the sensitivity of the technique, a single-bp mismatch was generated by site-directed mutagenesis, by elimination of a unique restriction enzyme site ***(12)***. A second known single-bp mismatch was donated from a patient with familial cortisol resistance ***(13)***.

2. Materials

All reagents not indicated in the text are from Sigma, St. Louis, MO. All H_2O used in these experiments was distilled and deionized.

1. Solution D (stock): 250 g guanidinium thiocyanate (Fluka, Glossop, Derbyshire, UK), 293 mL H_2O, 17.6 mL 0.75 *M* Na citrate, pH 7.0, 26.4 mL 10% sarcosyl. Heat to 65°C, and store for up to 3 mo.
2. 2 *M* Na acetate, pH 4.0. Store at 4°C.
3. Chloroform–isoamyl alcohol: 49:1 v:v. Store at 4°C.
4. Agarose sample buffer: 50% sucrose; 0.1 *M* ethylenediamine tetra-acetic acid (EDTA), pH 8.0; 0.025% Orange G.
5. 10X Glycine gel running buffer: 150 g glycine, 40 mL 0.5 *M* EDTA, 6 g NAOH. Make to 1 L with H_2O.
6. Denaturing sample buffer: Deionized formamide made 0.025% final concentration with bromophenol blue.
7. 10X RT-PCR buffer: 500 m*M* Tris-HCl, pH 8.0, 500 m*M* KCl, 50 m*M* dithiotreitol (DTT).
8. 4 *M* hydroxylamine hydrochloride: 4 *M* hydroxylamine hydrochloride (Aldrich, Gillingham, Dorset, UK) was titrated to pH 6.0 by addition of approx 0.3 vol of diethylamine (Aldrich). This solution must be made up fresh.
9. Osmium (Os) tetroxide: 2% Os tetroxide (Aldrich) in H_2O. This can be stored at 4°C.
10. Denaturing 6% polyacrylamide 8 *M* urea gel: 68 g urea; 24 mL acrylamide:*bis*-acrylamide mix 40% (w/v) (Northumbria Biologicals, Northumbria, UK); 16 mL 10X Tris-borate EDTA (TBE); 78.8 mL distilled deionized H_2O; 1 mL 10% ammonium persulfate; 200 µL *N',N',N',N'*-tetramethylethylenediamine.
11. 10X TBE, pH 8.3: 128 g Tris-base, 55 g boric acid, 40 mL 0.5 *M* EDTA, pH 8.0.

3. Methods

3.1. Subjects (2)

Monocytes were obtained from six CS and six CR asthmatic subjects. The two groups were matched in terms of age, gender, atopic status, cigarette smoking history, and baseline predicted forced expiratory volume (FEV). Both groups demonstrated a greater than 30% improvement in FEV, either spontaneously or after 400 µg of inhaled salbutamol via a metered-dose inhaler. The CR group demonstrated an improvement of only 3 ± 0.9% (mean ± SEM) after a 14-d course of 40 mg prednisolone, in contrast to the CS group, which demonstrated an improvement of 36 ± 2% (mean ± SEM) after a similar course of treatment (p = <0.0001).

3.2. Cell Separation

1. Monocytes were separated from heparinized venous blood by density centrifugation over Lymphoprep (Nycomed AS, Oslo, Norway) at 4°C, 800*g* for 20 min *(14)*.
2. Wash monocytes 3× in Hank's balanced salt solution without calcium or magnesium (Flow Laboratories, Irvine, Scotland).
3. Suspend at a concentration of 2 million/mL in Eagle's minimal essential medium (MEM), with Earle's salts and 2 m*M* glutamine (Gibco, Paisley, Scotland) supplemented with 25 m*M* HEPES and 0.1% bovine serum albumin (BSA) supplemented MEM (Sigma).
4. Add 2-mL aliquots of the cell suspension to 60-mm plastic plates (Cell Cult, Sterilin, Feitham, UK).
5. Incubate the plates in a humidified atmosphere of 5% CO_2 at 37°C for 60 min.
6. Nonadherent cells are aspirated off, and the plates washed twice with supplemented MEM without BSA.
7. After a 2-h incubation period, total RNA was immediately extracted from the adherent cells.

3.3. Preparation of Patient cDNA

3.3.1. Isolation of Patient RNA

RNA was extracted from monocytes using a modification of the acid-guanidinium-thiocyanate-phenol-chloroform method *(15)*.

1. 1 mL working solution D (stock solution D + 0.36 mL 2-mercaptoethanol (ME)/ 50 mL) was added to each 60-mm plastic Petri dish containing adhered monocytes from six CS and six CR asthmatic subjects.
2. Lysed cells were dislodged with a cell scraper and placed into a glass homogenizer.
3. 5 µL of *Escherichia coli* transfer RNA (tRNA) (Sigma) (1 µg/µL) was added as a carrier.

4. After homogenization add 1/10 vol Na acetate, pH 4.0; 1 vol water-saturated phenol, pH 3.7–4.5 (Gibco-BRL, Uxbridge, Middlesex, UK); 1/5 vol chloroform–isoamyl alcohol (24:1 v:v ratio).
5. Mix gently between each step.
6. Transfer samples to two 1.5 mL Eppendorf screw-top tubes.
7. Allow to cool for 20 min on ice, and centrifuged at 14,000*g* for 15 min at 4°C.
8. The upper aqueous phase containing the RNA is transferred to a 4-mL Sarstedt tube, and 1 mL isopropranol (BDH, Dagenham, Essex, UK) per original 1 mL solution D is added.
9. Precipitate at –20°C for 4–15 h.
10. Centrifuge at 14,000*g* for 15 min at 4°C to pellet the precipitated RNA.
11. The supernatant is decanted and the pellet dissolved in 300 µL solution D.
12. A second precipitation is performed by the addition of 30 µL 3 *M* Na acetate, pH 5.2 and 1 mL 100% ethanol, overnight at –20°C.
13. Centrifuge at 14,000*g* for 15 min at 4°C to pellet the precipitated RNA.
14. In order to remove any excess salt, the pellet is washed 4–5× with 70% ethanol, and allowed to dry at room temperature, after which it is dissolved in 24 µL of 5 m*M* 2-ME β-ME with 35 U RNase inhibitor (RNA guard, Pharmacia, Milton Keynes, UK).
15. The pellet is stored at –20°C, if not used immediately.
16. For quantification of total RNA 1 µL was added to 1 mL distilled, deionized H_2O, and the optical density at 260 n*M* is multiplied by 35 to give the amount of total RNA in µg.
17. The 5 µg tRNA added as carrier was then subtracted to give a working yield.
18. 1 µg was then added to 5 µL agarose sample buffer, in order to examine the integrity of the 28S and 18S human ribosomal band patterns on a 1% agarose gel in glycine buffer.
19. If the RNA appeared of good quality and was not degraded, it was immediately used for RT-PCR.

3.3.2. Reverse Transcription

Single-stranded cDNA is synthesized from mRNA by a specifically primed reverse transcription reaction using avian myeloblastosis virus-reverse transcriptase (AMV-RT) (Pharmacia).

1. 4 µg total RNA were reverse transcribed in the presence of 1X RT-PCR buffer and 1.125 m*M* each deoxynucleoside triphosphate (DNTP), 1.25 m*M* of a specific antisense primer (primers 4–6) (**Table 1**), 5 m*M* $MgCl_2$, 5 m*M* DTT, 25 ng BSA, and 17.5 U RNase inhibitor.
2. A mix containing total RNA, primers, and reverse transcriptase buffer was heated to 60°C for 5 min and allowed to cool to 42°C.
3. The AMV-RT was added for 30 min at 42°C, and the temperature adjusted to 50°C for a further 1 h.

3.3.3. Polymerase Chain Reaction

1. A 10 µL aliquot of reverse transcription products was used for first-round outer PCR in a reaction mixture.

Table 1
Sequence Data of Synthetic Oligonucleotide Primers Used for Overlapping PCR Amplification and for Site Directed Mutagenesis

Primer	Sequence	hGR cDNA site	Sense/ antisense
1.	GGC TCC TCT GCC AGA GTT GAT ATT CAC	114–130	Sense
2.	ATT TTG CAG GAT TTG GAG TTT TCT GG	709–737	Sense
3.	CTT CAG GCT GGA ATG AAC CTG GAA GCT CG	1576–1604	Sense
4.	CTT GGG GCA GTG TTA CAT TAC TGG GG	958–933	Antisense
5.	ACC TCC AAC AGT GAC ACC AGG GTA G	1745–1721	Antisense
6.	GCC CTC TAT AAA CCA CAT GTA GTG CG	2618–2559	Antisense
7.	TGA TGG ACT CCA AAG AAT CAT TAA CTC CTGG	131–161	Sense
8.	CAG GTA AAG AGA CGA ATG AGA GTC CTT G	742–770	Sense
9.	ACA GGA GTC TCA CAA GAA ACC TCT G	1645–1669	Sense
10.	CCA TTA TCC TTA ATT TTG GGT TTA GTG TCCG	914–884	Antisense
11.	GTG AGT TGT GGT AAC GTT GCA GGA AC	1718–1692	Antisense
12.	AAA CCT CTA CAG GAC AAA CTG ATA G	2551–2526	Antisense
13.	CGG GTA CC**G** **A**<u>**T**</u>**C** **T**CG AAT TCC GGT C	*Sac*I site MCS selection	Mutagenic
14.	ATG AGA GTC CTT <u>**A**</u>GA GAT CAG AC	758–780	

Oligonucleotide primers 1–12 were used in PCR amplification of overlapping segments of the hGR CDNA. Primer pairs 1 and 4 flank outer fragment A (844 bp); 2 and 5 flank outer fragment B (1036 bp); 3 and 6 flank outer segment C (1042 bp). Primer pairs 7 and 10 flank inner fragment A (784 bp); 8 and 11 flank inner fragment B (976 bp); 9 and 12 flank inner segment C (906 bp). The outer primer pairs are used for first-round PCR and the product serves as template for second-round nested PCR. The inner primer pairs are used for nested second-round PCR. Primers 13 and 14 were used as selection and mutagenic primers, respectively for site-directed mutagenesis. MCS, multiple cloning site on pGEM-3.

*All primers were synthesized by British Biotechnology, Abingdon, Oxon, UK, and were purified by high-pressure liquid chromatography.

2. This contained 1X RT-PCR buffer and a final concentration of 2 m*M* $MgCl_2$, 1.25 μ*M* of each dNTP, 0.5 U Perfect Match polymerase enhancer (Strategene, La Jolla, CA), 1.25 μ*M* outer sense primers (1–3) (**Table 1**), and 1 μ*M* outer antisense primers (4–6) (**Table 1**; *see* **Note 1**) and 2 U *Taq* DNA polymerase.
3. 10–20 cycles of PCR amplification were carried out under the following conditions: 90 s denaturation at 95°C; 120 s annealing at 60°C (10 min for the first four cycles), and 120 s primer extension at 72°C.
4. The initial denaturation period was 90 s, and the final extension time was 10 min.
5. A 2-μL aliquot of this reaction was added to a second round nested PCR mixture containing the above mixture and 1.25 μ*M* each of corresponding inner primers 7–12 (**Table 1**). Twenty cycles of PCR were carried out as above (*see* **Note 2**).
6. The amplified fragments were quantitated and dissolved at a final concentration of 2×10^{-13} mol/μL for use as patient substrate cDNA in subsequent CMA.

*3.4.1. Labeling of Primers for Nested PCR (*see ***Note 3****)*

200 ng (20 pmol) of each inner oligonucleotide primer (primers 7–12) (**Table 1**) were labeled using T4 polynucleotide kinase (PNK) (Promega, Madison, WI).

1. Add together 200 ng (20 pmol) primer with 50 μCi (10 pmol) [^{32}P] γ-adenosine triphosphate (ATP) (specific activity ≥5000 Ci/mmol; Amersham, Bucks, UK), 10 U T4 PNK in 20 μL 1X kinase buffer.
2. Incubate for 1 h at 37°C.
3. Inactivate the enzyme by incubation at 80°C for 15 min.
4. Make up the reaction mix to 200 μL with H_2O.
5. A chloroform extraction was then performed.
6. Primers were precipitated by adding 1/2 vol of 7.5 *M* ammonium acetate and 1 mL 100% ethanol on dry ice for 1–2 h.
7. Centrifuge at 4°C for 30 min.
8. Wash twice in 70% ethanol.
9. Dry under vacuum for 2 h.
10. Dissolve the labeled primers in water at a concentration of 0.5 μ*M* for use in subsequent annealing and PCR reactions (*see* **Note 4**).

3.4.2. Calculation of [^{32}P] Incorporation into Primers

1. 1 μL of the 200 μL reaction mix is diluted 1:10 in H_2O.
2. 2-μL aliquots of this mix applied to DE81 filter paper disks (Whatman, Maidstone, UK).
3. Unincorporated radioactivity is eluted with two washes with 0.5 *M* Na phosphate, pH 6.8, for two 5-min periods.
4. Filters were dried in a hybridization oven at 50°C for 30 min.

5. Add dried filters to 4 mL scintillation cocktail for β-spectrophotometry.
6. Incorporation of phosphate was calculated from the counts of radioactivity remaining on the filter disks as a percent of the total counts added.
7. The remainder of the reaction mix was extracted in an equal volume of phenol–chloroform.

*3.4.3. Generation of Labeled Probe Fragments (see **Note 5**)*

1. 1×10^9 copies of wild-type linearized hGR/pGEM-3/*Sac*I were used as substrate in the PCR.
2. PCR amplification was carried out under the following conditions: 90 s denaturation at 95°C, 120 s annealing at 60°C, 120 s extension at 72°C.
3. The reaction mixture contained RT-PCR buffer under the following optimal conditions: 2 m*M* $MgCl_2$, 125 μ*M* each of dNTP and 200 ng (20 pmol) each of labeled primer combinations encoding the inner fragments A, B, and C (**Table 1**), DNA substrate, and 2 U *Taq* polymerase in a final volume of 200 μL.
4. This is then divided into 5 × 40-μL aliquots for 20 cycles of PCR amplification.
5. An aliquot is resolved by denaturing polyacrylamide gel electrophoresis (PAGE), in order to estimate conversion to full-length fragment.
6. Total efficiency of conversion is calculated as the product of percentage incorporation × percentage conversion to full-length fragment × decay factor. The efficiency of conversion from primer to full-length fragment is between 50 and 90%.
7. The reaction mix is phenol–chloroform-extracted, Na-acetate-precipitated (*see above*), and an aliquot is diluted to 2×10^{-14} mol/μL for use as probe in subsequent CMA.

3.5. Chemical Mutational Analysis (see Note 6)

*3.5.1. Generation and Amplification of Mutated cDNA Fragments (see **Note 7**)*

In order to control for the sensitivity of mutational analysis, the authors generated an hydroxylamine-reactive A to G mutation at position 770 of the hGR cDNA, using site-directed mutagenesis, by elimination of a unique restriction enzyme site (in this case, *Sac*I) employing the Transformer Site-Directed Mutagenesis Kit (Clontech, Palo Alto, CA) ***(12)***. The manufacturer's instructions were carried out exactly as instructed (*see* **Note 8**).

An Os-reactive T to A mutation at position 2054 of the hGR cDNA from a patient with familial glucocorticoid resistance was kindly donated by Dr. George Chrousos, National Institutes of Health, Bethesda, MD (Mut_{2054}) ***(13)***. This substitution converts an aspartic acid residue for a valine at amino acid residue 641 (*see* **Fig. 1**).

Both mutants were linearized with the unique cutter *Kpn*I (Northumbria Biologicals).

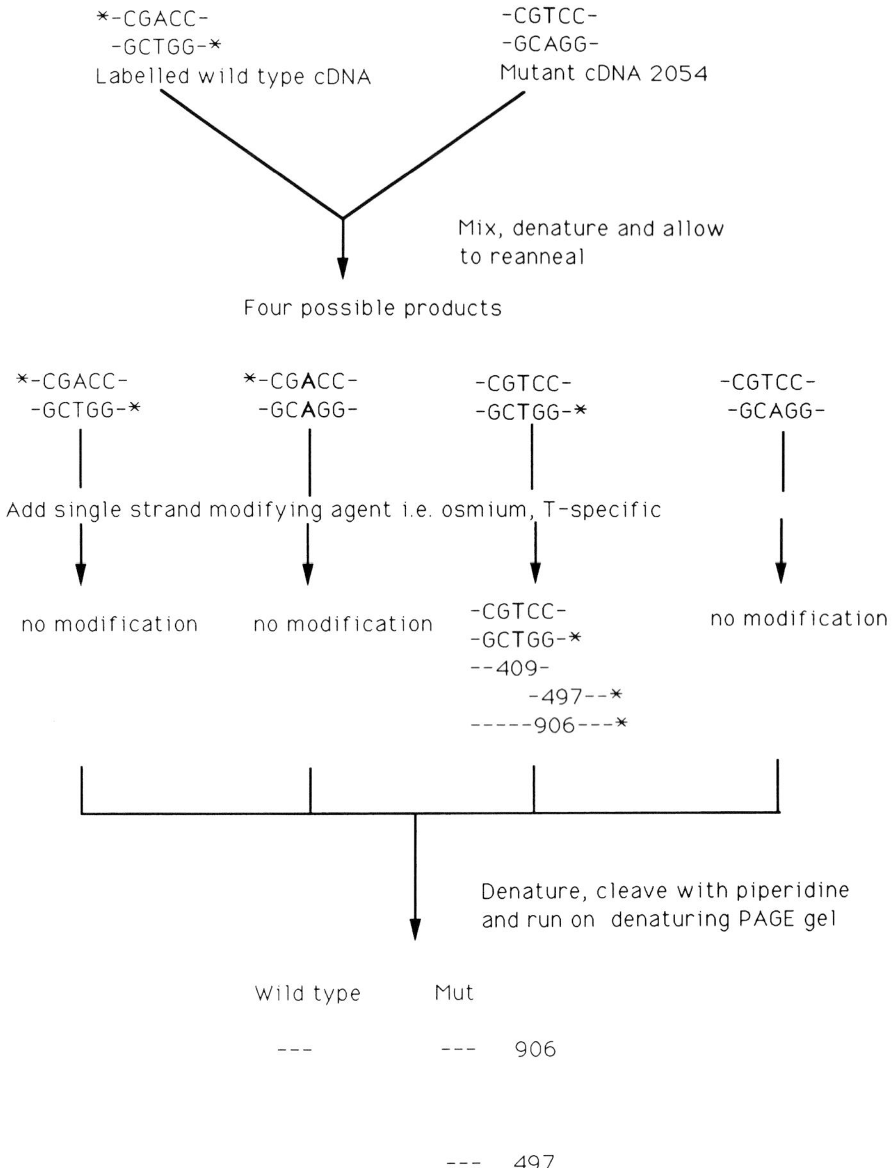

Fig. 1. Strategy for CMA; mutant C. Schematic representation of strategy for CMA of hGR cDNA, C mutant fragment, osmium-specific. The sequence shown is for A to T mutation at position 2054 of the C fragment (residues shown are 2052–2056). Asterisks denote the position of [γ-^{32}P]-ATP at the termini of end-labeled probe stands. The expected sizes of the products of heteroduplex cleaved by Os are shown below by the dotted lines: Only the uncleaved 906 bp and cleaved 497 bp bands are visualized, because the 409 bp is not radioactively labeled.

1. 500 pg cDNA were diluted into 10 μL H_2O containing 1 μL 10X buffer and 10 U enzyme.
2. The reaction mix was incubated for 60 min at 37°C.
3. The reaction was stopped by incubation at 60°C for 15 min.
4. 1×10^7 copies (approx 60 pg) used for second-round nested PCR.
5. The conditions used were the same as above, with 1.25 μ*M* inner sense primers 7/10(A) for Mut_{770} and 1.25 μ*M* 9/12(C) for Mut_{2054} (**Table 1**).
6. 20–24 cycles of PCR amplification were carried out under the above conditions, and the amplified fragments diluted to 2×10^{-13} mol/μL for use as mutant control substrate cDNA in subsequent CMA.

3.5.2. Heterodruplex Formation (see **Note 9**)

1. In order to minimize the formation of probe homoduplexes, hybridizations between labeled probe and corresponding target fragments are set up, in which the target (patients') cDNA is present in 10-fold molar excess more than probe cDNA.
2. 10 ng (1 μL 2×10^{-14} mol/μL) of [^{32}P]-labeled double-stranded cDNA probe fragments were added to 100 ng (1 μL 2×10^{-13} mol/μL) of corresponding patient or mutated cDNA fragment in 0.3 *M* NaCl, 0.1 *M* Tris-HCl, pH 8.0, in a final reaction volume of 10 μL.
3. Denature at 100°C for 5 min.
4. Incubate at 65°C for 10–16 h in 1.5-mL siliconized polypropylene tubes.
5. After hybridization, ethanol-precipitate the samples, with 80 μg mussel glycogen as a carrier (Boehringer-Mannheim UK, Lewes, UK), and resuspended in 14 μL 10 m*M* Tris-HCl, pH 8.0, 0.1 m*M* EDTA for subsequent chemical modification.

3.5.3. Hydroxylamine Modification

Incubate heteroduplex cDNA in 7 μL with 20 μL hydroxylamine solution (2.3 *M* final concentration) at 37°C for 2 h.

3.5.4. Osmium Modification

Incubate heteroduplex cDNA in 7 μL with a premix containing 5 m*M* Tris-HCl pH 8.0, 0.5 m*M* EDTA, 3% pyridine, and 2 μL of 2% Os tetroxide in a total volume of 25 μL at 37°C for 2 h.

3.5.5. Piperidine Cleavage

Hydroxylamine at pH 6.0 modifies the C5=C6 double bond in cytosine which then permits the ring to rearrange internally, and for cleavage to occur. Os tetroxide modification is a thymidine-specific reaction, in which the C5=C6 double bond is oxidized. Double-stranded DNA is attacked very slowly, and single-stranded regions are readily modified. At the mismatch site, the secondary structure of DNA is disrupted, which renders the corresponding bases susceptible to rapid chemical modification and sensitive to subsequent piperidine cleavage.

1. After modification, the heteroduplexes were ethanol-precipitated by addition of 1/10 vol 3 *M* Na acetate, pH 5.2, and 3 vol ethanol (–20°C).

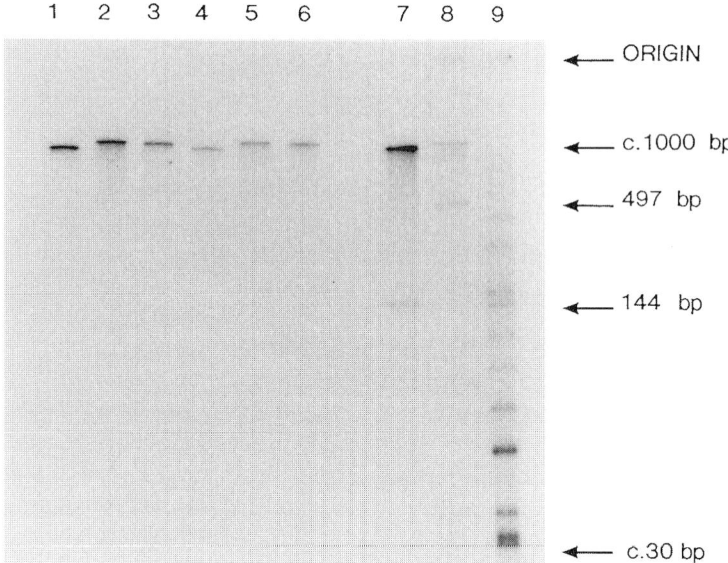

Fig. 2. CMA; CR asthma. Screening for mutations in CS sensitive asthma. A representative 6% denaturing PAGE gel of hydroxylamine and Os modification and subsequent piperidine cleavage of fragments A, B, and C generated from CR asthmatic subject. Patient cDNA was in 10-fold excess to labeled probe DNA. Lanes 1–3 represent fragments A, B, and C modified by hydroxylamine; lanes 4–6 represent fragments A, B, and C modified by Os; lane 7 is Mut A 770 modified by hydroxylamine; lane 8 is Mut C 2054 modified by Os; lane 9 is 5 ng of the labeled DNA mol wt marker *Hin*fI digest of Φ174. 12-h exposure at room temperature.

2. The pellet was washed 4× in 70% ethanol.
3. The pellet was resuspended in 50 µL of a fresh 1 *M* solution of piperidine (Aldrich) by vortexing for 30–60 s.
4. The mix was then incubated at 90°C for 30 min in a heating block.
5. Samples were ethanol precipitated (as above) and dissolved in deionized formamide (10 µL).
6. The samples were subsequently separated by electrophoresis on denaturing 6% polyacrylamide gels (*see* **Note 10**).
7. Gels were exposed from 4 to 20 h at –70°C using X-OMAT AR film (Sigma, Poole, UK).

The ability of the method to detect single base substitutions led to a search for new mutations in the hGR of six CS and six CR asthmatic subjects, employing this technique. Mismatch detection was carried out on the overlapping hGR cDNA fragments A, B, and C generated from six CS and six CR asthmatic subjects. **Figure 2** is representative of the CR group. In each experiment, the control mismatches were detected by hydroxylamine and Os tetroxide, but, no mismatch was detected in each of the six CS and six CR subjects studied. These results were confirmed by sequence analysis of the amplified products (*see* **Note 11**). Therefore, glucocorticoid resistance in chronic bronchial asthma cannot be explained on the basis of a consistent polymorphism within the hGR. This result indicates that the functional domains of the hGR are similar between the CS and the CR subjects, and that mismatches in these areas do not underlie glucocorticoid resistance in chronic bronchial asthma.

4. Notes

1. In combinations, A = primers 1 and 4, B = primer pairs 2 and 5, and C = primer pairs 3 and 6 (**Table 1**).
2. After 10–20 cycles of PCR amplification at optimal conditions, a background smear was obtained: 2 µL of this mix was then used as a substrate for second-round nested PCR. This produced sharp bands with very little background corresponding to overlapping fragments A, B, and C of the hGR, i.e., 784, 976, and 906 bp, respectively. The fragments were precipitated, washed, dissolved in 10 µL H_2O, and gel-quantitated. The range of concentrations obtained was 50–180 ng/µL. An aliquot was diluted to 2×10^{-13} mol/µL for use as patient substrate in subsequent hybridization reactions.
3. In this technique, wild-type cDNA is used as the reference template, against which corresponding patient cDNA is compared. In order to generate sufficient yields of hGR cDNA fragment substrate for CMA, it was necessary to perform nested PCR, using a second set of internal primers. Despite optimizing the annealing temperatures and Mg concentrations for each of the outer primers, it was not possible to generate sufficient cDNA to examine without decreasing the signal-to-noise ratio, so that the results could not clearly be interpreted. Because *Taq* polymerase can introduce mutations at a rate that is proportional to the number of cycles of amplification, it was critical to keep this number to a minimum. By using a second set of primers that lay directly internal to their corresponding counterparts, and, as template for this reaction, the products of the first round of PCR, 1–2 pg of each individual overlapping cDNA fragment was reproducibly obtained with little or no background interference.
4. A 1-µL aliquot was dissolved in 9 µL of denaturing sample buffer and a 2.5-µL aliquot denatured 95°C for 5 min and resolved by 8-*M* urea denaturing 6% PAGE, in order to examine the efficiency of conversion to full-length fragment. The incorporation range achieved was 12–44%. Primer 10 consistently demonstrated poor labeling, but this did not prove to be a problem in subsequent PCR amplification.
5. In the initial experiments, the wild-type cDNA overlapping fragments were amplified and radioactively labeled for use as probe in subsequent hybridization with corresponding patient fragments. By radioactively labeling a much smaller amount of primers (20 pmol vs 1.25 µ*M*), and using them for PCR amplification of wild-type fragments, the overall level of incorporation into the probe frag-

ments was more efficient. In order to increase the efficiency of the reaction, it was necessary to optimize the [Mg^{2+}] and annealing temperatures for each primer. The annealing temperature for each labeled primer was optimized by utilizing each primer in a linear elongation reaction at different temperatures for 30 min for one cycle. These experiments indicated that the optimal annealing temperature for each primer was 60°C and the optimum [Mg^{2+}] 2 m*M*. These experiments markedly increased the efficiency of the PCR, allowing generation of full-length labeled cDNA probes in large quantities for subsequent hybridization experiments.

6. The CMA method was developed out of the need for a screening method that detects 100% of mutations, so that direct sequencing of large stretches of DNA could be avoided. It is critical that any method of mutational analysis be sufficiently sensitive. The method is based on the fact that mismatched cytosine and thymidine bases are much more reactive to hydroxylamine and Os tetroxide, respectively, than Watson-Crick paired cytosine and thymidine. Hydroxylamine at pH 6.0 modifies the C5=C6 double bond in cytosine, which then labilizes the ring to internal rearrangement and cleavage. Os tetroxide modification is a thymidine-specific reaction, in which the C5=C6 double bond is oxidized. Double-stranded DNA is attacked very slowly, and single-stranded regions are readily modified. At the mismatch site, the secondary structure of DNA is disrupted, and it becomes single-stranded. This renders DNA susceptible to rapid modification and subsequent piperidine cleavage. The products are resolved by denaturing PAGE, and are detected by autoradiography. It is therefore critical to control for both hydroxylamine and Os modification, in order to be confident in the ability of the technique to detect single-bp mismatches.
7. This substitution converts a tryptophan residue to an amber stop codon at amino acid residue 212 (Mut_{770}). Briefly, the selection primer (no. 13 in **Table 1**) contains a T to G substitution at position 58 in the multiple cloning site of the plasmid pGEM-3, which renders *Sac*I, a unique cutter, unable to linearize the vector and hGR insert. The mutagenic primer 14 contains the desired bp substitution G for A (**Table 1**). The incorporated substitution was confirmed by dideoxy sequencing (Sequenase, United States Biochemical, Cleveland, OH).
8. A hydroxylamine-sensitive G to A substitution at position 770 of the hGR cDNA, which converts a tryptophan residue to an amber stop codon, was generated by means of site-directed mutagenesis by elimination of the unique restriction enzyme site *Sac*I in the multiple cloning site of the vector pGEM-3, which contains the hGR cDNA insert, using the method of Deng and Nickoloff ***(12)***. This method relies on the fact that plasmids containing the desired mutation will be resistant to *Sac*I linearization, and will therefore remain circular and be selected in preference to linearized plasmids in subsequent bacterial transformations. The presence of the mutation was confirmed by *Sac*I digestion and subsequent dideoxy sequencing using primer 2 (**Table 1**) as the sequencing primer.
9. Each experiment was controlled for modification by hydroxylamine and osmium, because the G to A mutation generated by site-directed mutagenesis is modified by hydroxylamine. An A to T mismatch at position 2054 of the hGR cDNA

from a patient with familial glucocorticoid resistance was used to control for Os sensitivity. Therefore, the crucial modification steps were controlled for in each experiment.

10. The products are resolved by denaturing PAGE and detected by autoradiography. The authors have applied a modification of this technique to detect mutations in amplified hGR cDNA by hybridizing labeled wild-type probe cDNA with a 10-fold excess unlabeled patient or mutated cDNA. Using double-stranded probes, with each strand labeled at the 5' end, both strands of the cDNA are screened for mutations simultaneously. This halves the number of reactions required to detect all possible mutations.
11. In order to confirm the sensitivity of the screening technique of CMA the overlapping cDNA fragments encoding the DNA-binding and transactivating domains of the hGR from a CR patient were cycle-sequenced. Base pairs 161–1692 were sequenced in both the sense and antisense direction, i.e., a total of 3390 bp. There was no difference between the 3390 bp of the patient sequenced and the published sequence, thus confirming the sensitivity of the mutational analysis.

References

1. Lane, S. J. and Lee, T. H. (1996) Mononuclear cells in corticosteroid-resistant asthma. *Am. J. Respir. Crit. Care Med.* **154,** S49–51.
2. Adcock, I. M., Lane, S. J., Brown, C. R., Peters, M. J., Lee, T. H., and Barnes, P. J. (1995) Differences in binding of glucocorticoid receptor to DNA in steroid-resistant asthma. *J. Immunol.* **154,** 3500–3505.
3. Cotton, R. G., Rodrigues, N. R., and Campbell, R. D. (1988) Reactivity of cytosine and thymine in single-base-pair mismatches with hydroxylamine and osmium tetroxide and its application to the study of mutations. *Proc. Natl. Acad. Sci. USA* **85,** 4397–4401.
4. Orita, M., Iwahana, H., Kanazawa, H., Hayashi, K., and Sekiya, T. (1989) Detection of polymorphisms of human DNA by gel electrophoresis as single-strand conformation polymorphisms. *Proc. Natl. Acad. Sci. USA* **86,** 2766–2770.
5. Sheffield, V. C., Cox, D. R., Lerman, L. S., and Myers, R. M. (1989) Attachment of a 40–base-pair G + C-rich sequence (GC-clamp) to genomic DNA fragments by the polymerase chain reaction results in improved detection of single-base changes. *Proc. Natl. Acad. Sci. USA* **86,** 232–236.
6. Myers, R. M., Larin, Z., and Maniatis, T. (1985) Detection of single base substitutions by ribonuclease cleavage at mismatches in RNA:DNA duplexes. *Science* **230,** 1242–1246.
7. Montandon, A. J., Green, P. M., Giannelli, F., and Bentley, D. R. (1989) Direct detection of point mutations by mismatch analysis: application to haemophilia B. *Nucleic. Acids. Res.* **17,** 3347–3358.
8. Green, P. M., Montandon, A. J., Ljung, R., Bentley, D. R., Nilsson, I. M., Kling, S., and Giannelli, F. (1991) Haemophilia B mutations in a complete Swedish population sample: a test of new strategy for the genetic counselling of diseases with high mutational heterogeneity. *Br. J. Haematol.* **78,** 390–397.

9. Little, M. H., Prosser, J., Condie, A., Smith, P. J., van Heymigen, V., and Hastie, N. D. (1992) Zinc finger point mutations within the WT1 gene in Wilms tumor patients. *Proc. Natl. Acad. Sci. USA* **89,** 4791–4795.
10. Coles, C., Condie, A., Chetty, U., Steel, C. M., Evans, H. J., and Prosser, J. (1992) p53 mutations in breast cancer. *Cancer Res.* **52,** 5291–5298.
11. Lane, S. J., Arm, J. P., Staynov, D. Z., and Lee, T. H. (1994) Chemical mutational analysis of the human glucocorticoid receptor cDNA in glucocorticoid-resistant bronchial asthma. *Am. J. Respir. Cell Mol. Biol.* **11,** 42–48.
12. Deng, W. P. and Nickoloff, J. A. (1992) Site-directed mutagenesis of virtually any plasmid by eliminating a unique site. *Anal. Biochem.* **200,** 81–88.
13. Hurley, D. M., Accili, D., Stratakis, C. A., Karl, M., Vamvakopoulos, N., Rorer, E., et al. (1991) Point mutation causing a single amino acid substitution in the hormone binding domain of the glucocorticoid receptor in familial glucocorticoid resistance. *J. Clin. Invest.* **87,** 680–686.
14. Lane, S. J. and Lee, T. H. (1991) Glucocorticoid receptor characteristics in monocytes of patients with corticosteroid-resistant bronchial asthma. *Am. Rev. Respir. Dis.* **143,** 1020–1024.
15. Chomczynski, P. and Sacchi, N. (1987) Single-step method of RNA isolation by acid guanidinium thiocyanate-phenol-chloroform extraction. *Anal. Biochem.* **162,** 156–159.

22

Histone Acetylation and Histone Deacetylation

Kazuhiro Ito, Peter J. Barnes, and Ian M. Adcock

1. Introduction

In the resting cell, DNA is tightly compacted to prevent transcription factor accessibility. During activation of the cell, this compact inaccessible DNA is made available to DNA-binding proteins, thus allowing the induction of gene transcription *(1,2)*. DNA is packaged into chromatin, a highly organized and dynamic protein–DNA complex. The fundamental subunit of chromatin, the nucleosome, is composed of an octomer of four core histones, an H3/H4 tetramer and two H2A/H2B dimers, surrounded by 146 bp DNA *(2,3)*. The packaging of DNA into nucleosomes acts as a barrier to the initiation of transcription by preventing the access of transcriptional factors, and RNA polymerase II, to their cognate recognition sequences *(4)*. Specific lysine residues in the *N*-terminal tails of the core histone can be post-translationally modified by acetylation of the ε-amino group. The dynamic equilibrium of core histone acetylation is established and maintained by histone acetyltransferase (HAT) and histone deacetylase (HDAC). Several transcriptional regulators possess intrinsic HAT and HDAC activities, strongly suggesting that histone acetylation and deacetylation play a causal role in regulating transcription *(5–8)*. There is compelling evidence that increased gene transcription is associated with an increase in histone acetylation; hypoacetylation of histone is correlated with reduced transcription or gene silencing (*2,7,8*; **Fig. 1**).

Therefore, analysis of the histone acetylation and deacetylation status of a cell gives a reflection on the cell activation status. In addition, histone acetylation and deacetylation are linked to cell cycle progression, and have been correlated with DNA repair and recombination events, as well as gene transcription *(9,10)*. This chapter describes a quantitative method for determination of transcription-dependent histone acetylation in culture cells and in vivo biopsies,

From: *Methods in Molecular Medicine, vol. 44: Asthma: Mechanisms and Protocols*
Edited by: K. F. Chung and I. Adcock © Humana Press Inc., Totowa, NJ

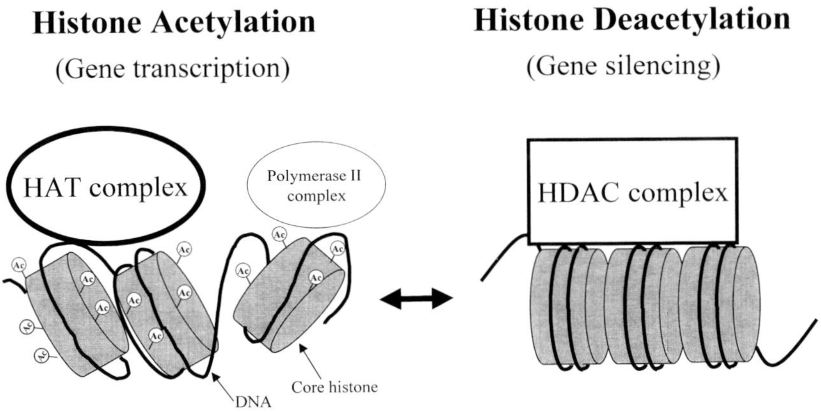

Fig. 1. Model of histone acetylation and histone deacetylation. HAT complex induces acetylation of core histone. Acetylation of internal lysines in core histones neutralizes the positive charge ($-NH_3^+ \rightarrow -NH-COCH_3$), and the affinity of histone *N*-terminal domains for DNA is significantly reduced, resulting in unwrapping DNA from core histone. In this situation, large molecules, such as RNA polymerase II, gain access to DNA, allowing gene transcription. In contrast, HDAC causes deacetylation of histones, increasing the positive charge, resulting in tightening up DNA coiling.

and a popular method that determines HAT and HDAC activity of the protein. This chapter provides detailed instructions for the method in A549 human bronchoalveolar epithelial cell line.

2. Materials

2.1. Histone Acetylation in A549 Cells

Except where stated, all regents are from Sigma (Poole, UK).

2.1.1. [^{3}H]-Acetate Incorporation

1. Hank's balanced saline solution (HBSS).
2. [^{3}H]-acetic acid (*see* **Note 1**).

2.1.2. Direct Histone Extraction

1. Lysis buffer: 10 m*M* Tris-HCl, pH 6.5, 50 m*M* Na bisulfite, 10 m*M* $MgCl_2$, 8.6% sucrose, 2% Triton X-100 (*see* **Note 2**), complete protease inhibitor cocktail (*see* **Note 3**), 100 ng/mL trichostatin A (TSA) (*see* **Note 4**).
2. Nuclei wash buffer: 10 m*M* Tris-HCl, pH 7.4, 13 m*M* ethylenediamine tetra-acetic acid (EDTA).
3. 5 *N* HCl.
4. Concentrated H_2SO_4.
5. Bradford protein assay kit (Bio-Rad Laboratories Ltd., Herts, UK).

2.1.3. Detection of Histone Acetylation

1. SDS-PAGE: 16% separating gel mix for two minigels: 4.0 mL of 40% acrylamide/*bis*-acrylamide solution (Anachem, Ltd., Luton, UK) (*see* **Note 5**), 3.75 mL of 1 *M* Tris-HCl, pH 8.8, 100 µL 10% (w/v) sodium dodecyl sulfate (SDS), and 4.05 mL distilled water. Add 10 µL of *N,N,N',N'*-tetramethylethylenediamine (TEMED) and 100 µL 10% (w/v) ammonium persulfate (APS) just prior to pouring the gel.
2. SDS-PAGE: 50% stacking gel mix for two minigels: 0.63 mL 40% acrylamide/*bis*-acrylamide solution (Anachem), 0.63 mL 1 *M* Tris-HCl, pH 6.8, 100 µL 10% (w/v) SDS solution, and 3.64 mL distilled water. Add 5 µL TEMED and 50 µL 10% (w/v) APS solution just prior to pouring the gel.
3. 4X SDS-polyacrylamide gel electrophoresis (PAGE) sample buffer (20 mL): 5 mL 1 *M* Tris-HCl, pH 6.8, 4 mL glycerol, 4 mL 10% (w/v) SDS solution, 40 mg bromophenol blue, and 7 mL distilled H_2O. Add 40 µL 2-mercaptoethanol (2-ME) to 1 mL 4X sample buffer just before use.
4. Prepare a stock of 10X SDS-PAGE running buffer; 30.3 g Tris-base, 144 g glycine, 10 g SDS in 1 L distilled H_2O. Store at room temperature (RT).
5. Liquid scintillation cocktail (ACSII, Amersham, UK).
6. Gel-staining solution: 0.2% (w/v) Coomassie brilliant blue R250 in 50% methanol and 10% acetic acid. Store at RT.
7. Gel-destaining solution: 33% methanol and 10% acetic acid. Store at RT.

2.2. Histone Acetylation Activity of Immunoprecipitated Protein

2.2.1. Immunoprecipitation

In this subheading, an example using rabbit anti-CBP antibody (Ab) is given.

1. HBSS.
2. 10X Immunoprecipitation (IP) buffer: 500 m*M* Tris-HCl, pH 8.0, 1.5 *M* NaCl, 50 m*M* EDTA, 5% NP-40; diluted on the day of the experiment with distilled H_2O. Add one complete protease inhibitor cocktail tablet to 10 mL IP buffer just before use (*see* **Note 3**).
3. 50 % Protein A-conjugated agarose slurry (*see* **Note 6**).
4. Normal rabbit immunoglobulin G (IgG) (*see* **Note 7**).
5. Relevant antibody (e.g., rabbit anti-CBP Ab).

2.2.2. IP-HAT Assay

1. [^{3}H]-acetyl coenzyme A (CoA) (*see* **Note 1**).
2. HAT buffer: 50 m*M* Tris-HCl, pH 8.0, 10% glycerol, 1 m*M* dithiothreitol, 0.1 m*M* EDTA. Store at 4°C (for up to 1 mo). Add complete protease inhibitor cocktail without EDTA (*see* **Note 3**) just before use.
3. P-81 phosphocellulose filter paper (Whatman, Maidstone, UK) 1 × 1 cm.
4. 1 *M* Na carbonate (pH 9.2), store at RT, and dilute with distilled H_2O to 20 m*M* (1:50) on the day of the experiment.

2.3. Histone Deacetylation Assay

2.3.1. Preparation of [^{3}H]-Labeled Histone

1. HBSS.
2. [^{3}H]-acetic acid (*see* **Note 1**).
3. Lysis buffer: 10 m*M* Tris-HCl, pH 6.5, 50 m*M* Na bisulfite, 10 m*M* $MgCl_2$, 8.6% sucrose, 2% Triton X-100, complete protease inhibitor cocktail, 100 ng/mL TSA (*see* **Notes 2–4**).
4. Nuclei wash buffer: 10 m*M* Tris-HCl, pH 7.4, 13 m*M* EDTA.
5. 5 *N* HCl.
6. Concentrated H_2SO_4.
7. TSA.
8. Cold acetone. Store at –20°C.

2.3.2. Preparation of HDAC Sample

1. HBSS.
2. HDAC A buffer : 15 m*M* Tris-HCl, pH 7.9, 450 m*M* NaCl, 0.25 m*M* EDTA, 10 m*M* ME, 10% glycerol. Store at 4°C (for up to 1 mo), and add complete protease inhibitor cocktail tablet, without EDTA, just before use.
3. HDAC B buffer: 15 m*M* Tris-HCl, pH 7.9, 0.25 m*M* EDTA, 10 m*M* ME, 10% glycerol. Store for up to 1 mo, and add complete protease inhibitor cocktail tablet, without EDTA, just before use.
4. HDAC C buffer: 15 m*M* Tris-HCl, pH 7.9, 10 m*M* NaCl, 0.25 m*M* EDTA, 10 m*M* ME, 10% glycerol. Store for up to 1 mo, and add complete protease inhibitor cocktail tablet, without EDTA, just before use.

2.3.3. HDAC Assay

1. HBSS.
2. Acid mixture (2.5 *N* HCl and 1 *N* acetic acid).
3. Ethyl acetate.
4. Liquid scintillation cocktail (ACSII).

3. Methods

3.1. Histone Acetylation in A549 Cells

3.1.1. [^{3}H]-Acetate Incorporation

1. Prepare 50% subconfluent (exponentially growing) cells in a six-well plate in supplemented Dulbecco's modified Eagle's medium.
2. Change to fetal calf serum (FCS)-free media approx 72 h before the experiment (*see* **Note 8**).
3. Cells are incubated with 0.005 mCi/mL of [^{3}H]-acetic acid in FCS-free medium for 10 min at 37°C before treatment.

*3.1.2. Histone Extraction (see **Note 9**)*

1. Wash the cells twice with ice-cold HBSS.
2. Add 500 μL ice-cold lysis buffer in each well, and scrape cells off quickly with a rubber policeman at 4°C.
3. Collect the cells into 1.5-mL Eppendorf tube, and keep them on ice for 10 min.
4. Wash the cells 3× with 200 μL ice-cold lysis buffer, or until the released nuclei are free of cytoplasmic tags, as judged by phase-contrast microscopy, and the supernatant is clear, each time centrifuged for 10 min at 10,000*g*.
5. After the last centrifugation, discard the supernatant, and wash the pellet once with nuclei wash buffer (10,000*g*, 4°C, 5 min) (*see* **Note 10**).
6. Resuspend the pellet in 150 μL ice-cold distilled H_2O, and mix vortex (*see* **Note 11**).
7. Add 6 μL 5 *N* HCl and 3 μL 18 *N* H_2SO_4 solution to nuclear suspension to give a concentration of 0.2 *N* and 0.36 *N* each (*see* **Note 12**).
8. Leave for 6–18 h at 4°C with rotating. Sonicate for 2 s ×2 ice, if necessary.
9. Centrifuge at 14,000*g* for 10 min at 4°C to remove acid-insoluble material.
10. Transfer 140 μL supernatant to new tube, and add 1.1 mL cold acetone to precipitate the histones.
11. Leave it at –20°C for overnight.
12. Centrifuge at 14,000*g* for 10 min at 4°C.
13. Wash the pellet with cold acetone by centrifugation, to remove acid.
14. Dry the final pellet under vacuum at RT.
15. Resolve in 50 μL distilled H_2O or HDAC C buffer (shown in **Subheading 2.3.2.**).
16. Determine the protein concentration by Bradford assay (Bio-Rad, Herts, UK).

*3.1.3. Detection of Histone Acetylation (see **Note 13**)*

1. Prepare the sample for SDS-PAGE (50 μg protein and 4X SDS-PAGE sample buffer) (*see* **Note 14**), and boil for 4 to 5 min, and then centrifuge at 14,000*g* for 20 s.
2. Set up SDS-PAGE apparatus according to the manufacturer's instructions.
3. Load the samples into appropriate wells on the 16% SDS-gel. The minigel should be run at 40 mA/gel for 30 min.
4. Stain the gel for 20 min with Coomassie brilliant blue staining solution.
5. Destain the gel in destaining solution for >6 h.
6. Cut out the band of core histones (**Fig. 2**), using a scalpel blade, and put into 3-mL scintillation vial.
7. Determine the radioactivity in excised core histones by liquid scintillation counting (see **Note 15**).
8. The data are shown following subtraction of baseline [^{3}H]-acetic acid incorporation. In this instance, [^{3}H]-acetic acid is added just before histone preparation (this shows nonspecific incorporation or contamination of free [^{3}H]-acetic acid while separating histone).

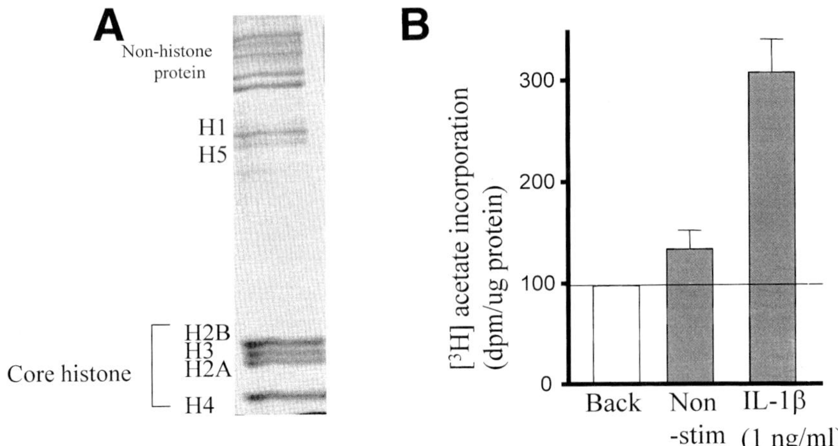

Fig. 2. **(A)** Representative results of 16% SDS-PAGE separation of histone extracted by acid. The gel was stained with Coomassie brilliant blue R-250. **(B)** Effect of interleukin (IL)-1β (1 ng/mL) on [^{3}H]-acetate incorporation (histone acetylation). Cells were incubated with IL-1β (1 ng/mL) for 6 h. Background shows nonspecific [^{3}H]-acetate incorporation and contamination of free [^{3}H]-acetic acid.

3.2. Histone Acetylation in Immunoprecipitated Protein

This method are applied to tissue- or cell-extracted protein, as well as to immunoprecipitates.

3.2.1. Immunoprecipitation

All steps should be performed at 4°C.

1. Collect the cells (1×10^7 cells) by scraping in 1 mL ice-cold HBSS, and gently pellet by centrifugation (5 min, 2000*g*).
2. The HBSS is aspirated, and the cells are resuspended into 500 µL IP buffer (*see* **Note 16**).
3. The lysis mixture is vortexed and incubated on ice for 15 min and centrifuged at 14,000*g* for 10 min at 4°C.
4. Transfer supernatant to a new tube.
5. Extracts are precleared with 10 µL 50% protein A agarose slurry and 2 µg normal IgG.
6. Incubate with rotation at 4°C for 2 h.
7. Centrifuge at 14,000*g* for 10 min at 4°C, and transfer supernatant to a new tube.
8. Relevant Abs (2–5 µg) are added to 500 µL extract, and incubate at 4°C for 2 h.
9. Protein-A agarose is added, and the mixture rotates slowly 6 h to overnight at 4°C.
10. The immune complexes are pelleted by gentle centrifugation (6000*g*, 5 min, at 4°C), and washed twice with 800 µL lysis buffer.

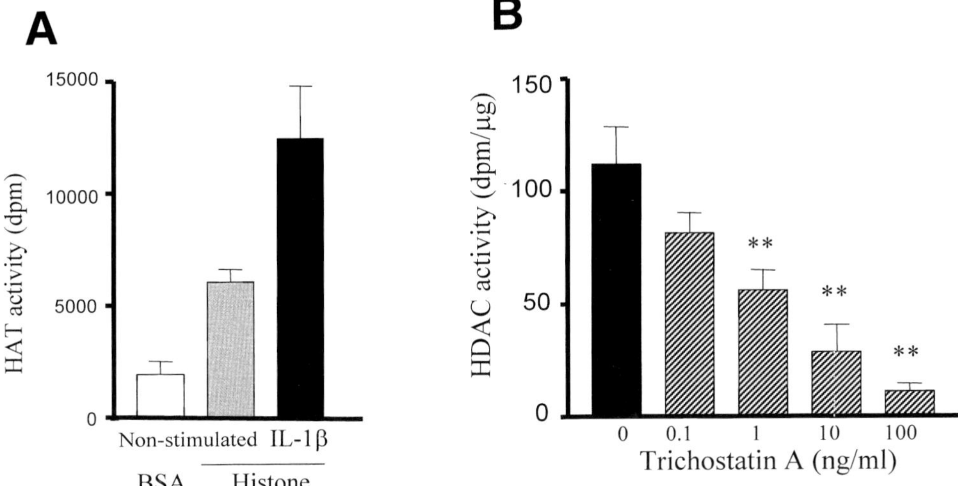

Fig. 3. **(A)** HAT activity of immunoprecipitated CREB binding protein (CBP). CBP HAT activity from A549 cells increased after IL-1β incubation (1 ng/mL, 6 h). As a control, BSA is used, instead of histone. **(B)** Inhibitory effect of TSA, a HDAC inhibitor, on HDAC activity extracted from A549 cells. TSA inhibited the HDAC activity in a dose-dependent manner, and the concentration of 100 ng/mL showed complete inhibition of HDAC activity.

11. Wash once with HAT buffer.
12. Aspirate supernatant completely, and add 150 μL HAT buffer.

*3.2.2. IP-HAT Assay (see **Note 17**)*

1. Add 20 μL 1 mg/mL crude extracted histone (*see* **Note 18**) and 1 μL [^{3}H]-acetyl-CoA (0.25 mCi) to IP sample (*see* **Note 19**).
2. Incubate at 32°C for 45 min.
3. To terminate the reactions, spot the reaction mixture onto Whatman P-81 phosphocellulose filter paper (1 × 1 cm).
4. Wash for 30 min with 0.2 *M* Na carbonate buffer (pH 9.2) at RT with 2–3 changes of the buffer.
5. Wash briefly with acetone and dry the filter.
6. Determine the radioactivity of dried filters in a liquid scintillation counter (*see* **Note 20**; **Fig. 3A**).

3.3. Histone Deacetylation

*3.3.1. Preparation of [^{3}H]-Labeled Histone (see **Note 21**)*

1. Prepare 80% subconfluent cells in 150-cm^2 flask.
2. Change medium FCS-free 24 h before the experiment.

3. Cells are incubated with 0.1 mCi/mL [^{3}H]-acetic acid in 10% FCS medium for 10 min.
4. Add 100 ng/mL TSA, and incubate for 6–8 h.
5. For extraction of histone, perform **steps 1–10** of **Subheading 3.1.2.**
6. Diluted with distilled water or HDAC C buffer to give a concentration of 1.5 mg/µL (150–200 dpm/µL).

3.3.2. Preparation of HDAC Sample

1. Wash the cell twice with cold HBSS.
2. Collect the cells by scraping into 1 mL ice-cold HBSS into Eppendorf tube.
3. Centrifuge at 10,000*g* for 5 min at 4°C.
4. Extract nuclei by cell lysis buffer (*see* **Subheading 3.1.2.**, **steps 1–5**).
5. Add 20 µL HDAC A buffer.
6. Vortex for 15 s vigorously, and leave it on ice for 20 min.
7. Collect supernatant and add 180 µL HDAC B buffer (*see* **Note 22**).

3.3.3. HDAC Assay

This method is applied to tissue extraction and immunoprecipitates, as well as to cell lysates.

1. Mix 15 µL [^{3}H]-labeled histone (1.5 mg/mL) with 25 µL crude HDAC extraction (*see* **Notes 22** and **23**).
2. Incubate at 30°C for 30 min.
3. Stop the reaction by addition of 10 µL acid mixture (2.5 *N* HCl and 1 *N* acetic acid).
4. Add 900 µL ethylacetate into reaction mixture.
5. Vortex vigorously, and leave for 5 min, then mix again.
6. Centrifuge at 14,000*g* for 5 min at 4°C.
7. Put a 600 µL aliquot of the upper organic phase into 3 mL liquid scintillation cocktail.
8. Determine the radioactivity of sample by liquid scintillation counter (*see* **Note 24**; **Fig. 3B**).

4. Notes

1. [^{3}H]-acetic acid and [^{3}H]-acetyl-CoA are currently supplied by New England Nuclear, Du Pont, UK. As [^{3}H]-acetyl CoA is kept frozen, place it at 4°C at least 1 h before use to thaw slowly.
2. Two percent of Triton X-100 is necessary for lysis of A549, HeLa, and MCF7 cells for rapid purification of nuclei. For U-937, mononuclear cells and other primary cultured cells 0.5–1% Triton X-100 is needed. These concentrations are relatively high; do not leave for more than 10 min. NP-40 (0.2–0.5%) can be used, instead of Triton X-100.
3. Complete protease inhibitor cocktail is supplied by Boehringer-Mannheim. For this lysis buffer, the tablet with EDTA is used. For other buffers containing EDTA described in this chapter, the tablet without EDTA is used.

4. TSA is obtained from Sigma (Poole, UK). The stock 100 μg/mL of 100% Ethyl alcohol should be stored at –20°C, and added to lysis buffer just before use.
5. Care should be taken with acrylamide and *bis*-acrylamide, because both have been reported to be neurotoxins. Care should be taken with SDS as well, because of its toxicity.
6. Antibodies bind with different affinities to protein A and G agarose. Normally protein A agarose is used for rabbit, goat Ab, and protein G for mouse, goat, and rat Ab. Protein A/G agarose can be used for any experiments.
7. Normal IgG, which matched to the animal of relevant antibody should be used.
8. In order to detect histone acetylation only by gene transcription, not by DNA recombination for proliferation (as a background), synchronization of cells is very important. A549 cells require 60–72 h for synchronization. Before the start of experiments, the synchronized timing should be checked by simple DNA content assay by fluorescence-activated cell sorter, using propidium iodide.
9. This method is adapted from the methods in **refs. *9*** and ***10***.
10. If you need to purify nuclei completely, final purification is achieved by pelleting the nuclei through a sucrose cushion. At first, resuspend the nuclei in approx 2 mL nuclei wash buffer with complete protease inhibitor cocktail. Overlay 2 mL of the nuclear suspension onto 5 mL sucrose cushion (30% [w/v] sucrose in nuclear wash buffer), and centrifuge at 2500*g* for 5 min at 4°C. Remove all the supernatant, and resuspend the pellet in the distilled water, then follow **steps 7–16** in **Subheading 3.1.2.**
11. If the nuclear pellet is difficult to resuspend, sonicate for 5 s on ice.
12. Instead of acid extraction, salt extraction procedures are also recommended. This method is advantageous, because the histones can be prepared in pure form, with little contaminating nonhistone proteins, and the core histone octamer can be readily isolated. The method relies on the differential affinities of histones and nonhistone proteins for DNA in varying salt conditions. Further details regarding this purification may be found in **ref. *13***.
13. If complete purification of core histone is not necessary, the 50 μL supernatant (**Subheading 3.1.2.**) can be added to 3 mL scintillant, and the radioactivity determined by liquid scintillation counting. In this case, 88–94% radioactivity is normally from histones, and 6–12% radioactivity from nonhistone protein or contamination of free [^{3}H]-acetic acid.
14. If the blue SDS sample buffer solution turns brown or yellow, then the sample is still acidic. Simply add approx 2–3 μL of 1 *M* Tris-base until the sample turns blue.
15. For visualization of the histone acetylation on the gel, the gel is stained with Coomassie solution and destained, and immersed and soaked in [^{3}H]-amplifier solution (Amersham, UK) for 15–30 min, and then the gel is dried onto Whatman 3MM filter paper under suction from an electric vacuum pump attached to a gel drier. Transfer the dried gel to a X-ray film cassette with containing Hyperfilm MP (Amersham, UK) and allow to autoradiograph at –80°C for an appropriate

time (normally 24–48 h). Instead of autoradiography of [^{3}H]-labeled histone, antiacetylated histone Abs are useful, which are available from Serotec (Oxford, UK) and Upstate (New York, NY).

16. This buffer is not too stringent, and is therefore useful for coimmunoprecipitation studies. Depending upon the object of experiment, strong buffer (e.g., radioimmunoprecipitation [RIPA] buffer) can be used; phosphate-buffered saline, pH 7.4, 0.5% NP-40, 0.15% SDS, 0.5% Na deoxycholate, complete protease inhibitor cocktail.
17. The following protocol is a modification of that given in **ref. *14***.
18. Calf thymus histone is also commercially available from Sigma.
19. In the case of biopsies (2 × 2 × 2 mm) or cells, add 100 μL HAT buffer with complete protease inhibitor cocktail and 0.1% NP-40, homogenize it with an A-type Dounce homogenizer (Wheaton, NJ) in 20 cycles, and sonicate for 5 s and 30 s-resting at three cycles on ice. Add 100 μL HAT buffer. Freeze and thaw once, and centrifuge at 14,000*g* for 10 min at 4°C. The supernatant is collected. Contamination of high concentration of detergent tends to inhibit HAT buffer. So keep the concentration of detergent under 0.05% for assay.
20. As the control, the following experiments are recommended.
    a. Total radioactivity (1 μL of [^{3}H]-acetyl-CoA).
    b. No IP protein, no histone, sample incubated with [^{3}H]-acetyl-CoA in HAT buffer.
    c. No IP protein, sample incubated with [^{3}H]-acetyl-CoA, histone in HAT buffer.
    d. Sample incubated with [^{3}H]-acetyl-CoA, IP protein, and bovine serum albumin (BSA), instead of histone in HAT buffer.
21. Labeled histones from red blood cells of chickens injected with phenylhydrazine (5 mg/mL iv) can also be used. Further details regarding this chicken-labeled histone may be found in **ref. *15***.
22. Salt concentrations above 200 m*M* increasingly inhibit HDAC activity. Therefore, dialysis may be necessary. Final salt concentration in assay is recommended to be 10–45 m*M*. In this protocol, final 22.5 m*M* of salt is used. This is a crude HDAC extraction. For partial purification of deacetylases, the deacetylase is precipitated by raising the concentration of $(NH_4)_2SO_4$ to 3.5 *M*. The dialysate is then loaded onto a diethylaminoethyl cellulose (Whatman DE52) column equilibrated with the HDAC C-buffer, and eluted with a linear gradient (0–0.6 *M*) of NaCl. A single peak of HDAC activity is eluted with 0.15 and 0.2 *M* NaCl. Further details regarding this partial purification may be found in **ref. *12***.
23. Instead of crude HDAC extracts, IP protein by following **steps 1–12** in **Subheading 3.2.2.** or biopsies sample extracted by following **steps 5–7** in **Subheading 3.3.2.** and **Note 19**, using HDAC buffer, instead of HAT buffer, can be used.
24. As the control, experiments described below are recommended.
    a. No HDAC protein (nonspecific release of [^{3}H] acetic acid).
    b. Sample incubated with [^{3}H]-labeled histone, HDAC sample, and TSA (100 ng/mL) (non-HDAC-dependent release of [^{3}H] acetic acid).
    c. Total radioactivity of labeled histone.

References

1. Beato, M. (1996) Chromatin structure and the regulation of gene expression: remodeling at the MMTV promoter. *J. Mol. Med.* **74,** 711–724.
2. Wolffe, A. P. (1997) Transcriptional control. Sinful repression. *Nature* **387,** 15–17.
3. Beato, M. and Eisfeld, K. (1997) Transcription factor access to chromatin. *Nucleic Acids Res.* **25,** 3559–3563.
4. Workman, J. L. and Buchman, A. R. (1993) Multiple functions of nucleosomes and regulatory factors in transcription. *Trends Biochem. Sci.* **18,** 90–95.
5. Gregory, P. D. and Horz, W. (1998) Chromatin and transcription-how transcription factors battle with a repressive chromatin enviroment. *Eur. J. Biochem.* **251,** 9–18.
6. Grunstein, M. (1997) Histone acetylation in chromatin structure and transcription *Nature* **389,** 349–352.
7. Kuo, M-H. and Allis, C. D. (1998) Roles of histone acetyltransferases and deacetylases in gene regulation. *BioEssays* **20,** 615–626.
8. Workman, J. L. and Kingston, R. E. (1998) Alteration of nucleosome structure as a mechanism of transcriptional regulation. *Annu. Rev. Biochem.* **67,** 545–579.
9. Kouzarides, T. (1999) Histone acetylases and deacetylases in cell proliferation. *Curr. Opin. Genet. Dev.* **9,** 40–48.
10. Taplick, J., Kurtev, V., Lagger, G., and Seiser, C. (1998) Histone H4 acetylation during interleukin-2 stimulation of mouse T cells. *FEBS Lett.* **436,** 349–352.
11. Turner, B. M. and Fellows, G. (1989) Specific antibodies reveal ordered and cell-cycle-related use of histone-H4 acetylation sites in mammalian cells. *Eur. J. Biochem.* **179,** 131–139.
12. Yoshida, M., Kijima, M., Akita, M., and Beppu, T. (1990) Potent and specific inhibition of mammalian histone deacetylase both in vitro and in vivo by Trichostatin A. *J. Biol. Chem.* **265,** 17,174–17,179.
13. Simon, R. H. and Felsenfeld, G. (1979) A new procedure for purifying histone pairs H2A+H2B and H3+H4 form chromatin using hydroxylapatite. *Nucleic Acid Res.* **6,** 689–696.
14. Ogryzko, V. V., Schiltz, R. L., Russanova, V., Howard, B. H., and Nakatani, Y. (1996) The transcription coactivators p300 and CBP are histone acetyltransferase. *Cell* **87,** 953–959.
15. Koelle, D., Brosch, G., Lechner, T., Lusser, A., and Loidl, P. (1998) Biochemical methods for analysis of histone deacetylases. *Methods Comp Methods Enzymol.* **15,** 323–331.

23

Genome-Wide Search for Asthma Genes

Adel H. Mansur and John F. J. Morrison

1. Introduction

In addition to important environmental factors, it is now well established that genetic factors contribute significantly to the development of asthma and atopy, accounting for between 30 and 60% of the predisposition ***(1–3)***. This genetic predisposition is likely to result from the inheritance of a multiple number of polymorphic or mutant genes ***(4)***. Over the past decade, numerous researchers have conducted genetic linkage and/or association studies that aimed to identify such genes. These two types of studies are fundamentally different. A linkage study compares the inheritance pattern of the disease phenotype to the inheritance pattern of a particular genetic marker in pedigrees, looking for coinheritance, and thus linking that particular marker locus to the disease. The association study, on the other hand, identifies candidate genes by comparing particular gene variant (allele) frequency in cases and controls, and therefore implicating that particular allele in the predisposition to the disease. Detecting genetic linkage usually indicates the presence of a gene within a genetic distance of approx 10 centimorgans (c*M*) around the linked locus. Genetic association tends to operate within a much shorter genetic distance (1 c*M*), but this distance varies, depending on the structure of the study population (relating to the ancestor founder effect).

Recent developments in understanding of the pathogenic mechanisms in asthma, at both cellular and molecular levels, provide a rich pool of biologically plausible candidate genes that could be studied directly, using what is termed the "candidate gene approach." However, in complex diseases, such as asthma, there are likely to be other, as yet unidentified genes. For this reason, genome-wide screens have been conducted to identify such genes by analyzing random markers, which are evenly distributed along the genome

From: *Methods in Molecular Medicine, vol. 44: Asthma: Mechanisms and Protocols*
Edited by: K. F. Chung and I. Adcock

(5,6). Identification of a linkage between a particular marker and asthma indicates the presence of a predisposing gene in the corresponding chromosomal region. This is the first step in asthma gene identification. Further analysis in the region is required to locate the culprit gene using an approach termed "positional cloning." This chapter outlines the steps required to conduct a genome screen study. The method described here reflects the experience of the authors and current knowledge. This field is developing rapidly both at the molecular level (e.g., the development of yet-denser genetic maps, using single nucleotide polymorphism [SNP] and full genotyping automation), and also at the statistical level. This chapter identifies recent developments in the field, and discusses areas of difficulty.

The first phase of conducting a genome screen study will require construction of a database, which could be either family-based or comprised of a case/control cohort of randomly recruited subjects. Individuals considered for the study will have detailed clinical characterization, which will include obtaining blood samples for DNA extraction. Having constructed a database, the next step will be to select and/or design panels of genetic markers that cover the genome in an evenly distributed fashion. This is followed by the process of genotyping, which comprises polymerase chain reaction (PCR) amplification of the selected markers, electrophoresis and sizing of the PCR products, assignment of alleles, and alleles binning. In the final stage, the clinical and genotypic data are compiled using specifically designed software that outputs the data in a format suitable for subsequent handling by linkage programs or other statistical packages.

2. Materials

2.1. Family Recruitment and Clinical Characterization

1. Ethical approval.
2. International Union against tuberculosis and lung disease (IUALTD) Bronchial Symptoms Questionnaire *(7)*.
3. Height and weight.
4. 10-mL tubes for clotted blood sample, and 10-mL ethylenediamine tetraacetic acid (EDTA)-containing tubes for anticoagulated blood sample.
5. Skin-prick testing (SPT) package (Dome/Hollister-Stier, Miles, Spokane, WA), with available resuscitation measures.
6. Bronchial challenge testing: Dry Bellows Spirometer (Vitalograph, Buckingham, UK). DeVilbiss hand-held nebulizers (De Vilbiss, Inc., Somerset, PA). Serial dilution of freshly made histamine solution *(8)*.

2.2. DNA Extraction

1. Red blood cell (RBC) lysis solution (8.3% w/v ammonium chloride, 0.037% (w/v) EDTA, and 1% potassium (K) hydrogen carbonate).

2. Phosphate-buffer saline (PBS): 0.8% (w/v) NaCl, 0.02% (w/v) KCl, 0.114% (w/v) disodium hydrogen phosphate, and 0.02% K phosphate, pH 7.4.
3. 0.6 *M* Na acetate, 10% w/v sodium dodecyl sulfate (SDS), 1 mg/mL proteinase K (Sigma, St. Louis, MO).
4. Phenol-chloroform:isoamyl alcohol:1 m*M* EDTA of 25:24:1 proportion, saturated in 10 m*M* Tris, pH 8.0 (Sigma).
5. 5 *M* ammonium acetate, 100% pure ethanol, 70% ethanol solution.

2.3. Genome Mapping Olignucleotide Primer Sets

Compatible sets of chromosome-specific, fluorescently labeled, microsatellite oligonucleotide primers ***(9)***. The ABI Prism Linkage Mapping Set (Applied Biosystems, Inc., Perkin Elmer, Branchburg, NJ) contains approx 350 markers, with an average distance between markers of 10 c*M*.

2.4. PCR Amplification

1. 10X thermobuffer, 500 m*M* KCl, 10 m*M* Tris-HCl, pH 8.3.
2. Deoxynucleotide triphosphates (dNTPs) mix: 10 m*M* each of deoxyadenosine triphosphate, deoxyoptosine triphosphate, deoxyguanosine triphosphate, and deoxythymidine triphosphate.
3. 25 m*M* $MgCl_2$.
4. Mineral oil.

2.5. Electrophoresis on ABI Prism 377

1. Access to Applied Biosystems (ABI) Prism 377 Genescanner.
2. 5 *M* ammonium acetate.
3. Loading buffer (5:1 deionized formamide: 25 m*M* EDTA with 50 mg/mL blue dextran). **Warning:** formamide is teratogenic.
4. 4.25% acrylamide/7 *M* urea gel mixture (Sequagel-4.25, National Diagnostics, Hessle Hull, UK). **Warning:** Acrylamide is a cumulative neurotoxic.
5. Genescan-500 Tamra (Applied Biosystems, Perkin-Elmer).

2.6. Computer Software

1. Genescan analysis software (Perkin-Elmer).
2. Genotyper software (Perkin-Elmer).
3. Genetic Analysis System (GAS) program, version 2.0, Alan Young, Oxford University, 1993–1995, available on Human Genome Mapping Project (HGMP) resource centre directory ftp.ebi.ac.uk pub/software/linkage-end-mapping.

3. Methods

3.1. Subject Recruitment and Characterization

For the purpose of genome screen study, families, rather than random subjects, are usually ascertained (*see* **Note 1**). Asthma usually presents at younger age, thus providing the advantage of recruiting families of asthmatic subjects with available parents. Previous asthma studies considered either nuclear families or extended families recruited from outbred populations, or families recruited from inbred populations. The commonest approach has been to study nuclear families recruited from outbred populations; such families are selected on the basis of the presence of multiple affected individuals, usually in the form of affected sibling pairs (sib-pairs).

The advantage of studying such families is that they are more likely to be representative of the general population at large. Additionally, affected sib-pairs are amenable to the robust nonparametric sib-pair linkage analysis, which effectively overcomes problems created by incomplete penetrance of genes or other parameters that confound the formal linkage analysis in complex disease ***(10)***.

However, studies on nuclear families drawn from outbred populations may suffer from lack of power caused by disease heterogeneity (different genes causing asthma in different subjects), and when only a fraction of the recruited families are affected by the genetic form of the disease. Extended pedigrees are generally considered to be a less attractive option in complex disease studies, since their analysis will often require formal parametric linkage analysis, which has proven to be controversial in complex traits. In contrast, inbred populations are likely to have been formed by a limited number of ancestors, thus reducing the confounding effect of heterogeneity. However, studying such populations may not be representative of the general population at large.

3.1.1. Recruitment of Affected Sib-Pairs

The sib-pair approach has been commonly used to study genetics of complex traits. To collect families with affected sib-pairs, the authors recommend the following recruitment criteria, to maximize both the informativeness and power of the data set.

1. Both of the affected (e.g., asthmatic) sibs should be at least 6 yr old. Younger children are usually difficult to characterize clinically, and conduction of specific tests, such as bronchial challenge test, may not be possible.
2. In any family, both parents should be available. Families with missing parental genotype or clinical data may compromise the informativeness of the data set (*see* **Subheading 3.8.1.**).
3. Select families with either zero or one affected parent. There is a small chance that the affected parents may carry two different disease-causing genes, which may reduce the power of the study by introducing heterogeneity ***(11)***.
4. The power of the study will depend mostly on the size of the sample obtained. The current state of knowledge does not allow accurate power measurement in complex trait studies, such as asthma, because the number of genes involved, their frequency, and their relative contribution, are not known. However, a rough

estimate of the suitable minimum number of sib-pairs required to identify a gene of certain effect may be provided by specifically designed simulation software, e.g., Simlink (Department of Public Health, University of Michigan, Ann Arbor, MI, or available online at http://www.hgmp.mrc.ac.uk/Registered/option/simlink.html) ***(12)***. Estimates have suggested that large sample sizes (500+ sib-pairs) are likely to be required to find genes of moderate effect, in a disease of relatively low heritability, such as asthma ***(13)***.

3.1.2. Clinical Characterization of Subjects

All recruited individuals should undergo detailed clinical characterization, which may include the following.

1. Following their identification, all recruited subjects should be given an identification number (ID), which should conform to the format of linkage programs, in which the first digit refers to the family number, followed by the subject ID (e.g., subject coded 10101 refers to the first member of family 101, and 10102 refers to the second member of the family, and so on).
2. Use a structured and validated questionnaire that covers asthmatic and atopic symptoms (e.g., the IUALTD questionnaire; *7*). Collected data should include age, country of birth, and racial origin. Details of asthmatic symptoms may include past history of wheeze, wheezing in the last 12 mo prior to the interview, nocturnal wheeze, severe attacks of wheeze (speech limited to only one or two words at a time), history of asthma, whether asthma was diagnosed by a doctor, age of onset, hospital admissions, rest and exercise-induced cough, and asthma medication current or past. Specific questions about atopic dermatitis may include history of itchy rash, itchy rash in the 12 mo prior to the interview, distribution of the rash, previous eczema diagnosis, age of onset, and current or recent medications. Allergic rhinoconjunctivitis questions may cover history of past or current sneezing, runny or blocked nose when not having a cold or flu; history of itchy, watery eyes; seasonal variations in the symptoms; established diagnosis of hay fever or rhinitis; and any recent or current medications, including desensitization courses. The questionnaire should also cover smoking history and familial history of allergic disease.
3. Bronchial reactivity may be measured in the subjects using the method of Yan et al. ***(8)***. The procedure details are beyond the scope of this chapter, but the following guidelines are required. Subjects should be instructed to abstain from using β-agonists, cromolyns, xanthines, and anticholinergics, for the appropriate length of time prior to the test. Spirometry (Vitalography) should be measured in all subjects. Individuals with more than 70% of predicted forced expiratory volume in one second (FEV_1) should be subjected to methacholine or histamine bronchial challenge. The bronchial reversibility status of subjects with less than 70% of predicted FEV_1 can be determined by FEV_1 remeasurement 15 min after inhalation of a β_2-agonist (e.g., 200 μg salbutamol). An increase in FEV_1 of more than 15% of predicted volume is usually taken to indicate a signifi-

cantly reversible obstructive airway ventilatory defect, consistent with the diagnosis of asthma.

4. Determine the atopic status of all subjects by SPT, total and specific serum immunoglobulin E (IgE) measurement, and eosinophil count. SPT by stylet can be performed using specific reagents of common allergens (because of risk of anaphylactic reactions, ensure that specific resuscitation measures are available prior to SPT). Clotted blood samples should be obtained for total and specific serum IgE measurement. Peripheral blood samples should be collected in EDTA-containing tubes, for DNA extraction and eosinophil counts.
5. Process the obtained clinical data carefully. Determine which phenotypes you intend to use as an end point in the analysis (*see* **Note 2**), and construct clinical data files in a linkage format suitable for subsequent handling by linkage programs (*see* **Subheading 3.7.**)

3.2. DNA Extraction

Numerous DNA extraction methods are available, which vary in efficiency, product purity, and time factor. The phenol–chloroform method has been widely used, and is described below.

1. Collect 10 mL peripheral venous blood in EDTA-containing tubes, then transfer the blood into 50-mL centrifuge tubes (Greiner, Labortechnik, Inc., Stonehouse, UK).
2. Add 3 vol RBC lysis solution (8.3% [w/v] ammonium chloride, 0.037% [w/v] EDTA, and 1% [w/v] K hydrogen carbonate), and mix the contents gently. Incubate the tubes at room temperature for 15 min. Collect the white cells by centrifugation at 12,000*g* for 10 min at room temperature (RT). Discard the supernatant, and repeat the process twice. At this stage, if whole RBCs are still present in the white cell pellet, then repeat the process of incubation in the RBC lysis solution one more time.
3. If the white cell pellet is free from RBC contamination, resuspend the cells in 500 μL sterile PBS (0.8% w/v NaCl, 0.02% w/v KCl, 0.114% (w/v) disodium hydrogen phosphate, and 0.02% K dihydrogen phosphate, pH 7.4, and transfer into 1.5-mL microcentrifuge tubes.
4. The peripheral blood leukocytes (PBLs) are lysed as follows: To each 500-μL sample of PBL suspension, add 500 μL of a 0.6 *M* solution of Na acetate (final concentration of 0.2 *M*), and mix the solutions gently. To this mixture, add 150 μL 10% (w/v) aqueous SDS (final concentration of 1% [w/v]), 150 μL 1 mg/mL solution of proteinase K (final concentration of 0.1 mg/mL) and 200 μL sterile H_2O. Mix the solutions again, gently. For proteinase K digestion, incubate the samples at 37°C for a period of 48 h.
5. Split the resultant viscous solution between two 1.5-mL microcentrifuge tubes, and remove the cellular protein by a phenol–chloroforom extraction. Add an equal volume of Tris-EDTA (10 m*M* Tris-HCl, pH 8.0, 0.5 m*M* EDTA) saturated phenol–chloroform (1:1 v/v), and mix the solutions.
6. Separate the aqueous and solvent layers by centrifugation in a microcentrifuge at 11,500*g* for 10 min at RT. Immediately remove the upper aqueous layer (contain-

ing the genomic DNA) by pipeting, place into a new microcentrifuge tube, and add a fresh equal volume of Tris-EDTA-saturated phenol–chloroform. Mix the solution again, and separate the aqueous and solvent layers again by centrifugation. Aspirate the upper layer, and place into another new microcentrifuge tube.
7. Add an equal volume of chloroform. Mix the solutions, and separate the aqueous and solvent layers by centrifugation. Aspirate, and place the aqueous layer into a new microcentrifuge tube.
8. Precipitate genomic DNA by adding a 1/10 vol 5 *M* ammonium acetate and 1 mL ice-cold 100% pure ethanol. Remove the precipitated genomic DNA from the mixture by spooling it onto a sealed sterilized glass Pasteur pipet.
9. Wash the DNA with 1 mL 70% ethanol in a microcentrifuge tube, and transfer into 500 µL sterile DNase-free water. Allow the DNA to resuspend overnight at 37°C. Once resuspended, the DNA concentration can be determined using DNA Fluorometer (Gene Quant, Pharmaci, Biotech, Cambridge, UK). Aliquot and code DNA, and store at –20°C in sequential order, according to subject's ID.

3.3. Linkage Mapping Sets and ABI Genescanners

Microsatellites are short lengths of DNA in which the nucleotide sequence consists of a variable number of repeats of specific base pairs (bps) (e.g., CA repeats), and are found scattered throughout the human genome. The variability in the length of the repeat sequence between the homologous chromosomes of an individual and among individuals' "allelic polymorphism," makes such markers valuable tools for following the transmission of marker alleles from one generation to another. Microsatellite marker polymorphism can be studied once the sequence flanking the microsatellite has been determined. PCR primers unique to this region are used to amplify the DNA obtained from the families. The amplified fragments are sized on nondenaturing polyacrylamide gels, using either radioisotope or fluorescent label technology. The ABI Genescanner machines detect fluorescent signaling in several colors, and perform semiautomated gel analysis, which efficiently reduces the time and labor required for large-scale microsatellite analysis (*see* **Note 3**). The ABI Prism 377 model has generally superseded previous models by gaining the advantage of speed, high resolution, and improved automated analysis modules.

For the purpose of a genome wide screen, sets of fluorescently labeled, chromosome-specific oligonucleotide primers have been developed ***(9)***. The sets are designed to allow multiplex PCR amplification or combined product electrophoresis on ABI Prism, by grouping microsatellites whose alleles could be distinguished by either size or fluorescent color label (*see* **Note 4**).

3.4. PCR Amplification

1. Obtain PCR primers for the region flanking the repeats chosen for the study.
2. Aliquot diluted DNA (2 µL containing 100 ng DNA) in 96-well microtiter plates in sequential order according to subjects ID.

3. Prepare a PCR master mix for 96 reactions, with an extra 5%, to allow for sampling error. PCR master mix for 100 reactions could be performed in 5-mL sterile tubes using 400 µL dH_2O, 200 µL 10X thermo buffer (Promega, Biosciences Inc., San Luis Obispo, CA), 200 µL dNTP mix (containing 150 µ*M* each dNTP/µL), 400 µL $MgCl_2$ (1.5–2.5 m*M*/µL), 400 µL (20 p*M*/µL) for oligonucleotide primer (forward), 400 µL (20 *p*M/µL) of oligonucleotide primer (reverse), and 20 µL (10 U/µL) of Ampli *Taq* polymerase.
4. Add 18 µL of PCR mix containing 2.0 µL 10X thermo buffer, 300 µ*M* of each dNTP, 20 p*M* of each primer, and 0.2 U *Taq* DNA polymerase (Promega), and 1.0–3.5 m*M* $MgCl_2$) (*see* **Note 5**). Add 40 µL mineral oil (Sigma) to the PCR mix.
5. Place the plate on a DNA thermal cycler, and perform amplification. The PCR cycling condition will vary, depending on the individual microsatellite (*see* **Note 5**).

3.5. Multiplex PCR Products Electrophoresis

Multiplex electrophoresis of PCR products of sets of microsatellites, which can be distinguished either by product size or color label, can significantly speed up the genotyping process. The steps mentioned below are those for electrophoresis on ABI Prism 377 (steps should be modified according manufacturer's instruction, if a different model used).

1. Combine 3–7 µL of PCR products of a compatible microsatellite panel obtained from one particular subject in 0.5-µL microcentrifuge tubes (*see* **Note 6**).
2. Precipitate the final mix (to remove excess salt and primers) by adding 1/6 vol 3 *M* ammonium acetate, and 2 vol 100% ethanol. Wash the pellet in 70% pure ethanol, dry by vacuum drier, and dissolve in 20 µL sterile dH_2O (*see* **Note 7**).
3. Use 0.5 µL of the coprecipitate, and add 1 µL loading solution (5:1 deionized formamide:25 m*M* EDTA with 50 mg/mL blue dextran). Add 0.5 µL Tamra-size standard ladder (500) (Perkin-Elmer). Vortex, then centrifuge briefly. Heat the samples at 90°C for 2 min. Place samples on ice, until ready to load.
4. Prepare 4.25% acrylamide–7 *M* urea gel on ABI Prism 377 gel cassette, using 36-cm well to read plates and 24- or 36-well comb, depending on the number of samples. Allow to set for 2 h.
5. While the gel is polymerizing, set up the ABI Prism 377 Genescanner. This includes setting up the analysis software, starting data collection software, setting default parameters, creating a sample sheet, and creating a run file (refer to ABI Prism 377 manufacturer's manual for details of these procedures).
6. Prepare the plates for loading on the instrument, and make sure the plates are clear of all dust or water spots, particularly in the laser reading region. Mount the gel cassette in the electrophoresis chamber. Scan the gel and plates before adding buffer and loading samples, by selecting the plate check option from the run window of the software. Fill the buffer chambers with freshly made 1X Tris-borate-EDTA and check for leaks. Place the gel in the designed place on the ABI Genescanner. Connect the front heat-transfer plate and electrode cables. Flush all

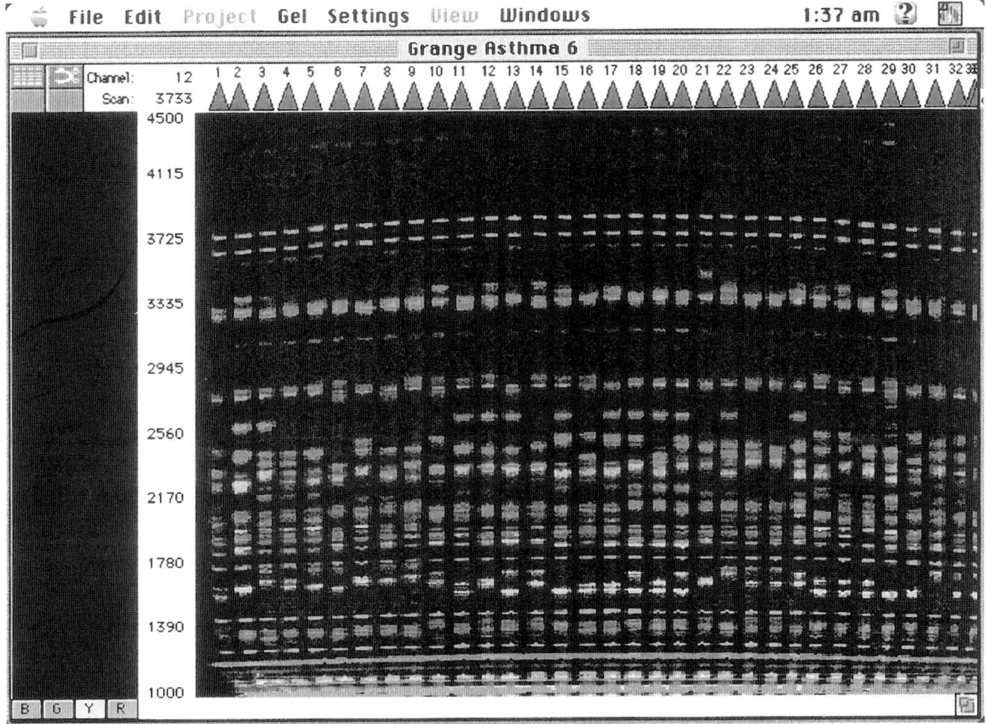

Fig. 1. Photograph of multiplex electrophoresis. A sample of an ABI 377 gel displaying multiplex fluorescently labeled PCR product electrophoresis. DNA from 33 individuals was amplified for 11 microsatellites that map to human chromosome14q (D14S50, TCRA, D14S49, D14S75, D14S978, D14S276, D14S750, D14S63, D14S251, and D14S267), in separate reactions. The PCR products of the 11 reactions from each individual were pooled together and run simultaneously. The 33 lanes are labeled at the top of the gel and each lane contains multiplexed PCR products from one individual. The Genescan analysis software calculates the microsatellite fragments size in relation to the Tamra standard, which overcomes any lane-to-lane variation. In this run, 363 genotypes were generated.

the wells with running buffer, using a needle and syringe, and choose the prerun module to equilibrate the temperature, and make sure all connections and components of electrophoresis system are working properly.

7. Pause the gel prerunning by clicking on *pause* in the run window. Flush all wells with running buffer. Immediately load 1.0 µL of samples in the lanes in the sequential order, as specified in the sample sheet. Click *cancel* in the run window, then click on *run* to start the electrophoresis (*see* **Note 8**; **Figs. 1** and **2**).

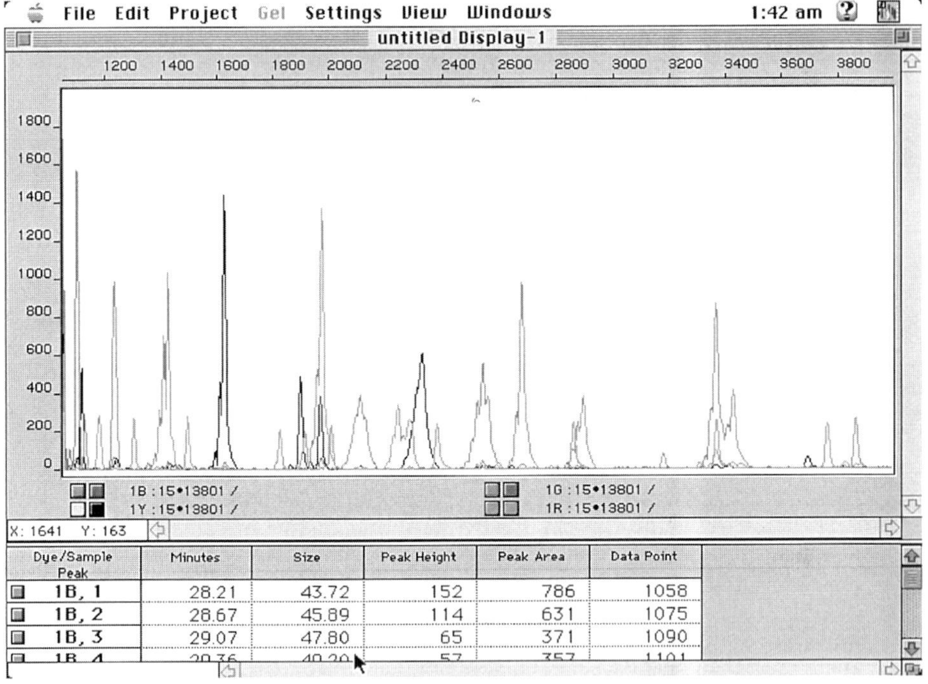

Fig. 2. Illustration of multiplex electropherogram. An example of multiplex electrophoresis of 11 microsatellite markers of an individual. All of the 11 markers are distinguishable either by size or fluorescent color.

3.6. Allelic Sizing and Semiautomatic Allele Calling

Analyze the electrophoresed gel, using ABI Prism 377 Genescan software, using the following specific procedures.

1. Examine the gel lane tracking, and correct any misalignment.
2. Check the Tamra-labeled standard at all lanes, and ensure that all DNA fragments of the Tamra standard are labeled by the correct corresponding size in bps (lane-to-lane variation may be encountered, which may lead to errors in sizing of some peaks (**Fig. 3**).
3. Export the data generated by the Genescan analysis software to the Genotyper software (ABI). This program allows allele sizing, up to two decimal digits. Alleles of specific marker are defined as the highest two peaks within the expected allele size range for that particular microsatellite. Use the filter label option and default parameters in allele sizing. Tabulate and check the genotype data generated by selecting and scrolling through multiple marker-specific electropherograms (**Fig. 4**). Finally, export the genotypes as tables containing allele sizes in

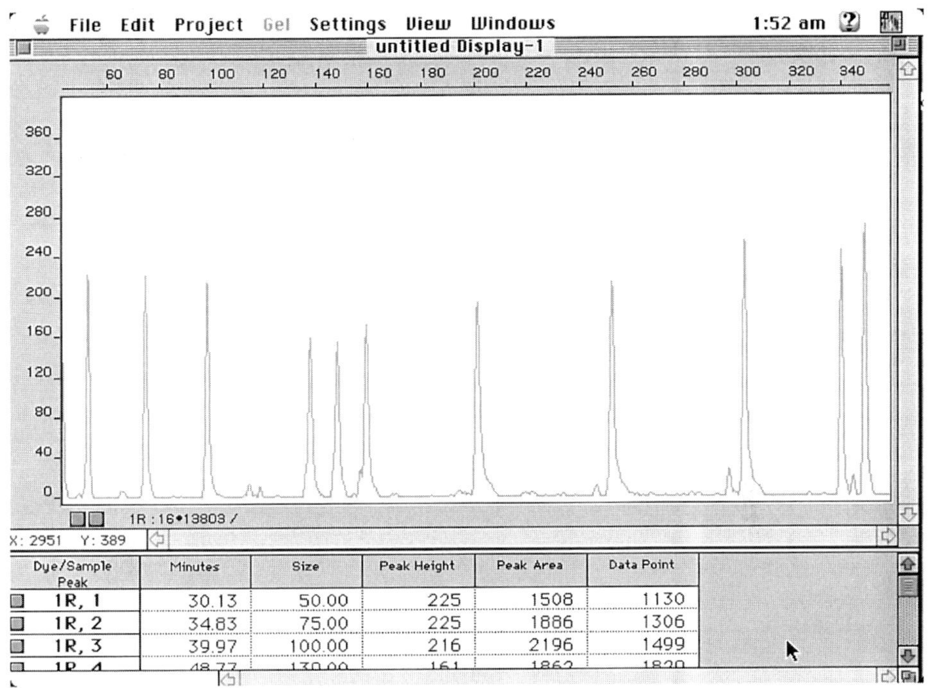

Fig. 3. Tamra-size standard marker. Tamra-size standard marker is included in each lane, to prevent variability in allele sizing within the gel and between different gels. The peaks seen represent DNA fragments of 50, 75, 100, 139, 150, 160, 200, 250, 300, 340, 350 bps, in sequential order from left to right with the corresponding scale in bp shown at the top of the plot.

bps which is accurate up to two decimal digits. At this stage, the generated data are suitable for handling by computer genetic analysis packages, such as Cyrillic (Cherwell Scientific, Ltd., The Magdalen Centre, Oxford, UK) and GAS.

3.7. Allele Binning and Pedigree/Genotype Data Construction

Prior to performing any statistical analysis, the raw genotype data need to be arranged in a format suitable for subsequent handling by linkage analysis programs. The GAS is able to read genotypic data given in terms of the lengths of microsatellite nucleotide repeats in bps (up to two decimal digits), and to process it into a form suitable for further analysis.

1. Obtain the GAS program and related manuals (in postscript format) (*see* **Subheading 2.6.**), and install it using either IBM PC DOS or Unix systems.
2. Prepare the genotype data file in a text format using database software (e.g., Excel). The file should have the following five-column format:

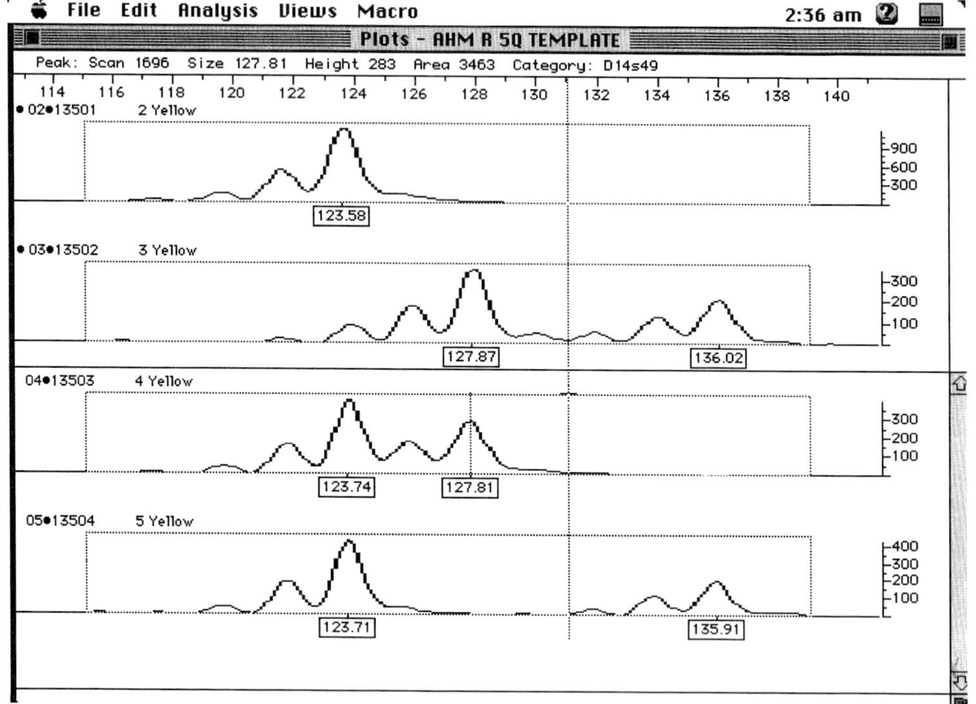

Fig. 4. Allele sizing of one family for marker D14S49 using Genotyper software. The plot displays genotyping of a family for a particular microsatellite (D14S49), as visualized on a Genotyper software. The scale in bp is given at the top of the plot. The graphs show a homozygous mother (13501) with genotype124/124, and a heterozygous father (13502) with genotype (128/136). The children genotypes are 124/128 for first offspring (13503), and 124/136 for the second offspring (13504).

locus-name pedigree subject allele1 allele2

3. Prepare pedigree data file(s) in a text format, using the following six-column format:

   pedigree number subject father mother sex affection status

   In the *affection status* column, enter either qualitative trait data, such as asthma (present or absent), or quantitative trait data, such as the log transformed total serum IgE (*see* **Note 2**).
4. Using the GAS program, examine allele sizes by constructing bar charts that illustrate allele clustering (**Fig. 5**).
5. Perform allele binning, using the global option of the *allsize* routine of GAS, in which a whole population is scored identically. Ambiguous alleles highlighted by the program need to be examined manually, and, if ambiguity is not resolvable, regenotyping is required.

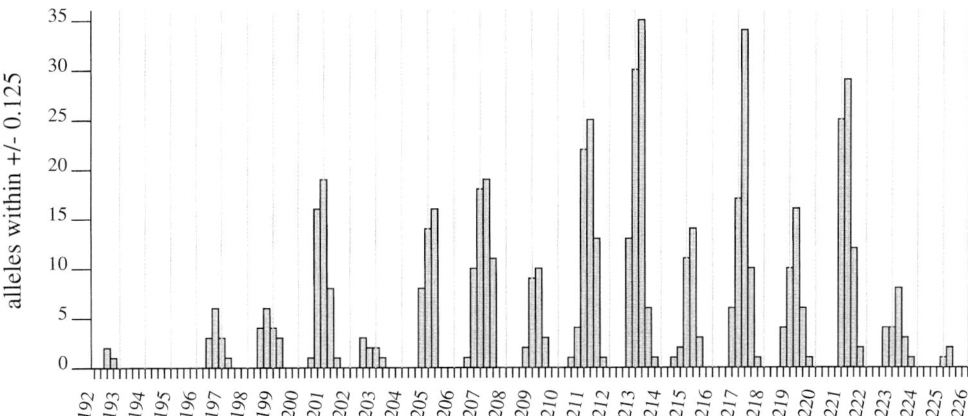

Fig. 5. Allele binning. A graph generated by GAS displaying allele clustering of a particular microsatellite (D14S267) typed using an ABI software that size alleles, which is accurate up to two decimal points. Data from markers with unambiguously defined alleles (as illustrated in this example) give rise to narrow peaks separated by broad, empty intervals. The horizontal axis represents size in bp, and the vertical axis represents allele frequency as encountered in the studied population.

6. GAS will also highlight any genetic inconsistency in the compiled data, i.e., each child should have a genotype consistent with that of their parents and any full siblings (*see* **Note 9**).
7. Using the *write* option of GAS, two files need to be created. The first will combine the pedigree and genotype data in the following format (*ped file*):

   pedigree subject father mother sex affection allele1 allele2 (for locus1)....

   The second file will contain loci description data (*dat file*), which include the affection locus and list of the genotyped microsatellites, listing their alleles number and frequency. GAS can *write* the two files (*ped.* and *dat*) in either GAS format or linkage format. The latter is preferred, because it can be handled by other linkage analysis software.

3.8. Statistical Analysis

3.8.1. Nonparametric Linkage Analysis

Allele-sharing methods are based on the principle that affected relatives inherit identical copies of the chromosomal region (containing the disease-causing gene) more often than expected by random Mendelian segregation. These are nonparametric tests, which do not require definition of the mode of inheritance of a disease, and hence are most suited to study complex diseases. This strategy is less prone to confounding factors, such as incomplete penetrance of a gene, genetic heterogeneity, or high frequency of disease alleles.

However, they may be less powerful than a formal parametric linkage analysis with correctly specified linkage model ***(10)***.

When the genotypes for the parents and siblings are available, the inheritance of the parental alleles can usually be followed unambiguously. If the two siblings can be seen to inherit the same allele from a parent, then they are said to be "identical by descent" (IBD) for this allele. However, when only the sibling genotypes are available so that parental origin cannot be deduced unambiguously, alleles that appear the same in siblings are termed "identical by state" (IBS).

3.8.1.1. Affected Sib-Pairs

Affected sib-pair analysis is the simplest form of these methods. Each affected sib-pair can show IBD sharing of zero, one, or two alleles of that marker (with 25, 50, 25% distribution expected under random segregation). Allele-sharing among all affected sib-pairs is measured statistically, using a simple χ^2 test. Excess sharing of a marker's alleles among affected sibs with a disease would indicate that this marker is linked to the disease-causing gene.

This analysis can be performed using the *SIBDES routine* of GAS. This routine performs basic IBD analysis on sib-pairs categorized according to affection status.

1. Operate GAS on a suitable system (e.g., UNIX).
2. Create GAS file, which should specify input (*read*) files, output (*write*) files, and use the following analysis routine:
   call sibdes (*locus locus-name options*);
   The input files are the *ped* and *dat* files generated in **step 7** of **Subheading 3.7.** Under *locus-name,* list the affection and marker loci to be analyzed, and, in the *options,* specify the weighting of the test by choosing either *strict* or *Hodge* (this function is employed to compensate for potential disproportionate effect of families contributing more than two siblings on the results ***[14]***).
3. Run GAS, and display results. The routine lists the various types of matings, the degree of allele sharing between sibs in each (and parental source), the 2-1-0 χ^2 scores, and associated probabilities.
4. The cutoff significance level required for declaring linkage remains a matter of controversy. Prior review of the published guides on interpretation of linkage results in complex disease is recommended ***(15–17)***.

The analysis may also be performed using the likelihood-based methods of sib-pair analysis or the affected-pedigree member methods. The choice of the suitable approach will depend on the pedigree structure and parental genotype data availability (*see* **Notes 10** and **11**).

3.8.1.2. Sib-Pair Analysis of Quantitative Traits

Rather than labeling individuals as affected or nonaffected, allele-sharing methods can be applied to quantitative traits, such as total serum IgE levels, bronchial hyperresponsiveness (BHR) slope, asthma, and atopy scores, as proposed by Haseman and Elston ***(18)***. This approach is based on the principle that phenotypic similarity between two relatives should be correlated with the alleles shared at a trait-causing locus. Regression analysis is performed for the squared difference in a trait between two relatives and the number x of alleles shared IBD at a locus. The widely used approach utilizes sib-pairs, but it can also be generalized to other relatives ***(19)*** and to multivariate phenotypes ***(20)***. The sib-pair-based approach could be performed using the *SIBIHE* routine built into the GAS program. This routine employs the Haseman-Elston algorithm in sib-pairs, and fits a slope using least-squares, in which allele sharing is the independent variable and the squared-trait difference as the dependent variable. A significantly negative slope would indicate linkage. The *SIBIHE* routine is more appropriate for a genome screen, because it combines the Elston-Haseman algorithm with interval mapping. This is a multipoint method, in which information from adjacent markers is used to infer missing or ambiguous allele-sharing. This method can be run as follows.

1. Run GAS, and prepare pedigree (*ped*) file, that contains affection status as a quantitative trait, and *dat* file specifying the quantitative trait alleles.
2. Specify the analysis module in the GAS file as follows:

   Call sibihe (locus *locus-names* theta *recom-fracs options);*

   Under *locus-names,* list the affection (quantitative) trait and marker loci to be analyzed in order.

   Under theta, list the genetic distance between adjacent markers in recombination fractions. This can be obtained either from published genetic maps (e.g., Genethon, Evry, France; http://www.genethon.fr/genethon.en_html ***[21]***), or generated from the data set by performing linkage analysis between the markers, using programs like Vitesse and Map (available on the web site http://www.hgmp.mrc.ac.uk, under the linkage analysis menu).

   Under options, include the weighting option *dfweight,* which compensates for families contributing disproportionate number of siblings.
3. Generate regression plots by activating the *graph* option. The data is generated in postscript format, which requires postscript graphic software for viewing or printing, e.g., ROPs Postscript interpreter, Giant Technologies Ltd.
4. GAS generates an output file, which contains the results of the sib-pair regression at the loci analyzed with probabilities.

   Multipoint sib-pair analysis of quantitative loci can also be performed using the Mapmaker/Sibs program (*see* **Note 10**).

3.8.2. Transmission Disequilibrium Test

In the transmission disequilibrium test (TDT), approach an association study can be performed on family-based data (***22***; *see* **Note 12**). In the TDT, a parent heterozygous for an associated allele A_1 and a nonassociated allele A_2 should more often transmit A_1 than A_2 to an affected child. This analysis can be performed using the *ASSTDT* routine of GAS. In this, all children are treated as independent observations, summing their transmitted and nontransmitted allele, and calculating the significance using the exact one-sided binomial distribution. The analysis can be performed by including only one child from each mating, as suggested by some authors, using fixed ascertainment criteria. To employ this strategy, other children need to be removed from the pedigree file before running *ASSTDT*.

1. Run GAS as above.
2. Specify the analysis module of GAS as below:
   Call asstdt (locus *locus-names options*); in *locus-names*, list affection and marker loci to analyze; *options*, use either *strict* or *Hodge* weight option, as in **Subheading 3.8.1.1.**
3. Display results in the output file.
4. Correct for multiple comparisons using appropriate statistical methods (e.g., Bonferroni correction).

TDT can also be performed using the ETDT program available on the web site http://www.hgmp.mrc.ac.uk, under the linkage analysis menu.

4. Notes

1. As an alternative to the sib-pair approach, families can be recruited as trios (parents and an affected offspring). This type of recruitment is suitable for the transmission disequilibrium testing (TDT), which analyzes alleles transmission from a parent to an affected offspring (*see* **Note 12**). Families with one affected child are easier to recruit than families with affected sib-pairs, and the TDT has been reported to have a higher power than the sib-pair analysis ***(23)***. However, successful application of TDT to genome screens requires the availability of highly dense genetic maps of polymorphic markers (covering the genome at 1-c*M* intervals). Currently, this is not possible, because of technical and statistical limitations (*see* **Note 3**). Nonetheless, TDT is currently considered by many researchers as the method of choice to study candidate genes.
2. Defining the allergic or asthmatic phenotype is a central issue in dissecting genetic components and their relationship to environmental influences. To date, there has been no uniform agreement on the phenotype defining asthma. Investigators have used different subjective or more concrete definitions of asthma, such as a physician's diagnosis of asthma, questionnaire data, the presence of BHR, or combinations of the above ***(24)***. Use of subjective clinical data alone, without objective assessment of the asymptomatic individuals, may lead to misclassification, which may add critical errors to the linkage analysis ***(25)***. Asthma is closely related to high total-serum IgE levels, atopy, and BHR ***(26)***. Both total serum IgE levels and BHR are useful measurements that can be analyzed as quantitative traits, thus allowing a more comprehensive utilization of the clinical data and

reduction of the risk of misclassification. Total serum IgE distribution in a general population is continuous and skewed. Logarithmic transformation, however, results in unimodal distribution of log IgE *(27)*. Total serum IgE levels vary widely amongst different populations and are significantly influenced by age, sex, and smoking *(28)*. Therefore, total serum IgE should be log transformed and corrected for age, sex, and smoking. Similarly, BHR, although often used in the literature as a dichotomous trait, can also be used as a continuous trait (BHR slope) *(29)*. Finally, both subjective and objective measurements of asthma can be combined in a quantitative asthma score, using a principal component analysis *(30)*.

3. In addition to the semiautomated genotyping approach described in this chapter, new approaches are being developed, which may provide a faster and simpler approach to genome screening. In case/control settings, pooled DNA, rather than performing individual genotyping, may be used *(31)*. Two pools of DNA are made by mixing equal quantities of DNA from all cases (pool 1) and controls (pool 2). Markers are typed in these pools, and the allele image patterns obtained on an ABI 377, compared for pattern differences, which reflect allele frequency differences between the two pools. An alternative developing approach depends on the automatic detection of SNPs, using microchips *(32)*. The development of DNA chips represents another major advance in DNA technology with enormous potential *(33)*.
4. Current linkage mapping sets contain between 250 and 350 microsatellites, spaced between 5 and 20 c*M* apart. Because of variation in the distance between neighboring markers, some chromosomal regions are poorly covered, which runs the risk of missing important linkage sites.
5. PCR amplification conditions for published microsatellites can be obtained from the genome database http://www.hgmp.mrc.ac.uk/gdb.
6. The number of microsatellite PCR products, which can be pooled together, will vary, depending on the ability to discriminate between the microsatellite products by either size or fluorescent label. Up to 12 markers (or more) may be combined. Depending on the efficiency of individual reactions, a volume between 3 and 7 μL of each PCR product from a compatible microsatellite set are pooled together. An approximation of the required volume can be estimated from the relative intensity of the product bands, as observed on an agarose gel. A smaller volume is used from concentrated products with intense bands.
7. This step may be omitted if only eight or less PCR products are combined, because the accumulated salt and primers in the solution is too low to influence the electrophoresis quality.
8. Dinucleotide repeats are peculiarly prone to replication slippage during PCR amplification, which can give rise to stutter bands when electrophoresed on a gel, making distinguishing between alleles hard to read, on some occasions. Tri- and tetranucleotide repeats give clearer results, but, so far, their number is limited. The authors advise the inclusion of PCR products of a control DNA, with known allele sizes, in the first and last lanes of gels of all intended runs, to confirm, throughout, consistency in allele-sizing. Runs with inconsistent control DNA allele sizes may indicate erroneous sizing, and may require repetition.

9. It is recommended that pedigrees containing marker haplotypes be constructed. The drawing of pedigrees can be performed by programs such as Cyrillic. Haplotyping of the analyzed markers may be performed manually by minimizing the number of recombinations between neighboring markers in each family. However, this is likely to be laborious and time-consuming. The Genehunter program can perform haplotyping using algorithms detailed in Kruglyak and Lander ***(34)***. Haplotyping allows examination of the accuracy of typing, by observing the number of double recombinants between adjacent markers. The observation of higher number of recombinants than expected in a given genetic distance would indicate typing errors. In addition, missing alleles for intervening markers of offspring could be inferred, when data for adjacent markers from parents and individuals indicated no recombination.
10. The affected sib-pair sample will usually provide a mixture of IBD and IBS data, because the genotypes for some, but not all, parents may be available. Such data may be analyzed by calculating the likelihood of the data, conditional on the IBD probabilities being different from 0.25, 0.5, 0.25, rather than using χ^2 tests. One program that uses this approach was written by Kruglyak and Lander, and is called Mapmaker/Sibs (NIH, Bethesda, MD) ***(35)***.
11. Analysis can be generalized to involve all affected pedigree members (APM). This method is most suited for studying larger pedigrees. Initially the APM approach was based on studying allele-shared IBS ***(36)***. In the IBS based allele-sharing methods, an estimation of the correct allele frequency of the marker loci is essential. Relatives are more likely to share common alleles of a marker by chance alone, and, if the frequency of such alleles was misspecified as a rare allele, a spurious increase in IBS allele sharing will be observed, leading to a false-positive linkage result. In families with more complete parental genotype data, analysis can be performed using IBD-based APM ***(34)***. Such analysis can be performed for dichotomous traits using the nonparametric LOD score (NPL score) approach built into the Genehunter software package. This program allows estimating the IBD allele sharing in all affected relatives in a pedigree, rather than just sib-pairs. It handles multigeneration families (i.e., more than two generations), and extracts maximum information from pedigrees of average size. It tests whether the affected relatives share allele IBD more often than expected under the random segregation. The statistic reported (NPL score) will represent the observed deviation from Mendelian expectation, and will roughly follow the normal distribution.
12. Linkage analyses can detect gene effect over long distances of the genome (up to 20 c*M*); however, they usually have low resolution, with subsequent difficulty in narrowing the linked region. Association studies, on the other hand, are based on the principle that linkage disequilibrium may be generated because of a "founder effect," which occurs when a large proportion of people affected by a disease in a population is descended from a common ancestor who carried the mutation. As the gene carrying the mutation is transmitted through subsequent generations, the meiotic process of crossover and recombination means that the surrounding alle-

les will gradually become unlinked, and only the markers close to the disease gene, with very low probability of recombination, will still be associated with the disease. This approach of analysis can therefore be very useful in narrowing areas of interest in a genome (e.g., linked regions), and also in examining candidate genes. It has also been postulated that this approach is more powerful in detecting genes with moderate effect in complex traits than linkage analysis *(23)*.

References

1. Duffy, D. L., Martin, N. G., Battistutta, D., Hopper, J. L., and Mathews, J. D. (1990) Genetics of asthma and hay fever in Australian twins. *Am. Rev. Respir. Dis.* **142,**1351–1358.
2. Nieminen, M. M., Kaprio, J., and Koskenvuo, M. (1991) A population-based study of bronchial asthma in adult twin pairs. *Chest* **100,** 70–75.
3. Harris, J. R., Magnus, P., Samuelsen, S. O., and Tambs, K. (1996) No evidence for effects of family environment on asthma: a restrospective study of Norwegian Twins. *Am. J. Respir. Crit. Care Med.* **156,** 43–49.
4. Barbee, R. A., Brown, W. G., Kaltenborn, W., and Halonen, M. (1981) Allergen skin-test reactivity in a community population sample: correlation with age, histamine skin reactions and total serum immunoglobulin E. *J. Allergy Clin. Immunol.* **68,** 15–19.
5. Daniels, S. E., Bhattacharrya, S., James, A., et al. (1996) A genome-wide search for quantitative trait loci underlying asthma. *Nature* **383,** 247–250.
6. Collaborative Study on the Genetics of Asthma (1997) A genome-wide search for asthma susceptibility loci in ethnically diverse populations. The Collaborative Study on the Genetics of Asthma (CSGA). *Nat. Genet.* **15,** 389–392.
7. Burney, P. G., Laitinen, L. A., Perdrizet, S., Huckauf, H., Tattersfield, A. E., Chinn, S., et al. (1989) Validity and repeatability of the IUATLD (1984) Bronchial Symptoms Questionnaire: an international comparison. *Eur. Respir. J.* **2,** 940–945.
8. Yan, K., Salome, C., and Woolcock, A. J. (1983) Rapid method for measurement of bronchial responsiveness. *Thorax* **38,** 760–765.
9. Reed, P. W., Davies, J. L., Copeman, J. B., et al. (1994) Chromosome-specific microsatellite sets for fluorescence-based, semi-automated genome mapping. *Nat. Genet.* **7,** 390–395.
10. Lander, E. S. and Schork, N. J. (1994) Genetic dissection of complex traits. *Science* **265,** 2037–2048.
11. Spence, M. A., Bishop, D. T., Boehnke, M., Elston, R. C., Falk, C., Hodge, S. E., et al. (1993) Methodological issues in linkage analyses for psychiatric disorders: secular trends, assortative mating, bilineal pedigrees. Report of the MacArthur Foundation Network I Task Force on Methodological Issues. *Hum. Hered.* **43,** 166–172.
12. Ploughman, L. M. and Boehnke, M. (1989) Estimating the power of a proposed linkage study for a complex genetic trait. *Am. J. Hum. Genet.* **44,** 543–551.
13. Scott, W. K., Pericak-Vance, M. A., and Haines, J. L. (1997) Genetic analysis of complex diseases. *Science* **275,** 1327–1327.

14. Hodge, S. E. (1984) Information contained in multiple sibling pairs. *Genet. Epidemiol.* **1,** 109–122.
15. Lander, E. and Kruglyak, L. (1995) Genetic dissection of complex traits: guidelines for interpreting and reporting linkage results. *Nat. Genet.* **11,** 241–247.
16. Swift, M. (1995) Subjective attacks on statistical significance. *Nat. Med.* **1,** 1134.
17. Curtis, D. and Sham, P. C. (1995) Model-free linkage analysis using likelihoods. *Am. J. Hum. Genet.* **57,** 703–716.
18. Haseman, J. K. and Elston, R. C. (1972) The investigation of linkage between a quantitative trait and a marker locus. *Behav. Genet.* **2,** 3–19.
19. Blackwelder, W. C. and Elston, R. C. (1985) A comparison of sib-pair linkage tests for disease susceptibility loci. *Genet. Epidemiol.* **2,** 85–97.
20. Amos, C. I., Wilson, A. F., Rosenbaum, P. A., Srinivasan, S. R., Webber, L. S., Elston, R. C., and Berenson, G. S. (1986) Approach to the multivariate analysis of high-density-lipoprotein cholesterol in a large kindred: the Bogalusa Heart Study. *Genet. Epidemiol.* **3,** 255–267.
21. Dib, C., Faure, S., Fizames, C., et al. (1996) A comprehensive genetic map of the human genome based on 5,264 microsatellites. *Nature* **380,** 152–154.
22. Spielman, R. S., McGinnis, R. E., and Ewens, W. J. (1993) Transmission test for linkage disequilibrium: the insulin gene region and insulin-dependent diabetes mellitus (IDDM). *Am. J. Hum. Genet.* **52,** 506–516.
23. Risch, N. and Merikangas, K. (1996) The future of genetic studies of complex human diseases. *Science* **273,** 1516, 1517.
24. Xu, J., Panhuysen, C., Taylor, E., Wiesch, D., and Meyers, D. (1997) Empirical evaluation of genome scans for linkage of a quantitative trait associated with a complex disorder. *Genet. Epidemiol.* **14,** 927–932.
25. Xu, J., Wiesch, D. G., and Meyers, D. A. (1998) Genetics of complex human diseases: genome screening, association studies and fine mapping. *Clin. Exp. Allergy* **28(Suppl.),** 1–5; 26–28.
26. Sears, M. R., Burrows, B., Flannery, E. M., Herbison, G. P., Hewitt, C. J., and Holdaway, M. D. (1991) Relation between airway responsiveness and serum IgE in children with asthma and in apparently normal children. *N. Engl. J. Med.* **325,** 1067–1071.
27. Barbee, R. A., Halonen, M., Lebowitz, M., and Burrows, B. (1981) Distribution of IgE in a community population sample: correlations with age, sex, and allergen skin test reactivity. *J. Allergy Clin. Immunol.* **68,** 106–111.
28. Burrows, B., Halonen, M., Barbee, R. A., and Lebowitz, M. D. (1981) The relationship of serum immunoglobulin E to cigarette smoking. *Am. Rev. Respir. Dis.* **124,** 523–525.
29. Cockcroft, D. W., Murdock, K. Y., and Mink, J. T. (1983) Determination of histamine PC20. Comparison of linear and logarithmic interpolation. *Chest* **84,** 505, 506.
30. Lawrence, S., Beasley, R., Doull, I., Begishvili, B., Lampe, F., Holgate, S. T., and Morton, N. E. (1994) Genetic analysis of atopy and asthma as quantitative traits and ordered polychotomies. *Ann. Hum. Genet.* **58,** 359–368.
31. Daniels, J., Holmans, P., Williams, N., Turic, D., McGuffin, P., Plomin, R., and Owen, M. J. (1998) A simple method for analyzing microsatellite allele image

patterns generated from DNA pools and its application to allelic association studies. *Am. J. Hum. Genet.* **62,** 1189–1197.

32. Wang, D. G., Fan, J. B., Siao, C. J., et al. (1998) Large-scale identification, mapping, and genotyping of single-nucleotide polymorphisms in the human genome. *Science* **280,** 1077–1082.
33. Castellino, A. M. (1997) When the chips are down. *Genome Res.* **7,** 943–946.
34. Kruglyak, L. and Lander, E. S. (1996) Limits on fine mapping of complex traits. *Am. J. Hum. Genet.* **58,** 1092, 1093.
35. Kruglyak, L. and Lander, E. S. (1995) Complete multipoint sib-pair analysis of qualitative and quantitative traits. *Am. J. Hum. Genet.* **57,** 439–454.
36. Weeks, D. E. and Lange, K. (1988) Affected-pedigree-member method of linkage analysis. *Am. J. Hum. Genet.* **42,** 315–326.

Index

H

I

L

M

N